INTERROGATING GENDERED PATHOLOGIES

INTERROGATING GENDERED PATHOLOGIES

EDITED BY
ERIN A. FROST AND MICHELLE F. EBLE

UTAH STATE UNIVERSITY PRESS
Logan

Published by Utah State University Press
An imprint of University Press of Colorado
245 Century Circle, Suite 202
Louisville, Colorado 80027

 The University Press of Colorado is a proud member of
the Association of University Presses.

The University Press of Colorado is a cooperative publishing enterprise supported,
in part, by Adams State University, Colorado State University, Fort Lewis College,
Metropolitan State University of Denver, Regis University, University of Colorado,
University of Northern Colorado, University of Wyoming, Utah State University, and
Western Colorado University.

∞ This paper meets the requirements of the ANSI/NISO Z39.48–1992 (Permanence of
Paper).

ISBN: 978-1-60732-984-8 (paperback)
ISBN: 978-1-60732-985-5 (ebook)
https://doi.org/10.7330/9781607329855

Library of Congress Cataloging-in-Publication Data

Names: Frost, Erin A., editor. | Eble, Michelle F., 1974– editor.
Title: Interrogating gendered pathologies / edited by Erin A. Frost and Michelle F. Eble.
Description: Logan : Utah State University Press, an imprint of University Press of Colo-
    rado, [2020] | Includes bibliographical references and index.
Identifiers: LCCN 2020004847 (print) | LCCN 2020004848 (ebook) | ISBN
    9781607329848 (paperback) | ISBN 9781607329855 (ebook)
Subjects: LCSH: Women—Health and hygiene. | Women's health services. |
    Feminism—Health aspects.
Classification: LCC RA564.85 .I579 2019 (print) | LCC RA564.85 (ebook) | DDC
    613/.04244—dc23
LC record available at https://lccn.loc.gov/2020004847
LC ebook record available at https://lccn.loc.gov/2020004848

The University Press of Colorado gratefully acknowledges the generous support of East
Carolina University toward the publication of this book.

Cover illustrations:
Light bulb © Athanasia Nomikou/Shutterstock; stethoscope © RikoBest / Shutterstock

For everyone who has questioned, intervened in, and advocated for people despite challenging pathologies.

CONTENTS

List of Figures and Tables   ix

Acknowledgments   xi

Introduction: Interrogating Gendered Pathologies

Erin A. Frost and Michelle F. Eble   3

SECTION I: SENSORY EXPERIENCES

1   Corporeal Idioms of Distress: A Rhetorical Meditation on
Psychogenic Conditions

Cathryn Molloy   27

2   Art-i-facts: A Methodology for Circulating Infertility
Counternarratives

Maria Novotny and Elizabeth Horn-Walker   43

**SECTION II: PATIENTHOOD AND PATIENT-PROVIDER
COMMUNICATION**

3   "We're All Struggling to Be a Complete Person": Listening to
Rhetorical Constructions of Endometriosis

Leslie R. Anglesey   67

4   Simulating Gender: Student Learning in Clinical Nursing
Simulations

Lillian Campbell   83

5   "I Felt Very Discounted": Negotiation of Caucasian and Hispanic/
Latina Women's Bodily Ownership and Expertise in Patient-
Provider Interactions

Leandra H. Hernández and Marleah Dean   101

SECTION III: SOCIAL CONSTRUCTION OF ILLNESS/ BIOMEDICALIZATION OF BODIES

6   Orgasmic Inequalities and Pathologies of Pleasure
    Colleen A. Reilly   121

7   From the Margins to the Basement: The Intersections of Biomedical Patienthood
    Caitlin Leach   138

8   Women and Bladder Cancer: Listening Rhetorically to Healthcare Disparities
    Kerri K. Morris   157

SECTION IV: DIGITAL MEDICAL RHETORICS

9   Bras, Bros, and Colons: How Even the Mayo Clinic Gets It Wrong Gendering Cancer
    Miriam Mara   171

10 Interrogating Race-Based Health Disparities in the Online Community Black Women Do Breastfeed
    Lori Beth De Hertogh   188

11 Gendered Risk and Responsibility in the American Heart Association's Go Red for Women Campaign
    Mary K. Assad   205

SECTION V: TEXTUAL EXAMINATIONS

12 Pathologizing Black Female Bodies: The Construction of Difference in Contemporary Breast Cancer Research
    Jordan Liz   223

13 Overcoming Postpartum Depression: Individual and Social Gendered Pathology in Self-Help Discourse
    Beth L. Boser   239

14 Making Bodies: Medical Rhetoric of Gendered and Sexed Materiality
    Sage Beaumont Perdue   256

About the Authors   273
Index   277

FIGURES AND TABLES

FIGURES

2.1 "My Consent" by Meg 50

2.2 "Bloodlines" by Meg 51

2.3 "Failed IVF #1" by Sara 53

2.4 "Picture Your Fertility: An Interactive Art Event" 60

2.5 Meg's "My Consent" at "Picture Your Fertility: An Interactive Art Event" 60

2.6 Michigan Exhibit at Local Fertility Clinic 61

2.7 Exhibit at the Examined Life Conference 61

4.1 Air force medical personnel practice patient care on a male manikin similar to the one used by nursing students in this study. 87

4.2 Nursing instructors often use wigs to transform a male manikin into a female for the simulation. 92

TABLES

5.1 Participant Demographics 114

9.1 Incidence and Mortality Rates from CDC 175

ACKNOWLEDGMENTS

The idea for this collection began through discussion of our own experiential knowledge related to interactions with healthcare and medical providers. We were absolutely thrilled when our call for proposals and vision for this collection garnered so much research on the intersection of gender and biomedicine. We are grateful to the brilliant contributors to this collection who shared both their lived experiences and intellectual understandings over the course of proposing, writing, and revising their chapters. We were excited, frustrated, saddened, and invigorated by some of what is documented within these pages. Mostly, though, we are encouraged by the advocacy and interventions discussed here for interrogating pathologies that marginalize and oppress specific bodies based on sex and gender. We are grateful especially to scholars who are women, queer, trans, and nonbinary; if submissions to this collection are any indication, they represent the overwhelming majority of academics paying attention to this kind of work. We're also very grateful to Rachael Levay, acquisitions editor at Utah State University Press, who believed in this collection from the very beginning. She worked with us and the reviewers to make this collection strong and compelling. Thanks also to Laura Furney, assistant director and managing editor, Daniel Pratt, production manager, and everyone else at Utah State University Press who worked tirelessly during the pandemic to meet the original publication date. We also appreciate the support we received for this collection from the Department of English and the Thomas Harriot College of Arts and Sciences at East Carolina University. Finally, thanks to you, readers, who we feel confident will build on the scholarship of this collection and work toward more socially just practices within biomedicine.

***

This project was imagined, revised, (reimagined, rerevised) and ultimately born over the course of several years. My undying thanks to Michelle for her vision, guidance, and friendship. I'm grateful to our contributors for trusting us with their intellectual work and for their faith and patience, and to Rachael Levay for seeing the potential of this manuscript. Angela Haas, Kellie Sharp-Hoskins, Marie Moeller, Nikki Caswell, Barbi Smyser-Fauble, Will Banks, Matt Cox, Alana Baker,

Carleigh Davis, Cecilia Shelton, Temptaous Mckoy, Gina Kruschek, Abigail Morris, and Andy Frost are always ready to bounce ideas when the writing gets tough; thanks, friends, for being part of my feminist network. Finally, all my love to my family who supported me during good times and hard times over the course of the making of this collection: Andy, Caroline, Sammy, Mom, Dad, Rachel, Ty, Dory, Melody, Sebastian, and Sharky. —Erin

***

A collection like this one takes many years, many conversations, lots of writing, editing, revising, and lots of patience. This project is a testament to creating original, collaborative scholarship that is generated through the process, and I'm indebted to Erin and the contributors for this experience. My heartfelt gratitude to Erin for her keenness and vision for collaborative projects and scholarship; her intellectual curiosity and execution; but most of all, her friendship. I'm grateful to my students who have taught me so much about embodiment and knowledge-making practices and how to move from theoretical frameworks to rhetorical interventions and practices. I am lucky to have a very large network of folks (too numerous to list) who support and inspire me professionally and personally, and I appreciate every single one of them. Special thanks to my friends who have become family, Will, Andy, Erin, Nikki, James, Matt, Josh, and Angela, for all the laughter and good food! And, finally, thanks and love to Shane, Mara, and Lagniappe (Yap), who support, celebrate, and love me in all I do. —Michelle

ACKNOWLEDGMENTS

The idea for this collection began through discussion of our own experiential knowledge related to interactions with healthcare and medical providers. We were absolutely thrilled when our call for proposals and vision for this collection garnered so much research on the intersection of gender and biomedicine. We are grateful to the brilliant contributors to this collection who shared both their lived experiences and intellectual understandings over the course of proposing, writing, and revising their chapters. We were excited, frustrated, saddened, and invigorated by some of what is documented within these pages. Mostly, though, we are encouraged by the advocacy and interventions discussed here for interrogating pathologies that marginalize and oppress specific bodies based on sex and gender. We are grateful especially to scholars who are women, queer, trans, and nonbinary; if submissions to this collection are any indication, they represent the overwhelming majority of academics paying attention to this kind of work. We're also very grateful to Rachael Levay, acquisitions editor at Utah State University Press, who believed in this collection from the very beginning. She worked with us and the reviewers to make this collection strong and compelling. Thanks also to Laura Furney, assistant director and managing editor, Daniel Pratt, production manager, and everyone else at Utah State University Press who worked tirelessly during the pandemic to meet the original publication date. We also appreciate the support we received for this collection from the Department of English and the Thomas Harriot College of Arts and Sciences at East Carolina University. Finally, thanks to you, readers, who we feel confident will build on the scholarship of this collection and work toward more socially just practices within biomedicine.

***

This project was imagined, revised, (reimagined, rerevised) and ultimately born over the course of several years. My undying thanks to Michelle for her vision, guidance, and friendship. I'm grateful to our contributors for trusting us with their intellectual work and for their faith and patience, and to Rachael Levay for seeing the potential of this manuscript. Angela Haas, Kellie Sharp-Hoskins, Marie Moeller, Nikki Caswell, Barbi Smyser-Fauble, Will Banks, Matt Cox, Alana Baker,

Carleigh Davis, Cecilia Shelton, Temptaous Mckoy, Gina Kruschek, Abigail Morris, and Andy Frost are always ready to bounce ideas when the writing gets tough; thanks, friends, for being part of my feminist network. Finally, all my love to my family who supported me during good times and hard times over the course of the making of this collection: Andy, Caroline, Sammy, Mom, Dad, Rachel, Ty, Dory, Melody, Sebastian, and Sharky. —Erin

***

A collection like this one takes many years, many conversations, lots of writing, editing, revising, and lots of patience. This project is a testament to creating original, collaborative scholarship that is generated through the process, and I'm indebted to Erin and the contributors for this experience. My heartfelt gratitude to Erin for her keenness and vision for collaborative projects and scholarship; her intellectual curiosity and execution; but most of all, her friendship. I'm grateful to my students who have taught me so much about embodiment and knowledge-making practices and how to move from theoretical frameworks to rhetorical interventions and practices. I am lucky to have a very large network of folks (too numerous to list) who support and inspire me professionally and personally, and I appreciate every single one of them. Special thanks to my friends who have become family, Will, Andy, Erin, Nikki, James, Matt, Josh, and Angela, for all the laughter and good food! And, finally, thanks and love to Shane, Mara, and Lagniappe (Yap), who support, celebrate, and love me in all I do. —Michelle

INTERROGATING GENDERED PATHOLOGIES

Introduction

INTERROGATING GENDERED PATHOLOGIES

Erin A. Frost and Michelle F. Eble

The goal of this collection is to point out, interrogate, and formulate tactics to intervene in unjust patterns of pathology. In doing this work, we assemble a transdisciplinary approach from/to technologies, rhetorics, philosophies, epistemologies, and biomedical data that surround and construct the medicalized body, and we seek to reattach them to bodies and to corporeal experience. In other words, this collection's purpose is to consider the lived effects of biomedicine's gendered norms on embodied experiences—on people's lives. This collection must necessarily rearticulate disciplinary contexts/territories/categories, utilizing a variety of inter/multi/transdisciplinary[1] approaches so the whole work taken together forms a transdisciplinary way of reimagining embodied data. This collection resists notions of embodiment as separate from or necessarily in opposition to biomedical knowledge. It interrogates gendered pathologies.

PART 1: WHY PATHOLOGIES?

Research that attempts to address health disparities and/or inequalities tends to focus on technology and biology despite the fact that pathology—the process by which causes and symptoms of diseases are determined—clearly has rhetorical, social, and cultural components that are just as significant. Even when health-disparities research addresses social determinants, it tends to focus on patient compliance, language barriers, environmental factors, geographic areas, or socioeconomic levels rather than on the relationship between gendered biomedical discourse and how bodies are defined and categorized.

We use the concept of pathology because it provides us with a theoretical lens through which to examine how bodies are marked, diagnosed, and categorized. Pathology has several meanings in biomedical

DOI: 10.7330/9781607329855.c000

discourse. It can refer broadly to the study of disease or illness, or more specifically to the causes of a disease or examination of tissue, blood, or fluid samples toward diagnosing a disease while also being used in other contexts to refer to something abnormal or deviant, as in pathological fear or pathological liar. Outside biomedical discourse, scholars sometimes use pathology as a metaphor for indicating how groups of people are represented in discourse. For example, Nadine Hubbs (2014) talks about "pathologizing the working class through the queer" (157) in *Rednecks, Queers, and Country Music.* Hubbs's treatment of country music works across class, gender, and sexuality (among other characteristics) to show that tolerance and acceptance of difference rests upon the middle class's desire to separate itself from the working class, and vice versa. Thus, pathologizing—or stereotyping, categorizing, mocking, and pushing away—particular kinds of people serves as a way to reinforce class divisions.

We draw on these multiple meanings—both the literal and metaphorical—of pathology; in fact, this collection takes its exigence from the intersection of these two definitions. We are concerned not only with conditions, syndromes, disorders, and diseases that have been defined but also with how *pathologies* and *pathological* are terms used to define, identify, and categorize particular bodies in juxtaposition to the androcentric body. Female bodies in particular are disproportionately pathologized—which in this case means medicalized, labeled as nonnormative, and brought under surveillance and disciplined by the biomedical sphere. This should concern not just women but everyone: "Indeed, we are all more or less abnormal in some way or another, and thus we are all potential targets for psychiatric power" and medical power (Taylor 2015, 264). This relationship among gender, pathologies, and inequalities is deeply rooted in the patriarchal and hierarchical context of biomedicine and the types of knowledge (and bodies) privileged in those spaces. Gendered pathologies are perpetuated by divorcing women's embodied experiences from technical and scientific information or knowledge generated about them by others. This sort of rhetorical move is not new and is predicated upon a (false) assumption that experiential data are not empirical. Feminists have long valued experiential data as a way to resist this separation—and these experiential data have long been dismissed within the realm of biomedicine when attached to or emerging from female bodies.[2]

Feminist technoscience scholars in particular provide a foundation for this collection of essays in at least two ways: first, they question how socially constructed notions about sex, gender, and sexuality "influence the production of medical knowledge about sex and sexed bodies in ways that affect subsequent research . . . and lived experiences" (Fishman, Mamo, and Grzanka 2017, 397). Second, they call us to examine and resist knowledges that "produce and reflect inequalities through epistemological frames such as binary logics of normal/pathological" (400). Feminist technoscience scholars, as well as this collection, are concerned with how biomedical knowledge is produced, what that knowledge means for particular kinds of bodies, and challenging any inequalities that happen—and are reified—as a result.

Donna Haraway (1990) and Sandra Harding (2005), among other feminist technoscience scholars, question objectivity and neutrality within science, technology, and biomedical spheres, as these contexts are political, socially constructed, and gendered despite dominant narratives and claims to the contrary. Haraway's cyborg imagery suggests "a way out of the maze of dualisms"—actor and agent, subject and object—"in which we have explained our bodies and our tools to ourselves" (181). For Haraway, embodied knowledge is essential to finding meaningful explanations for our bodies. The material body must be present for us to learn about and through it and to take "responsibility for difference in material-semiotic fields of meaning" (92). For Harding, the subjects or agents of knowledge are "embodied and visible, because the lives from which thought has started are always present and visible in the results of that thought" (63). Subjects of knowledge are not different from objects of knowledge in that "the same kind of social forces that shape objects of knowledge also shape knowers and their scientific projects" (64). In other words, classifications, categorizations, and pathologizations of bodies in modern biomedicine often depend on notions of knowledge incorrectly understood as universal, objective, and disembodied—failing to account for embodied knowledges so important in these contexts for specific bodies.

Intervening within the gendered nature of biomedicine and its knowledge, assumptions, and technologies requires an understanding of pathologies as "working machines" and how these machines have been used to separate the material body and its experiences from prevailing understandings and knowledges about the body. To explain, Judy Wajcman (2004) argues that "gender relations can be thought of as materialized in technology, and masculinity and femininity in turn acquire their meaning and character through their enrollment and embeddedness in working machines" (107). These machines—whether articulated as technology, biomedicine, or biomedicine-as-technology[3]—are "a socio-material product—a seamless web or network combining artefacts, people, organizations, cultural meanings and knowledge" that operates within a set of assumed gender power relations (106). Wajcman's theoretical approach, technofeminism, "shares the constructivist conception of technology as a sociotechnical network, and recognizes the need to integrate the material, discursive and social elements of technoscientific practice" (46). In other words, we must return experience—culture, embodied data, subjectivity—to the body.[4]

Biomedicine often tries to separate women's unruly bodies and experiences, specifically, from the official information or data collected or assumed about them. Only considering the "standard" data about the body eliminates the context necessary in understanding how diverse bodies respond to disease and illness and, as a result, how they might be diagnosed and treated. According to N. Katherine Hayles (1999), "Information, like humanity, cannot exist apart from the embodiment that brings it into being as a material entity in the world; and embodiment is always instantiated, local, and specific" (54). While data about bodies allow us to have a broader view and generalize among groups and categories of bodies, they can also be limiting and exclusionary if embodied experiences aren't also accounted for. For example, Alana Baker (2017) discusses the importance of considering the "numerous embodiments that are involved in the construction of the data bodies in medical technical communication that display differences" since focusing on centric epistemologies excludes other bodies. As one possible solution, she calls for clinical researchers to report findings that account for biological sex and gender, among other identity markers, in an effort to "create more inclusive, more accurate definitions of health and disease" (86–87). The ways biomedicine currently categorizes and defines certain diseases and illnesses based on specific data—or lack thereof—ultimately pathologize certain bodies already at risk or in groups disadvantaged in some way. We agree with Maureen Johnson et al. (2015) when they ask that scholars "approach embodiment through these complex relationships to emphasize the role of the physical body in all rhetorics, to complicate the ways bodies are understood to work and perform as rhetorical agents, and to intervene in the ways bodies both inscribe and are inscribed upon" (42). Rather than focusing on data and pathologies as separate from bodies or ways to categorize bodies, we want to reconcile data within the context of embodied experiences, as this gives us a diverse view of multiple bodies and how they are constructed. In response to decades of work on technoscience and health disparities, this collection interrogates, disrupts, and complicates the pathologies often marked on female bodies while also calling into question the binary categories of gender often defaulted to and perpetuated as normal.

PART 2: BIOMEDICINE IS GENDERED

The flattening of gendered experience into two singular and supposedly dimorphic narratives happens commonly in language about reproduction and should be critiqued (Ritz 2017). Robert Martin (2018) refers to the common understanding that sperm race to penetrate an egg—an anthropomorphization of embedded gender roles—as "the macho sperm myth" and cautions that such "incorrect science" and "biased information" can have material consequences for fertility treatments. Robert Martin is drawing on Emily Martin's (1991) "The Egg and the Sperm: How Science Has Constructed a Romance Based on Stereotypical Male-Female Roles," which points out that female reproductive elements have a much more active role in the reproductive process than is normally represented; the uterus constricts to move the sperm along and "the egg traps the sperm and adheres to it so tightly that the sperm's head is forced to lie flat against the surface of the zona" (493). Despite these biological realities, the active role of female reproductive agents still does not represent dominant understandings of reproductive biology. Obviously, cultural and social understandings of sex and gender influence scientific and biomedical explanations. Biomedicine is gendered. Science is not neutral. This is, in part, because medical researchers and practitioners are charged with responding to the needs of a wide diversity of bodies. In responding to so many needs, institutions tend to focus on the needs of a few, behaving as though one standard idealization of a body can be used as a referent for all people.

Unfortunately, this limitation means "female patients' symptoms are less likely to be taken seriously by doctors, and women are more likely to be misdiagnosed, have their symptoms go unrecognized, or be told what they're experiencing is psychosomatic" (Adler 2017, para. 6). In fact, this is true for nonbinary-, genderqueer-, trans-, and/or intersex-identified people as well as those who are queer, disabled, or identify as a racial/ethnic minority. While this collection takes gender as an organizing principle, for reasons we explain below, it also strives to point out the many inequalities (including intersectional inequalities) pathologies enact in biomedicine. (In particular, the chapters in this collection often refer to women's health and experiences but may also describe the experiences of transmen and nonbinary patients.) No institution could ever be "neutral" in its treatment of human beings; however, institutions are often not only unequal in such treatment but also inequitable. Biomedicine and public health as institutions also have historical patterns of responding to particular kinds of bodies in unjust and inequitable ways. These differences exist along lines of gender, race, sexual orientation, and ability—and they can only be remedied with a transdisciplinary, intersectional approach. In an example that evokes race as its organizing principle, Dr. Mary Bassett accepted Columbia University's Frank A. Calderone Prize in Public Health in October 2016 with this directive: "We must explicitly and unapologetically name racism in our work to protect and promote health—this requires seeing the ideology of neutral public health science for what it is and what it does. We must deepen our analysis of racial oppression, which means remembering some uncomfortable truths about our shared history. And we must act with solidarity to heal a national pathology from which none of us—not you and not me—is immune" (*Huffington Post*, February 8, 2017). As Bassett points out, some bodies are well served by the existing institution of biomedicine and its attendant norms, priorities, and cultures. Some are not.

Women are categorically denied access to the same kinds of healthcare men receive. This is true of everything from access to prescription medication to treatment of pain to the seriousness with which medical personnel assess women's claims about their embodied experiences. "Nationwide, men wait an average of 49 minutes before receiving an analgesic for acute abdominal pain. Women wait an average of 65 minutes for the same thing" (Fassler 2015). Joe Fassler (2015) wrote about his wife's treatment for ovarian torsion by an emergency room in which the hospital personnel simply didn't believe she was in agony. "Pain without lesion" (Zhang 2017)—or symptoms without clearly observable causes—presents a problem for medical professionals, who then must accomplish their work based on their experiences *with* the patient rather than their observations *of* the patient. As Michel Foucault (1973) says in *The Birth of the Clinic*, lacking "a science in which the visible and the describable [are] caught up in a total adequation," complete and accurate description—as in that of physician to physician, or, we might extrapolate, patient to physician—is impossible (116). In those situations in which "the [clinical] gaze is confronted by obscure masses, by impenetrable shapes, by the black stone of the body," the physician becomes reliant not only upon what is describable (by the patient) but also by what is believable (by the physician) (117). What is believable by the physician is, of course, constrained by the physician's beliefs about the patient—which, we know, are dependent upon the identity characteristics of both parties.

Historically, the subject of reliance upon (women's) experience has been taken up in feminist scholarship precisely because it is so often and so roundly discredited elsewhere. Evidence of this bias in healthcare is overwhelming. Depression in women is "misdiagnosed between 30 and 50% of the time" (Johnson 2013). Women are treated less aggressively by healthcare practitioners until they prove they are as deserving of care as male patients, a practice colloquially called "Yentl Syndrome." Baker (2017) shows that medical education materials privilege visualizations of male bodies as standard. Gender bias exists in diagnosis and suggested treatment options, especially when it comes to certain health conditions like heart disease, knee replacement, and critical care (Kent, Vital, and Varela 2012). Johnson's (2013) explanation of heart disease (the leading killer of women in the United States) diagnoses is instructive. She explains that men typically experience discrete blockages in their arteries, while women's arteries more often retain plaque in diffuse, even patterns; thus, a typical man may have a single, large blockage while a typical woman may experience a narrowing of the coronary artery. This narrowing is more difficult to see via cardiac catheterization—which is the standard test to diagnose heart disease, regardless of the patient's sex.[5] An intracoronary ultrasound would be a more useful "gold standard" for women patients, and its widespread usage would reflect an equitable approach to healthcare. However, this test is not considered the gold standard because of the focus on a singular (male) pathology of the disease.

While diseases are often treated as if they affect only the "standard" body, the history of pathologizing women based on their bodily differences to men extends back centuries (Ehrenreich and English 2010; Tuana 1993) and resonates in modern analyses of biomedical discourse within contemporary scientific and medical establishments. In late 2016, the popular press began to report that a study on male birth control had been cancelled due to side effects. According to NPR ("Male Birth Control" 2016), researchers "gave shots to 320 men every eight weeks, in different countries around the world" and the trial was very effective—initial results said 96 percent—at preventing pregnancy. The most common side effects were acne and mood swings, and most participants said they would use the product if it were commercially available. Nevertheless, the study was cancelled. Many people critiqued the choice to cancel, and the concern of a number of feminist critics was that when women report the very same side effects, they are not taken seriously. Women in similar trials decades ago were not warned about side effects, were not told the drug was experimental in the first place, or (in the case of incarcerated women) were not given a choice about participating. After women reported side effects similar to those reported in the recent male study, the drugs were still approved and distributed. In fact, subsequent studies of the side effects of female birth control then ceased, meaning women's complaints and experiences taking these drugs were ignored for decades until the first major study correlating hormonal contraception and depression came out—devastatingly late—in 2016 (Skovlund et al. 2016). It is worth noting that women—who are more typically responsible for birth control—are 70 percent more likely to experience depression than men (Johnson 2013). In addition, men are twenty-two times more likely than a woman to have a physician recommend a total knee replacement given the same symptoms (Borkhoff et al. 2008). A report by the Connors Center for Women's Health & Gender Biology (Brigham and Women's Hospital 2014) identifies and discusses four diseases (cardiovascular disease, lung cancer, depression, and Alzheimer's disease) for which sex differences and inequities exist in how men and women experience these illnesses and in the treatment for them. And these are just a few examples.

Further, evidence of gender- and race-based health disparities continues to exist despite numerous legislative attempts to eradicate them. The National Institutes of Health (NIH) Revitalization Act of 1993 requires the inclusion of women and minorities in clinical research (National Institutes, "NIH Policy," n.d.). The designation of the Center for Minority Health and Health Disparities as an NIH institute in 2010 evidences acknowledgment of these issues (National Institutes, "National Institute," n.d.). In 2000, the Healthy People program (originally established in 1979) transitioned from reducing health disparities to achieving health equity and eliminating health disparities by 2020, suggesting some progress (Healthy People 2020, "Disparities," n.d.). More recently, the Centers for Disease Control and Prevention Office of Public Health Scientific Services (2013) released the *CDC Health Disparities and Inequalities Report—United States, 2013*, which documents the factors that lead to health disparities and inequities in an effort to make healthcare more equitable across a variety of social groups. Partially in response to these failed legislative attempts to move toward equity, the field of health and medical rhetorics has produced numerous studies over the past fifteen years showing continuing disparities in health (Agne, Thompson, and Cusella 2000; Bennett 2009; Berg and Mol 1998; Britt 2001a, 2001b; Brueggemann et al. 2001; Dutta and Kreps 2013; Eggly et al. 2015; Kevles 1998; Lynch and Dubriwny 2005; Sankar et al. 2004; Zoller and Meloncon 2013).

Simply increasing attention to gender-based disparities is not enough. It is important to pay attention to other identity characteristics that put certain types of people at risk for less-than-adequate care (Sauer 2002; Scott 2003; Grabill and Simmons 1998; Kreps 2005). In addition, health-care professionals and scholars of health and medical rhetorics must complicate the notion of sex as a determining category, as well as the collapsing of sex and gender in many contexts. A recent article from *Pharmacy Practice* notes that "it has been recommended that sex and gender be examined as separate effects, especially when considering potential differences in diagnosis and treatment options between men and women" (Liu and Dipietro Mager 2016). Both sex and gender are independently complicated; for example, medical discourses do not often make apparent the experiences of either intersex or transgender bodies. Reliance upon a binary system—failure to recognize diverse types of bodies and how they experience illness and disease—has real consequences for people attempting to receive medical care. For example, as noted above, Johnson (2013) reports that heart disease presents differently in women than it does in men. While this information is important in better diagnosing women (who historically have been measured against male norms), it also risks not accounting for the fact that not all women (or men) present in the same way; some women might experience symptoms "like a man" or vice versa—to say nothing of those who do not identify according to either of our culture's simplistic sexually dimorphic gender categories.

One of our responses to the gendered nature of biomedicine is this collection, which advocates for intersectional approaches to dealing with gendered pathologies and healthcare disparities while utilizing gender as a primary lens. We chose gender as our main approach because (1) it is an identity characteristic directly and overwhelmingly related to reduced quality of care and (2) it is the organizing category through which we (as cisgender white women) can most directly offer experience-based critiques of our own—and, as we can never remove the lens of our own bodies from research, this is important to acknowledge. Choosing gender as an organizing category for this collection called forth certain types of responses; while it did not prevent our contributors from discussing intersectional approaches, the chapters do constellate around particular types of experiences. In other words, this introduction and the chapters in this collection problematize particular pathologies. The essays in this collection contribute to the burgeoning field of health and medical rhetorics by rhetorically and theoretically intervening in what are often seen as objective and neutral decisions related to the body and scientific and medical data about it.

PART 3: ON THE IMPORTANCE OF A COLLECTIVE APPROACH

This collection, then, is a space for multiple disciplinary approaches to recovering the value of experiential data and putting it into conversation with a variety of other methods for gathering and making sense of data—some revered by biomedicine and some less so—to create a fuller picture of embodied experiences related to pathologies. The essays challenge notions of evidence-based medicine as the only data relevant to medical orthodoxy (Derkatch 2016) and engage the field of health and medical rhetorics in more actively reorienting ourselves toward recognition of the whole body—including attendant embodied experiences—in context. As a result, this collection examines how "this theoretical re-orientation is itself a disruption, which expands beyond one view of embodiment, and encourages listening to multiple voices" (Johnson et al. 2015, 42).

As contributors to this project, we resist the notion, however, of returning data to a single body. A single author—or a single disciplinary approach—attempting to do this work could easily contribute to narrow understandings of what this recovery work might look like. Instead, we have conceptualized this work as a transdisciplinary collection for this very reason: herein are represented a number of different perspectives on what it might look like to return health and medical data to embodied experience, to consider the effects of gendered and intersectional biomedical norms on lived realities, to subvert the power of institutions in ways that move us toward biomedical justice. We do not want to construct a single body, so we must employ a multiplicity of perspectives and voices. The authors in this collection operate from similar ideologies but from different (trans)disciplinary epistemologies. That is, we all operate from the belief that biomedicine as an institution treats some bodies unjustly based on identity characteristics, but we come to this central idea with different theoretical commitments, epistemologies, and approaches. Our ways of thinking about and responding to this shared belief are different.

We situate this collection within the field of health and medical rhetorics. Drawing on the work of both medical rhetoricians (Heifferon and Brown 2008; Keränan 2010; Koerber 2013; Scott 2003; Segal 2008) and technoscience scholars (e.g., Haraway 1990; Harding 2005; Hayles 1999; Wajcman 2004), this collection reunites technological and biological information with the lived, social, cultural, and gendered realities of the bodies said information belongs to—including valuing data that operate outside the schema of traditional dimorphic gender identifications. This collection responds to Lisa Meloncon and Erin Frost's (2015) call to consider how "feminist perspectives reveal insights into ideological perspectives of the other that are extremely important in a health-care industry that maintains persistent hierarchies and classes" and explore what a "feminist orientation can offer to the way we research in the rhetorics of health and medicine" (11). Part of the impetus for a collection like *Interrogating Gendered Pathologies* is that scholarship is extremely limited on rhetoric, gender, and intersectional theories as a lens through which to reunite technological and biological data with embodied data toward more complete and just approaches to health and medical rhetorics.

The field of rhetorics of health and medicine is a relatively newly established field; the books published to date have helped form a foundation. Still, much of this work focuses on in-depth studies of specific diseases or medical illnesses rather than taking thematic approaches that might reveal patterns across contexts of care. This collection follows in the vein of work like Barbara Heifferon and Stuart Brown's *Rhetoric of Healthcare: Essays Toward a New Disciplinary Inquiry* (2008), Joan Leach and Deborah Dysart-Gale's *Rhetorical Questions of Health and Medicine* (2010), and Meloncon and J. Blake Scott's *Methodologies for the Rhetoric of Health and Medicine* (2018), which brings together chapters that offer approaches and analyses of a variety of health and medical topics. Since the early 2000s, other publications (see for example Page Smith, Bernice Hausman, and Miriam Labbok's 2012 *Beyond Health, Beyond Choice: Breastfeeding Constraints and Realities*; Meloncon's 2013 *Rhetorical Accessability: At the Intersection of Technical Communication and Disability Studies*; Christa Teston's 2017 *Bodies in Flux: Scientific Methods for Negotiating Medical Uncertainty*; and Elizabeth L. Angeli and Richard Johnson-Sheehan's 2018 special issue of *Technical Communication Quarterly* aimed at forging ties between rhetorics of health and medicine, the medical humanities, and biomedicine) have addressed medical and health rhetoric topics and contributed to legitimizing and establishing this field, which makes books like *Interrogating Gendered Pathologies* possible. More recently, scholars in the field have produced monographs on particular medical topics—such as brain tumors, diabetes, HIV, breast-feeding, alternative medicine, hysteria, infertility, pregnancy, and cancer care (Arduser 2017; Bennett 2009; Britt 2001a; Derkatch 2016; Graham 2015; Jensen 2016; Keränen 2010; Koerber 2013, 2018; Seigel 2014).

This collection, however, brings together scholars addressing health and medical topics along the axis of a particular critical perspective using a range of complementary and intersectional theoretical approaches. The work that follows builds on the promise of the field while capitalizing on a unique and important concept—pathologies—toward investigating how a wide variety of theories and methodologies can help us interrogate the important issues we identify in health and medical rhetorics.

PART 4: CONTENTS OF THIS COLLECTION

This collection is organized into five sections that each focus on a particular concept or on a mode of communication. Those five sections are sensory experiences, patienthood and patient-provider communication, social construction of illness/biomedicalization of bodies, digital medical rhetorics, and textual examinations. The chapters in this collection are interconnected in myriad ways, and we could have chosen many approaches to constellating them. We chose this approach for several reasons: (1) by beginning with sensory experiences and moving to modes of communication, we enact our feminist argument in favor of framing experiential knowledge as foundational; (2) we believe this approach places chapters into manageable chunks that will be conceptually legible to students; and (3) by including different kinds of categories (e.g., concepts and media) as organizing principles, we draw attention to the messiness of arrangement work and create openings for readers to imagine other vectors of possibility. Although we have grouped the chapters according to the overarching categories mentioned above, each chapter contains elements that would allow it to move across those categories. We encourage readers to consider what different possibilities might emerge by paying attention to the transcategorical nature of many of these chapters and imagining the organization of this collection differently.

We also want to draw attention to what is not present in this collection. In soliciting chapters, we called for examinations of gendered approaches to pathologies, noting that female bodies, nonwhite bodies, queer bodies, and differently abled bodies are often marked as particularly risky and more frequently become subjects of damaging pathologies. We said, "This collection will focus especially on gender issues—in part because of a dearth of work in this area—but we also seek to recognize the intersectionality of health disparities across race, ethnicity, sexual orientation, and (dis)ability." While some of the chapters in this collection engage intersectionality and take on important inclusionary and relationship-building work, the overall pattern of proposals we initially received in response to our call largely centered and/or made most apparent women's experiences. This result is somewhat unsurprising, particularly given our choice to use gender (though, notably, not sex) as an organizing principle. However, we would be remiss if we did not note the prevalence with which any engagement with the term *gender* is read as female oriented.[6] Further, it is important we make apparent that this collection is representative of the proposals we received (and larger patterns in the field) in that it is almost exclusively women, queer, and nonbinary individuals who do the hard work of interrogating gendered pathologies.

We follow Julie Jung and Amanda Booher (2018) in their attention to "important exclusions" (6), as well as in their application of theoretical approaches aimed toward furthering responsible academic practices. This collection—its impetus, orientation, inclusions, and ultimate shape—and the feminist technoscience work it builds on owes much to indigenous and decolonial epistemologies (Haas 2012; Sandoval 2000; Smith 2012); in particular, the following chapters should be read within the context of thinking about the ways scholar-practitioners can make philosophies matter differently, the ways interdependence and intersectionality are "ontological fact[s] of human existence" (Jung and Booher 2018, 6), and the ways our theoretical commitments insist upon resisting "the subject/object dichotomy and the mind/body dichotomy as well" (Rìos 2015, 65).

Section 1 ("Sensory Experiences") highlights this collection's promise to value experiential data—as many feminist traditions have—by privileging those data in the same way traditional medical knowledge is often privileged. In the first chapter, "Corporeal Idioms of Distress: A Rhetorical Meditation on Psychogenic Conditions," Cathryn Molloy develops a theoretical lens, "corporeal idioms of distress," in order to account for both the psychogenic and physiological symptoms that contribute to understanding and treating symptoms, disorders, and disease. She points out that clinical rhetorical listening and recognizing patient ethos might provide insight for those patients often marginalized in the medical encounter due to unknown etiologies or because their symptoms don't seem to have an apparent cause. Maria Novotny and Elizabeth Horn-Walker's "Art-i-facts: A Methodology for Circulating Infertility Counternarratives" offers their community-engaged methodology in order to disrupt the tendency in our pronatalist culture that links femininity with fertility and, as a result, pathologizes infertility. They see this public-pedagogy approach as a way to make "visible the gendered constructions of biomedicine" (44) and to circulate counternarratives in response to the dominant gendered experiences of women given an infertility diagnosis. In doing so, they help create a community of support, make apparent the experiences of their participants, and help reduce the shame, silence, and stigma often associated with infertility.

In section 2 ("Patienthood and Patient-Provider Communication"), the authors describe, critique, and offer avenues of action related to the communication that occurs between physicians and female patients. Leslie R. Anglesey, in "'We're All Struggling to Be a Complete Person': Listening to Rhetorical Constructions of Endometriosis," uses her personal experiences as a patient with endometriosis in order to illustrate how women are not believed or taken seriously when communicating their pain to physicians, which can cause delays in diagnosis of serious conditions. Drawing on narrative medicine, Anglesey provides suggestions for how physicians might listen to how their patients make sense of their pain over time and work collaboratively as partners in these healthcare encounters. Drawing on field research, including observations and interviews with nursing students completing clinical simulations, Lillian Campbell's "Simulating Gender: Student Learning in Clinical Nursing Simulations" discusses the gendered nature of nursing simulation training. Using a rhetorical material approach, Campbell concludes that the simulations and the debriefings after could benefit from discussions related to intersectionality in order to resist reifying stereotypical gendered interactions. Leandra H. Hernández and Marleah Dean, in "'I Felt Very Discounted': Negotiation of Caucasian and Hispanic/Latina Women's Bodily Ownership and Expertise in Patient-Provider Interactions," explore how physicians dismiss female patients' concerns through the (re)construction of the historical, pathologized, neurotic female patient, as well as physicians' outright rejection of patients' experiential knowledge. They conclude that attention to the relationship between language and power in patient-provider interactions might make for more productive relationships in which patients feel heard.

The third section ("Social Construction of Illness/Biomedicalization of Bodies") offers perspectives on sociocultural elements of pathologization practices. In "Orgasmic Inequalities and Pathologies of Pleasure," Colleen Reilly examines the ways in which the female orgasm (or lack thereof) is pathologized by analyzing the debates in the medical literature pertaining to the vaginal orgasm. Reilly points out the inadequate information regarding female pleasure on popular websites (WebMD and the Mayo Clinic) that perpetuates the idea that the androcentric model of sex has contributed to orgasmic inequalities. The pathologizing of women who may not find pleasure in this way are told something is wrong with them. Reilly concludes by describing female sexual dysfunction as the new hysteria. In "From the Margins to the Basement: The Intersections of Biomedical Patienthood," Caitlin Leach argues for intersectional inquiry into how gender and health are constructed in US-based cardiovascular and sexual dysfunction research. Leach suggests that current medical discourse "problematically implies biomedicine alone can overcome the institutional structures of racism, sexism, cissexism, classism, and ableism as they intersect to impact women's cardiovascular and sexual health" (138–139). Leach further argues that one common solution to practices of exclusion—inclusion—can actually compound injustice when actors do not pay attention to the effects of their practices as they exist within unjust systems. We must instead look to intersectional approaches to enact large-scale, institutional reform in order to resist inequitable effects of biomedicalization. Like Leach, Kerri K. Morris also raises concerns about exclusionary practices as a result of sociocultural understandings of illness in "Women and Bladder Cancer: Listening Rhetorically to Healthcare Disparities." Drawing on her own experience of being—finally—diagnosed with bladder cancer, Morris examines the ways in which identification leads to misdiagnosis and/or missed diagnoses. By grounding her work in specific experience and calling attention to the ways her experience does not stand in for the experiences of all people or all women—"At the same time, I was going through perimenopause, *for me* a time of unpredictable menstrual cycles" (167)—Morris demonstrates the importance of personalizing medicine beyond socialized understandings of gendered disease: "It is a matter of listening in the gaps and acknowledging that women's and men's diagnoses diverge in ways that harm women. It is a way of listening rhetorically for nonidentification" (167).

The common characteristic of the collection's fourth section is digital medical rhetorics. Miriam Mara's chapter "Bras, Bros, and Colons: How Even the Mayo Clinic Gets It Wrong Gendering Cancer" examines how even an altruistic, prestigious organization like the Mayo Clinic can reinforce the pathologized gendering of illness. Mara examines the Mayo Clinic website to point out rhetorical patterns in which the organization implies (or even outright suggests) that women's bodies are weak and that their reproductive organs will turn on them, thus justifying efforts to surveil and discipline female bodies to excess. Mara points to the ways this digital artifact reinforces problematic notions about women's embodiment, and she questions those biases about women's bodies. Lori Beth De Hertogh turns to community-generated digital artifacts in her examination of how *Black Women Do Breastfeed*, an online breastfeeding community, resists historical/biomedical tendencies to code African American women as unwilling or unable to care for their children. "Interrogating Race-Based Health Disparities in the Online Community *Black Women Do Breastfeed*" engages race-based health disparities related to breastfeeding and offers recommendations for more inclusive research. More specifically, De Hertogh traces histories of African American women breastfeeding, while acknowledging her subject position as a "heterosexual, white, middle-class woman," and engages in a deep "interrogation of the ways pathology operates as a form of meaning making that shapes women's health experiences" (190). De Hertogh also cautions that even unofficial activist health texts can reify health disparities—as when documentation suggests formula feeding is somehow deficient—and that rhetoricians must be diligent about reframing these tendencies. In "Gendered Risk and Responsibility in the American Heart Association's Go Red for Women Campaign," Mary K. Assad likewise critiques rhetorical patterns that overgeneralize, recognizing the complexity when advocacy accomplishes a goal of greater awareness but also contributes to troubling cultural patterns that could counteract the positive effects of that awareness. Assad examines the web-based messages of the Go Red for Women campaign, critiquing its role in using heart disease as a site for reinforcing traditional roles. For example, Assad points out that Go Red for Women's attention to self-care positions the campaign to advocate for more equal gender roles, but the campaign instead "reinforces them by urging a woman to perform self-care *so that* she can continue to occupy the caregiver role" (217). Assad complicates attention given to gender-based risk factors rather than sex-specific risk factors derived from a woman's physiology.

The final section ("Textual Examinations") offers critiques of literature about health and medicine. Jordan Liz offers a critical philosophical examination of two recent case studies about breast cancer. Liz's "Pathologizing Black Female Bodies: The Construction of Difference in Contemporary Breast Cancer Research" critiques the pathologization of African American women in breast cancer research, articulating "a series of assumptions regarding race, gender and disease susceptibility operative in these studies" (224). By parsing the ways race and class are taken up in these examples of medical literature, Liz points out that concern over cancer rates in white women motivates the study of African American women, that these studies shift responsibility related to public health campaigns in worrisome ways, and that whiteness is falsely constructed as normal. While this chapter examines two case studies, those studies engage in rhetorical patterns that are familiar and widespread. Beth L. Boser also focuses on rhetorical patterns in health literature in "*This Isn't What I Expected: Overcoming Postpartum Depression*: Individual and Social Gendered Pathology in Self-Help Discourse," which analyzes the rhetorics of postpartum disorder in relation to medical discourses. Boser is concerned with how gender and motherhood intersect with mental health and pathology and conducts a critical rhetorical analysis of the book *This Isn't What I Expected: Overcoming Postpartum Depression* to point out the importance of revising such texts when their assumptions rely upon old-fashioned constructions of gender to the detriment of their readers. Boser astutely points out the importance of differential care and intersectional awareness in the self-help genre, as well as the necessity of resisting assumptions that equate "real" problems with biological problems. Boser ultimately advocates holistic and experience-based approaches as a way forward. The final chapter of this section—and the collection—builds on the importance of differential, experience-based, and material approaches to medical rhetoric. Sage Beaumont Perdue's philosophical exploration "Making Bodies: Medical Rhetoric of Gendered and Sexed Materiality" argues for (and provides) a more thoughtful examination of medical rhetoric's uptake of gender and sex. Perdue points out that biomedicine limits gendered possibilities while eliding the role of performativity and asks how medical rhetorics engender epistemological and ontological truths of materiality. This chapter "concerns itself with the ways medical rhetoric and fixed notions of bodily appearance reduce materiality as both *site* and *sight*, evading particular phenomenological experiences of the clinical encounter and nonnormative ways of being-in-the-world" (256). This chapter shifts the collection toward new lines of inquiry, centering transgender, nonbinary, and gender-nonconforming embodiment and questioning gendered and sexed norms in clinical and cultural encounters. Perdue ends with a plea "to not only honor stories of illness but also to honor stories and narratives of becoming and being gendered and sexed" (267).

In sum, these many diverse chapters offer a multiplicity of approaches to interrogating and intervening in the gendered pathologies that construct and limit our lives and health. By considering these perspectives in concert and by allowing them to exist in conversation and in tension with one another, we both model options and create openings for interventions in entrenched pathological patterns. We hope others might take up similar approaches with different orientations as guiding principles, and we hope this collection provides starting points for such work.

NOTES

1. Many of the chapters in this collection take multidisciplinary approaches, which we understand to mean they draw on and speak back to more than one discipline. Some also take inter- or transdisciplinary approaches; we have resisted labelling them individually because disciplinary boundaries and definitions are dependent upon individual (contributor and audience) perceptions. We leave this, then, as a jumping-off point for conversations about what constitutes inter/multi/transdisciplinarity. We see this collection as a whole as a transdisciplinary project, meaning that the sum of the parts demonstrates a way—beyond and across existing disciplines—of approaching rhetorics of health and medicine.
2. We purposely resisted adding citations to this sentence in order to challenge the notion that such common, mundane experiences for female and feminist scholars must be evidenced.
3. Francesca Bray (1997) argues that technologies include social and cultural systems.
4. Some scholars argue that data and the body have never been and never could be separated—that the nature-culture split is manufactured. We agree but also point to the political-scientific world in which we live, wherein agents of biomedicine and everyday culture behave as if that split is "real" (for more, see Barad 2007.)
5. These differences in disease presentation may explain why men and women tend to experience heart attack symptoms differently. Education surrounding heart attack symptoms is a parallel pathology. Education about heart attack symptoms has typically identified chest pain and pain in the left arm as warning signs. However, women more commonly experience jaw and neck pain, stomach pain, and fatigue.
6. Further, "women's health" is often reductively read as "female reproductive health" (See, for example, Frost, Gonzales, Moeller, Patterson, and Shelton's forthcoming *Technical Communication Quarterly* special issue on Unruly Bodies).

REFERENCES

Adler, Kayla Webley. 2017. "Women Are Dying Because Doctors Treat Us Like Men." *Marie Claire, April 25.* http://www.marieclaire.com/health-fitness/a26741/doctors-treat-women-like-men.

Agne, Robert R., Teresa L. Thompson, and Louis P. Cusella. 2000. "Stigma in the Line of Face: Self-Disclosure of Patients' HIV Status to Health Care Providers." *Journal of Applied Communication Research* 28 (3): 235–261.

Angeli, Elizabeth L., and Richard Johnson-Sheehan. 2018. "Introduction to 'Medical Humanities and/or the Rhetoric of Health and Medicine.'" Special issue, *Technical Communication Quarterly* 27 (1): 1–6.

Arduser, Lora. 2017. *Living Chronic: Agency and Expertise in the Rhetoric of Diabetes.* Columbus: Ohio State University Press.

Baker, Alana F. 2017. *Pragmatic Feminist Empiricism: An Original Analytical Framework.* PhD diss., East Carolina University.

Barad, Karen. 2007. *Meeting the Universe Halfway: Quantum Physics and the Entanglement of Matter and Meaning.* Durham, NC: Duke University Press.

Bennett, Jeffrey A. 2009. *Banning Queer Blood: Rhetorics of Citizenship, Contagion, and Resistance.* Tuscaloosa: University of Alabama Press.

Berg, Marc, and Annemarie Mol, eds. 1998. *Differences in Medicine: Unraveling Practices, Techniques, and Bodies.* Durham, NC: Duke University Press.

Borkhoff, Cornelia M., Gillian A. Hawker, Hans J. Kreder, Richard H. Glazier, Nizar N. Mahomed, and James G. Wright. 2008. "The Effect of Patients' Sex On Physicians' Recommendations for Total Knee Arthroplasty." *Canadian Medical Association Journal* 178 (6): 681–687.

Bray, Francesca. 1997. *Technology and Gender: Fabrics of Power in Late Imperial China.* Berkeley: University of California Press.

Brigham and Women's Hospital. 2014. "A Report of the Mary Horrigan Connors Center for Women's Health & Gender Biology at Brigham and Women's Hospital." http://www.brighamandwomens.org/Departments_and_Services/womenshealth/Connors Center/Policy/ConnorsReportFINAL.pdf.

Britt, Elizabeth C. 2001a. *Conceiving Normalcy: Rhetoric, Law, and the Double Binds of Infertility.* Tuscaloosa: University of Alabama Press.

Britt, Elizabeth C. 2001b. "Medical Insurance as Biopower: Law and the Normalization of (In)Fertility." In *Body Talk: Rhetoric, Technology, Reproduction,* edited by Mary Lay, Laura Gurak, Clare Gravon, and Cynthia Mynti, 207–225. Madison: University of Wisconsin Press.

Brueggemann, Brenda Jo, Linda Feldmeier White, Patricia A. Dunn, Barbara A. Heifferon, and Johnson Cheu. 2001 "Becoming Visible: Lessons in Disability." *College Composition and Communication* 52 (3): 368–398.

Centers for Disease Control and Prevention Office of Public Health Scientific Services. 2013. "CDC Health Disparities and Inequalities Report—United States, 2013." *MMWR: Morbidity and Mortality Weekly Report* (supplement) 2 (3). https://www.cdc.gov/mmwr/pdf/other/su6203.pdf.

Derkatch, Colleen. 2016. *Bounding Biomedicine: Evidence and Rhetoric in the New Science of Alternative Medicine.* Chicago: University of Chicago Press.

Dutta, Mohan J., and Gary L. Kreps, eds. 2013. *Reducing Health Disparities: Communication Interventions.* New York: Peter Lang.

Ehrenreich, Barbara, and Deirdre English. 2010. *Witches, Midwives and Nurses: A History of Women Healers.* New York: Feminist Press.

Eggly, Susan, Ellen Barton, Andrew Winckles, Louis A. Penner, and Terrance L. Albrecht. 2015. "A Disparity of Words: Racial Differences in Oncologist–Patient Communication about Clinical Trials." *Health Expectations* 18 (5): 1316–26.

Fassler, Joe. 2015. "How Doctors Take Women's Pain Less Seriously." *Atlantic,* October 15. https://www.theatlantic.com/health/archive/2015/10/emergency-room-wait-times-sexism/410515/?utm_source=atlfb.

Fishman, Jennifer R., Laura Mamo, and Patrick Grzanka. 2017. "Sex, Gender, and Sexuality in Biomedicine." In *The Handbook of Science and Technology Studies,* 4th ed., edited by Rayvon Fouché, Clark Miller, Laurel Smith-Doerr, and Ulrike Felt, 393–419. Cambridge: MIT Press.

Foucault, Michel. 1973. *The Birth of the Clinic: An Archaeology of Medical Perception.* New York: Vintage Books.

Frost, Erin A., Laura Gonzales, Marie Moeller, GPat Patterson, and Cecilia Shelton, eds. Forthcoming Spring 2021. Special Issue on Unruly Bodies, Intersectionality, and Marginalization in Health and Medical Discourse. *Technical Communication Quarterly.*

Grabill Jeffrey T., and W. Michele Simmons. 1988. "Toward a Critical Rhetoric of Risk Communication: Producing Citizens and the Role of Technical Communicators." *Technical Communication Quarterly* 7 (4): 415–441.

Graham, S. Scott. 2015. *The Politics of Pain Medicine: A Rhetorical-Ontological Inquiry.* Chicago: University of Chicago Press.

Haas, Angela. 2012. "Race, Rhetoric, and Technology: A Case Study of Decolonial Technical Communication." *Journal of Business and Technical Communication* 26 (3): 277–310.

Haraway, Donna. 1990. *Simians, Cyborgs and Women: The Reinvention of Nature.* New York: Routledge.

Harding, Sandra. 2005. "Rethinking Standpoint Epistemology: What Is 'Strong Objectivity'?" In *Feminist Theory: A Philosophical Anthology,* edited by Ann E. Cudd and Robin O. Andreason, 218–236. Oxford: Blackwell.

Hayles, N. Katherine. 1999. *How We Became Posthuman: Virtual Bodies in Cybernetics, Literature, and Informatics.* Chicago: University of Chicago Press.

Healthy People 2020. n.d. "Disparities." Last modified November 9, 2018. https://www.healthypeople.gov/2020/about/foundation-health-measures/Disparities.

Heifferon, Barbara, and Stuart C. Brown, eds. 2008. *Rhetoric of Healthcare: Essays Toward A New Disciplinary Inquiry.* New York: Hampton.

Hubbs, Nadine. 2013. *Rednecks, Queers, and Country Music.* Oakland: University of California Press.

Jensen, Robin E. 2016. *Infertility: Tracing the History of a Transformative Term.* University Park: Pennsylvania University Press.

Johnson, Maureen, Daisy Levy, Katie Manthey, and Maria Novotny. 2015. "Embodiment: Embodying Feminist Rhetorics." *Peitho Journal* 18 (1): 39–43.

Johnson, Paula. 2013. "His and Hers . . . Healthcare." TEDWomen video, 14:30. https://www.ted.com/talks/paula_johnson_his_and_hers_healthcare?language=en.

Jung, Julie, and Amanda Booher, eds. 2018. *Feminist Rhetorical Science Studies: Human Bodies, Posthumanist Worlds.* Carbondale: Southern Illinois University Press.

Kent, Jennifer A., Vinisha Patel, and Natalie A. Varela. 2012. "Gender Disparities in Health Care." *Mount Sinai Journal of Medicine* 79 (5): 555–559.

Keränan, Lisa. 2010. *Scientific Characters: Rhetoric, Politics, and Trust in Breast Cancer Research.* Tuscaloosa: University of Alabama Press.

Kevles, Bettyann H. 1998. *Naked to the Bone: Medical Imaging in the Twentieth Century.* New Brunswick, NJ: Rutgers University Press.

Koerber, Amy. 2013. *Breast or Bottle? Contemporary Controversies in Infant-Feeding Policy and Practice.* Columbia: University of South Carolina Press.

Koerber, Amy. 2018. *From Hysteria to Hormones: A Rhetorical History.* University Park: Pennsylvania University Press.

Kreps, Gary L. 2005. "Narrowing the Digital Divide to Overcome Disparities in Care." In *Health Communication in Practice: A Case Study Approach,* edited by Eileen Berlin Ray, 357–364. Hillsdale, NJ: Lawrence Erlbaum.

Leach, Joan, and Deborah Dysart-Gale. 2010. *Rhetorical Questions of Health and Medicine.* Lanham, MD: Lexington Books.

Liu, Katherine A., and Natalie A. Dipietro Mager. 2016. "Women's Involvement in Clinical Trials: Historical Perspective and Future Implications." *Pharmacy Practice* 14 (1): 708–716.

Lynch, John, and Tasha Dubriwny. 2005. "Drugs and Double Binds: Racial Identification and Pharmacogenomics in a System of Binary Race Logic." *Health Communication* 19 (1): 61–73.

"Male Birth Control Study Killed after Men Report Side Effects." 2016. *All Things Considered.* National Public Radio. http://www.npr.org/sections/health-shots/2016/11/03/500549503/male-birth-control-study-killed-after-men-complain-about-side-effects.

Martin, Emily. 1991. "The Egg and the Sperm: How Science Has Constructed a Romance Based on Stereotypical Male-Female Roles." *Signs* 16 (3): 485–501.

Martin, Robert D. 2018. "The Macho Sperm Myth." Aeon. https://aeon.co/essays/the-idea-that-sperm-race-to-the-egg-is-just-another-macho-myth.

Meloncon, Lisa, ed. 2013. *Rhetorical Accessability: At the Intersection of Technical Communication and Disability Studies.* Amityville, NY: Baywood.

Meloncon, Lisa, and Erin Frost. 2015. "Charting an Emerging Field: The Rhetorics of Health and Medicine and Its Importance in Communication Design." *Communication Design Quarterly* 3 (4): 7–14.

Meloncon, Lisa, and J. Blake Scott, eds. 2018. *Methodologies for the Rhetoric of Health and Medicine.* New York: Routledge.

National Institutes of Health. n.d. "NIH Policy and Guidelines on the Inclusion of Women and Minorities as Subjects in Clinical Research." Last modified November 9, 2018. https://grants.nih.gov/grants/funding/women_min/guidelines.htm.

National Institutes of Health. n.d. "National Institute on Minority Health and Health Disparities (NIMHD)." Last modified November 9, 2018. https://www.nih.gov/about-nih/what-we-do/nih-almanac/national-institute-minority-health-health-disparities-nimhd.

Ríos, Gabriela Raquel. 2015. "Cultivating Land-Based Literacies and Rhetorics." *Literacy in Composition Studies* 3 (1): 60–70.

Ritz, Stacey A. 2017. "Complexities of Addressing Sex in Cell Culture Research." *Signs: Journal of Women in Culture and Society* 42 (2): 307–327.

Sauer, Beverly. 2002. *Rhetoric of Risk: Technical Documentation in Hazardous Environments.* Mahwah, NJ: Lawrence Erlbaum.

Sandoval, Chela. 2000. *Methodology of the Oppressed.* Minneapolis: University of Minnesota Press.

Sankar, Pamela, Mildred K. Cho, Celeste M. Condit, Linda M. Hunt, Barbara Koenig, Patricia Marshall, Sandra Soo-Jin Lee, and Paul Spicer. 2004. "Genetic Research and Health Disparities." *Journal of the American Medical Association* 291 (24): 2985–2989.

Scott, J. Blake. 2003. *Risky Rhetoric: AIDS and the Cultural Practices of HIV Testing.* Carbondale: Southern Illinois University Press.

Segal, Judy. 2008. *Health and the Rhetoric of Medicine.* Carbondale: Southern Illinois University Press.

Seigel, Marika. 2014. *The Rhetoric of Pregnancy.* Chicago: University of Chicago Press.

Skovlund, Charlotte Wessel, Lina Steinrud Mørch, Lars Vedel Kessing, and Øjvind Lidegaard. 2016. "Association of Hormonal Contraception with Depression." *JAMA Psychiatry* 73 (11): 1154–1162.

Smith, Linda Tuhiwai. 2012. *Decolonizing Methodologies: Research and Indigenous Peoples.* London: Zed Books.

Smith, Paige Hall, Bernice L. Hausman, and Miriam Labbok. 2012. *Beyond Health, Beyond Choice: Breastfeeding Constraints and Realities.* New Brunswick, NJ: Rutgers University Press.

Taylor, Chloë. 2015. "Female Sexual Dysfunction, Feminist Sexology, and the Psychiatry of the Normal." *Feminist Studies* 41 (2): 259–292.

Teston, Christa. 2017. *Bodies in Flux: Scientific Methods for Negotiating Medical Uncertainty.* Chicago: University of Chicago Press.

Tuana, Nancy. 1993. *The Less Noble Sex: Scientific, Religious and Philosophical Conceptions of Women's Nature.* Bloomington: Indiana University Press.

Wajcman, Judy. 2004. *TechnoFeminism.* Malden, MA: Polity.

Zhang, Sarah. 2017. "The Long History of Discrimination in Pain Medicine." *Atlantic*, February 28.

Zoller, Heather, and Lisa Meloncon. 2013. "The Good Neighbor Campaign as a Communication Intervention to Reduce Health Disparities." In *Communication and Health Disparities,* edited by Gary L. Kreps and Mohan J. Dutta, 436–456. New York: Hampton.

SECTION I

Sensory Experiences

1

CORPOREAL IDIOMS OF DISTRESS
A Rhetorical Meditation on Psychogenic Conditions

Cathryn Molloy

INTRODUCTION

During high school, Emily Deaton (2015) struggled with joint pain, dizziness, and fatigue—symptoms her doctors assured her were almost certainly psychogenic, as high school is quite a stressful time. However, Deaton's symptoms persisted. Repeatedly, she faced mistrust from her physician. As she explained in her narrative published on the website The Mighty, Deaton later discovered her symptoms stemmed from "a form of dysautonomia called postural orthostatic tachycardia syndrome, or POTS[1] for short" (para. 6). Considering her ignored pleas for a medical rather than a mental-health diagnosis, Deaton opined, "Ultimately, doctors need to realize that patients know their bodies best" (para. 9). Rachel Fassler (2015) encountered similar suspicion when she arrived in a Brooklyn emergency room writhing in abdominal pain. For hours, she was told to wait her turn before being diagnosed with an ovarian torsion—an extremely painful medical emergency requiring immediate surgery.

Similarly, Lorraine Boissoneault's (2015) doctors dismissed her complaints of unusual depressive symptoms as graduate-school stress. Tests later confirmed what Boissoneault had suspected: her thyroid condition was causing her symptoms. Unlike the course of treatment that had been suggested to her for the stress-related depression from which she did not happen to suffer, a simple tweak to her thyroid-medications regimen brought immediate relief. Reflecting on this experience, Boissoneault eloquently observed, "As frustrating as it was to have my physiological symptoms dismissed as pyschosomatic, the real tragedy is how regularly this bias occurs. Study after study has shown that women's symptoms and their pain are more likely to be downplayed or dismissed outright by physicians than similar complaints voiced by male patients" (para. 5). These women were mislabeled with what are variously referred to as *psychosomatic symptoms*, *psychogenic symptoms* (the term used most in

DOI: 10.7330/9781607329855.c001

this chapter), *somatic symptoms,* or *somatizations.* Collectively, such terms demarcate assemblages of symptoms believed to be etiologically psychological; these symptoms are thought to originate not in the patient's body but in their mind. Unfortunately, such cases are far from unique. The examples above resulted in an eventual diagnosis and some relief. Other cases end quite tragically.

Lisa Smiril was a thirty-six-year-old professor and mother living in Leeds, England, when she began to experience shortness of breath, wheezing, and pain in her arms (Philipson, *The Telegraph,* March 8, 2013). Several physicians assured Smiril her symptoms were the result of anxiety and stress; they prescribed antidepressants and sent her on her way. Over the course of a year, however, Smiril developed additional symptoms, including visual migraines and temporary vision loss. Eventually, Smiril was able to convince a reluctant physician to order a thoracic x-ray, which revealed metastatic lung cancer. Had her cancer been detected sooner, it would not have spread to her liver and bones. Despite this daunting news, Smiril took her diagnosis with grace and dignity, expressing immense relief and vindication at finding a physical reason for her symptoms. However, by the time her cancer was detected, it was too late for any existing treatments to save her life. In a blog post composed near her death, Smiril bluntly describes the stakes of inaccurate psychogenic-symptoms labels and their relevance in interrogating gendered pathologies: "I can't prove it, and this is just my opinion, but I have no doubt in my own mind that my misdiagnosis was in large part due to the fact that I was a middle aged female and that my male doctors were preconceived towards a psychological rather than a physiological diagnosis."

Research seems to support Smiril's hunch; biases abound in well-intentioned clinical exchanges (Chapman, Kaatz, and Carnes 2013; Hoffman and Tarzian 2001). Indeed, Leandra Hernández and Marleah Dean's (chapter 5, this collection) interview study "revealed two connected themes: (1) the (re)construction of the pathologized, neurotic, exaggerating female patient who needs to be 'fixed' and (2) the denial of patients' experiential knowledge" (106). If physicians are more likely to attribute women's symptoms to psychogenic etiologies, efforts to more fully comprehend the nature of psychogenic symptoms where they do (and perhaps more important, do not) appear are pressing. This research must take place on a number of fronts, but rhetoricians of health and medicine are well situated to make substantial contributions to such work since subjective patient reports and clinical conversations constitute a rather wide swath of diagnostic terrain. Seeking out theory-driven linguistic interventions through which psychogenic symptoms might be better illuminated is the topic of this chapter.

To begin this work, I briefly discuss biases in diagnostics. From there, recent changes to psychogenic conditions diagnostic criteria in the fifth edition of the *Diagnostic and Statistical Manual of Mental Disorders* (*DSM-5*) are examined from a rhetorical perspective. Next, I further examine inaccurate and imprecise psychogenic-symptoms diagnoses to pave the way for the argument that the cultural psychiatric term *idioms of distress* might be a useful theoretical concept to serve as a starting point to further unpack the disparities in psychogenic-symptoms diagnoses. After explaining major themes in idioms-of-distress research, those themes are used alongside theories in rhetorical and ethical listening scholarship to propose the new term *corporeal idioms of distress*—a concept that assumes all manifestations of illness and disease are both psychogenic and physiological in nature and that physicians should, thus, listen to subjective patient reports with heightened sensitivity to complexity and context if they wish to mitigate potential biases. I argue that *corporeal idioms of distress* might elucidate assumed psychogenic conditions and their diagnoses (and thus clarify biases in diagnostics). The chapter concludes with a call for more research on psychogenic-conditions diagnostics, with emphasis on the need for medical rhetoricians to undertake related field-based studies in patient ethos in diverse clinical exchanges.

BIASES IN DIAGNOSTIC PRACTICES

When one gender is disproportionately diagnosed with a controversial disorder, interrogating the biases in the diagnostic process should be a high priority. Just as those suffering from symptoms with mostly organic causes are best identified as such when courses of treatment are designed, those suffering from psychogenic symptoms must be identified as such, lest they put themselves and their doctors through tedious, costly medical testing that might, ironically, make the somatizations/psychogenic symptoms worse. Moreover, perhaps a serious consequence of the poorly understood nature of instances in which mostly psychogenic physical symptoms present themselves is the attendant misdiagnosis of those suffering from complaints for which other explanations are discernable—if the physician is willing to consider and look for them, which requires a careful and methodical consideration of context and a capacity for especially creative inquiry. Given time constraints on medical professionals and the soaring costs of diagnostic testing for consumers, finding rhetorical interventions through which patients suffering with difficult-to-diagnose symptoms might make themselves better understood is crucial.

As Lisa Keränen (2014) explains, "A rhetorical approach to illness and disease calls attention to the role of language in shaping meaning and action" (48). It is thus not surprising that rhetoricians of health and medicine have concerned themselves with controversial medical and psychiatric conditions—especially when etiology is opaque, unknown, or contested, as it frequently is in cases in which physicians wonder whether the patient is suffering from psychogenic symptoms. Medical rhetoricians take as a given that significant social and cultural components drive deliberations on pathologies. Likewise, rhetoricians—in the business of examining patterns of persuasion—are a natural fit for examining such things, particularly when the subjective patient report supplements empirical evidence in most diagnostic practice. One question rhetoricians might ask in the interest of patient advocacy is whether there is a way to describe a physical complaint as either purely psychogenic or purely physiological.

The complex ontologies at play in the manifestation of illnesses and diseases make the strictly binary articulation of symptoms virtually impossible, and corporeal idioms of distress, as its attributes are delineated below, is a concept that begins with this assertion.

As the narratives cited above make clear, when symptoms are considered separable into discrete categories of "in the body" or "in the mind," many women suffering from difficult-to-diagnose medical conditions are told their symptoms are psychogenic and have no basis in their bodies per se, and the suffering might continue unabated. In fact, women are much more likely than men to suffer such indignities. As Karl-Heinz Ladwig et al. (2001) explain, "One of the most enduring and poorly explained findings about somatization disorder is the preponderance of women with the disorder," but their research finds "that low social class and high emotional distress impart a significant confounding influence on the gender relationship" to somatization (517). Similarly, Yessenia Castro, Joyce Carbonell, and Joye Anestis (2012) found that gender rather than biological sex often determine patterns of somatization. However, while researchers have shown that women have higher rates of somatization, etiological inquiries into this phenomenon have been relatively scant (Wool and Barsky 1994). There is consensus among psychiatric and related researchers, in fact, that the literature on psychogenic conditions is inadequate and that research in this area is infrequent (Skovenborg and Shröder 2014).

Relatedly, S. Scott Graham (2015) finds the binary thinking that too often separates bodies and minds to be largely to blame for the "pervasive distrust of so-called subjective patient report" (118). Indeed, binary thinking pervades discussions of psychogenic symptoms, as the assumption that a symptom is either in the body or "all in your head" is widespread. The idea that the complexity of the human person would allow for such neat parsing is worth further interrogation. The psychiatric community is not unaware of the myriad controversial issues surrounding the diagnoses of disorders related to somatization—including a concern for ineffectual binaries.

The DSM-5 on Psychogenic Conditions

In 2013, the field of psychiatry ushered in several controversial changes in the form of the *DSM-5*, including significant shifts in the definition of psychogenic disorders or somatization disorder. As the *DSM-5* factsheet on the newer coinage "somatic symptoms disorder" (SSD) explains, "While medically unexplained symptoms were a key feature for many of the disorders in *DSM-4*, an SSD diagnosis does not require that the somatic symptoms are medically unexplained. In other words, symptoms may or may not be associated with another medical condition" (American Psychiatric, "Somatic Symptoms" n.d., para. 3). The *DSM-5* thus makes a concerted effort to move away from language that specifically mentions no organic cause for complaint as a diagnostic criterion. Instead, the emphasis in the *DSM-5* SSD diagnostic criteria is placed on the individual's *reaction* to symptoms. For a diagnosis of SSD, one must exhibit "disproportionate and persistent thoughts about the seriousness of one's symptoms," including "persistently high level of anxiety about health or symptoms" and "excessive time and energy devoted to these symptoms or health concerns" (American Psychiatric, "What is Somatic Symptom Disorder" n.d., para. 3). Similar changes were implemented for related disorders. Now, a patient with excessive worry over health concerns with some physical symptoms is diagnosed SSD, while a patient with high levels of health anxiety without symptoms (formerly hypochondriasis) is diagnosed with illness anxiety disorder. The American Psychiatric Association ("Highlights" n.d.) offers the following explanation for these revisions: "The reliability of medically unexplained symptoms is limited, and grounding a diagnosis on the absence of an explanation is problematic and reinforces mind-body dualism."

This shift thus marked an important rhetorical move on the part of the psychiatric professionals responsible for these revisions; references to a lack of a physical cause for complaint are conspicuously absent from the *DSM-5*. This move is logical, as the newer SSD diagnostic criteria expand the range of SSD and related disorders while avoiding potential claims of misdiagnosis should an organic cause eventually be found. These changes seem to be positive in the sense that a diagnosis of SSD would not necessarily foreclose on the possibility of continued inquiries into a patient's complaints. However, SSD and related disorders as they are delineated in the *DSM-5* are still quite controversial, as it is now possible to diagnose more people with a mental disorder if they happen to be preoccupied with health concerns. Health issues—particularly if one is suffering greatly—would, out of necessity, lead to some amount of preoccupation (Katz, Rosenbloom, and Fashler 2015). When diagnostic categories proliferate in each successive iteration of the *DSM*, rhetoricians point out that the use of this manual leads to pathologizing normal behaviors (Reynolds 2008). The psychiatric community's well-intentioned move to avoid binary thinking is not without its pitfalls; ironically, it might reify the very binary it attempts to nullify.

INACCURATE AND IMPRECISE DIAGNOSES

As the women's stories in the beginning of this chapter demonstrate and as the literature cited above substantiates, even post-*DSM* revisions, psychogenic conditions are widely attributed to psychological disturbance with emphasis on anxiety and depression. Once these factors are identified as the source of physical discomfort, other potential etiologies are underexplored or flat-out ignored. Nonetheless, the landscape is further muddied in the context of incompatibility between symptoms and observations. If a physician, in other words, wants to see some sign of injury to substantiate a claim of, say, ankle pain, but a patient claims her ankle is in pain without discernable "proof," the physician might become convinced that such a cause does not exist and that the pain is "in her head."

Granted, the assumption that psychogenic symptoms can present themselves is not without valid precedent. Anxiety and depression can, in fact, lead to a host of physical symptoms that can masquerade as serious diseases. Chest pain, for instance, can be a symptom of extreme stress but can also indicate heart attack. Dizziness—a classic anxiety symptom—can also indicate serious inner-ear pathology. Lethargy and fatigue could indicate depression but could also be a matter of anemia or signs of an autoimmune disorder. As Harvard Medical School's (2008) "Harvard Women's Health Watch" page explains, "Anxiety . . . plays a role in somatoform disorders, which are characterized by physical symptoms such as pain, nausea, weakness, or dizziness that have no *apparent* physical cause" (para. 4; emphasis added). Even though the argument can be made that "no apparent physical cause" does not automatically equate to no physical cause, the question remains: If psychogenic symptoms do sometimes occur, what is to be done to avoid overextending scant medical resources on expensive tests for those who are suffering from psychogenic symptoms while simultaneously avoiding circumstances in which serious medical concerns are dismissed as "all in your head"?

Physician Steven Novella (2009) describes the conundrum: "Psychogenic symptoms often mask underlying physiological disease. And the risks of both false positives and false negatives are high" (para. 2). Graham (2015) cautions that "psychogenic pain" is too often "a diagnosis for the undiagnosable" (63). Such insights are vital. If psychogenic symptoms stand in for more intricate explanations for suffering, the courses of treatment that follow them will do the same. Such complexity requires multiple pathways toward effective diagnosis—many of which will hinge not on exhaustive testing but on creative, attentive, insightful exchanges between diagnosing physicians and their patients and a sensitive perception of body/mind connection. Medical rhetoricians are well suited to suggest related theoretical frameworks designed to cut down on biases in diagnostics, and the term *corporeal idioms of distress* constitutes such an attempt.

THE IDIOMS OF DISTRESS AS GENERATIVE ORIGIN
FOR A NEW THEORETICAL FRAMEWORK

Before further explicating *corporeal idioms of distress*, it is important to unpack the dominant themes in idioms-of-distress research. One way to carve out an effective scheme for addressing difficult clinical cases is to examine patterns of real and imagined somatization through the lens of the cultural psychiatric term *idioms of distress*. Research on this highly rhetorical concept looks specifically at how sociocultural factors give way to idiomatic expressions through which groups of people attempt to communicate their psychic suffering (see, for example, Durà-Vilà and Hodes 2012; Hinton et al. 2010). Idioms of distress are "social, cultural, and interpersonal ways (i.e., symbols, behaviors, language, or meanings) of expressing, explaining, and coping with distress and suffering" (Morrison, Gregory, and Thibodeau 2011, 517). Conceptually, idioms of distress drive research efforts—many of which are ethnographic—meant to uncover the specific linguistic choices a given population might make to describe psychological suffering; it focuses on how these idioms might be understood in context. As Mark Nicther (2010) compellingly explains,

> Being attentive to idioms of distress led me to examine more closely interpersonal, social, political, economic and spiritual sources of distress, to appreciate tacit communication and to pay attention to cultural dimensions of illness experiences as well as responses to therapeutic interventions, from nosology to treatment to sick and risk role identities. (402)

Idioms of distress, thus, are lenses that lead researchers to be especially sensitive to context and complexity in their attempts to better understand patients' psychiatric complaints. Researchers examining idioms of distress often find patients' expressions of suffering are heavily influenced by past and current events, shaped by beliefs, core values and cultural norms (Keys et al. 2012).

Moreover, some researchers point out that idioms of distress serve as discursive vehicles through which patients "relate their individual suffering in a metaphorical way to suffering on a collective level" (de Jong and Reis 2010, 314). Idioms of distress, in other words, allow for the possibility that a patient's report of suffering might have a metonymic relationship to wider swaths of suffering on a cultural level. For example, Gulf syndrome—a condition found in the 1980s among Indian migrant workers in the Arabian Gulf—was characterized not by a similar set of symptoms but by "types of behavior that articulated subjective states of vulnerability and distress" (Nichter 2010, 407). After returning to South India, workers and their wives would check into clinics and undergo a battery of diagnostic tests; they then "used the results of tests as traces of some truth about how they had been treated abroad (for the worker) or at home and at the mercy of in-laws (for the spouse) and the toll that hard work or neglect had taken on their bodies" (407). Thus, the care-seeking behavior of these men and women led to diagnostic tests, and they used results to process and articulate their suffering.

Likewise, idioms-of-distress researchers are committed to finding ways to bring relief to suffering born of cross-cultural misunderstanding, expressing explicit concern for health complaints that are ignored or disregarded (Núñez 2009). In sum, idioms-of-distress research hones in on relational, collective, socioeconomic, and even spiritual sources of distress. They seek out the implicit; they take everyday utterances in clinical exchanges as potentially metaphoric and as perhaps influenced by a host of temporally situated, complex factors. Meditating on idioms-of-distress research, thus, leads to questions like: what if psychogenic symptoms in women are at least partially physical manifestations of anguish born of deep inequality, or misogyny even? In that vein, couldn't other marginalized groups similarly experience symptoms at least partially influenced by the inequalities that surround their lived experiences? Important, though, does that mean no part of these physical complaints has organic origins of any kind?

I argue that idioms-of-distress research, in its focused attention on context, allows for the possibility of building a theory of a corporeal idiom of distress—an expression that represents a symptom (or set of symptoms) for which myriad etiologies are at play. In considering corporeal idioms of distress, a single causal relationship between symptom and cause would, therefore, need to be rejected in favor of painting a more complex portrait of suffering and an attendant multifaceted course of treatment.

The word *idiom*, of course, refers to "the specific character or individuality of a language," to "the manner of expression considered natural to or distinctive of a language" (*Oxford*, "idiom," n.d.). Adding *corporeal* calls attention to the "nature of the animal body as opposed to the spirit," the "physical," the "bodily," the "mortal," and the body's ability to communicate psychic suffering (*Oxford*, "corporeal," n.d.). The concept of corporeal idioms of distress takes its lead from traditional definitions of idioms of distress in its careful consideration of context but parts ways in its expansion into physical symptoms both of the body *and* of the mind. Calling idioms of distress *corporeal*, in fact, is not without precedent in the literature. While idioms-of-distress researchers mostly approach their work within psychiatric frameworks as in the literature cited above, a few address psychogenic components directly, noting there is a possibility of "a culturally mediated illness where an individual suffering from psychological issues expresses distress in the form of physical symptoms and somatic complaints, with no known organic cause" (So 2008, 170).

Weighing in on this complex theoretical terrain in a similar fashion, Arthur Kleinman (1986), in a strikingly eloquent turn of phrase, explains, "Somatization indicates the processes of communication and exchange through which a bodily idiom of distress signifies and negotiates social and personal problems" (500). In other words, for Kleinman, multifaceted subjective symptoms reports could be better understood if care providers were well versed in the social and personal problems with which their patients suffer. Kleinman's approach, thus, highlights the importance of psychosocial suffering in unpacking psychogenic symptoms. Even with these notable exceptions to idioms-of-distress research as mostly limited to psychiatric symptoms, *corporeal* is added to highlight the importance of bodily symptoms and the relevance of such concepts beyond psychiatry itself.

Thinking of psychogenic symptoms or somatizations as potentially communicating social or personal issues—as, in fact, idiomatic—reframes the conversation on psychogenic symptoms by giving them an explicit sociocultural precursor and thus taking the burden and blame from the patient herself and rendering it as a logical bodily response to inequalities. Important, these bodily responses need not be purely psychogenic; in their complexity, they might have etiological origins in the kind of psychosocial suffering that leaves an organic trace.

For example, as medical doctor Donald Barr (2014) has observed, "Most of the variability in health status we find in the United States and other developed countries . . . has everything to do with one's position in the social hierarchy" (1). Work like Barr's highlights the pervasive evidence that social status is a significant determinant of health outcomes. That is, disenfranchised populations are more likely than those with elite social status to suffer from debilitating illnesses and death. Such insights help substantiate the idea that bodies can make sociocultural suffering manifest in more ways than one. If a body, say, develops type 2 diabetes due to the inadequate availability of healthy foods, it can also develop, for instance, vertigo from being regularly treated like a second-class citizen. There is no way to know for sure this dizziness, though, does not also stem from some physical manifestation of social suffering that leaves an organic trace on the body, as well as on the mind.

Following Kleinman's creative usage and those idioms-of-distress researchers who have explored somatizations in relation to the term, I am thus drawn to *idioms of distress* as a rhetorical lens through which to meditate on the ways bodies make sociocultural suffering visible and, more important, on the dense and layered materializations of suffering that are both psychogenic and physiological in etiology and in expression—the thick and stratified ontologies that comprise a disease (Mol 2003). Given this density, it is quite possible most complaints have physical components and psychological components—particularly in the way diagnoses are reached. That is, since medical diagnostics rely on empirical evidence as well as on patient reports, there is always already a subjectivity at play. This subjective element manifests in obvious ways in the form of subjective patient reports. However, the highly subjective nature of examining empirical signs of disease indicate that these things are also highly contingent. I call the concerted attention to the conflation of physiological and psychological symptoms *corporeal idioms of distress* to highlight the subjective nature of suffering and to call attention to the potential for the body and mind to be simultaneously and equally implicated in the expression of illness and disease—and for neither the body nor the mind to be able to separate one from the other or escape the thick milieu from which their bodily complaints emerge.

Such an approach, of course, dismisses the mind/body dualism the *DSM-5* is also attempting to move away from in its description of SSD and related disorders. However, rather than leaving organic etiologies by the wayside, corporeal idioms of distress conceptually frame patients' symptoms as both/and. In other words, corporeal idioms of distress allow for the possibility that any articulation of symptoms involves both the body and the mind, so attempts to separate the one from the other in diagnostics can ultimately lead to confusion, mistrust, and inaccurate diagnoses.

Corporeal idioms of distress could be useful, but they presuppose rhetorical and ethical listening habits and strong patient ethos. For such a complex view of illness and disease to come to the fore, rhetorical rather than more traditional clinical listening habits—those tuned in to the possibility of corporeal idioms of distress—might provide better insights into patient care, might give way to robust studies of psychogenic etiologies, and eventually could lead to fewer cases of misdiagnosis. In attempting this argument, I call on health researchers in rhetoric to frame inquiries in ways that honor medicine as offering "not a knowledge of isolated bodies, but a range of diagnostic and therapeutic interventions into lived bodies, and thus into people's daily lives" (Mol and Law 2004, 58). Corporeal idioms of distress offer a lens through which such listening habits might be cultivated.

CORPOREAL IDIOMS OF DISTRESS: RHETORICAL LISTENING AS ALTERNATIVE TO POSITIVIST CLINICAL LISTENING HABITS

Considering symptoms to be corporeal idioms of distress also means allowing for the possibility that symptoms are metonyms for social inequalities of one form or another. Making this ontological leap would require care providers to alter their listening habits from clinical—which I define as those listening habits that pay homage to the medical-industrial complex—to rhetorical. Rhetorical listening is operationalized by relying on Krista Ratcliffe's (2005) landmark work with the term, which emphasizes the term's widespread usability in rhetorical study, noting that "as a trope for interpretive intervention, rhetorical listening signifies a stance of openness that a person may choose to assume in relation to any person, text, or culture" (17). Julie Jung (2005), in line with Ratcliffe, explains that in efforts to listen rhetorically, we must "continually interrogate our processes of identification, examining how we both connect with and disconnect from our discursive construction of self and others" (345). In the same way, I suggest physicians might gain insight into patient suffering by examining patterns of somatization as they relate to patterns of disenfranchisement and to issues of intersectionality in their local communities—vantage points that assume corporeal idioms of distress over and against binary explanations for suffering. That is, overlapping and interdependent sociocultural realities make the oversimplified nature of binary thinking where health and medical diagnostics are concerned with an issue that deserves more attention than it has traditionally received.

Further, framing clinical exchanges in ways that take as a given that all symptoms are both psychological and physiological will yield more productive conversations and could lead to more equitable distribution of empirical diagnostic testing. Rhetorical listening habits as articulated here bear some resemblance to "ethical listening" habits. As Rachel Snow et al. (2013) explain, "Ethical listening recognizes that good listening is utterly receptive, non-judgmental, silent, and bodily still, and in so being frees the speaker to establish her/his own subjective presence for the listener" (57).

In uneven power dynamics such as clinical spaces, such postures toward patients could lead to more full-bodied accounts of the minutia of contextual factors that lead to symptoms. Considering corporeal idioms of distress as a theoretical framework in clinical exchanges is an ideal, and it would rely heavily on a physician's willingness to cultivate rhetorical and ethical listening habits and especially acute cross-cultural communication skills; it would make it incumbent on diagnosing physicians to explore physiological possibilities alongside psychogenic ones without summing up the situation via psychogenic lenses prematurely. In some ways, then, corporeal idioms of distress are a sleight of hand that erases the notion of a patient having symptoms that are "all in their head" from the equation. Such a move sidesteps biases in diagnostic practices by highlighting the potential for all patients to present with symptoms worth further empirical *and* sociocultural investigation.

CONCLUSION: PATTERNS OF SOMATIZATION, PATTERNS OF DISENFRANCHISEMENT

As J. Blake Scott, Judy Segal, and Lisa Keränen (2013) have suggested, "If our work is to fulfill its aims, it must reach and influence its multiple audiences, which include the range of stakeholders and publics tied to the practices we examine" (3). Likewise, Maria Novotny and Elizabeth Horn-Walker (chapter 2, this collection) "see this work as imperative to engaging in public rhetoric by blurring the lines of who such scholarship is for: academics or communities we work with" (62).

In line with such thinking, and considering the wide-scale adoption of a corporeal-idioms-of-distress framework in clinical settings unlikely in the short term, I wonder what kinds of moves patients could make on their own in clinical exchanges that would promote rhetorical, ethical listening and attention to corporeal idioms of distress. Rhetorical/ ethical listening habits on the part of the diagnosing physician would be ideal, but how can these listening habits be actively encouraged or even insisted upon by the patient?

In some ways, the biases that characterize clinical exchanges are not easily undone. Women often have their symptoms treated with suspicion, and cisgender men are most likely to have their symptoms, instead, taken seriously and their complaints met with compassionate, timely, and rigorous diagnostic testing. However, that assertion is thrown into crisis when issues of intersectionality are brought into the fray. Is a cisgender homeless man, for example, likely to get that kind of care? Does someone with a long history of mental illness receive prompt attention for claims of physical distresses? Issues of intersectionality make it impossible to stick to the binary assertion that men's symptoms and complaints lead to quality care and women's are roundly dismissed. Leslie Anglesey (chapter 3, this collection) addresses this very issue, noting that "increased attention to medical discourses of endometriosis, and female pelvic pain more broadly, is fraught with social assumptions and consequences" (68) and that "reports of pain by women are not dismissed only because of the ways female bodies are expected to experience pain but also because of the longstanding rhetorical figure of the hysterical woman, which is still prevalent in medical discourse today." (70).

Thinking of symptoms as corporeal idioms of distress is a modest attempt to build a linguistic-based theoretical intervention that might sidestep the binary of psychogenic and physiological conditions in homage to the interpretive nature of, the infinite imprecision of, diagnostic practices, but it is also an approach I hope can lead to fruitful conversations on how myriad markers of credibility—or lack of credibility—can be successfully navigated in clinical exchanges if the patient is prepared to advocate for themself. Gender biases aside, as K. H. Ladwig et al. (2001) suggest, other aspects of perceived credibility might influence whether or not a person is diagnosed as suffering from psychogenic symptoms. Examining psychogenic conditions' overdiagnosis in women from a rhetorical perspective calls up issues of rhetorical ethos in subjective patient reports and how the patient's perceived credibility (or not) influences the diligence with which diagnosing physicians perform aggressive testing—and ethos, of course, includes, but also supersedes, biological sex.

Likewise, corporeal idioms of distress as presented in this chapter take as a primary motivation the misdiagnosis of women with psychogenic symptoms, but examining such inequities through intersectional lenses is also worth parsing. When a patient has any number of stigmas, of course, they might not be trusted in clinical exchanges, and their physical complaints are more likely to be taken as psychogenic than if the patient were considered more credible.

Somatic symptom disorder (SSD) and related disorders stand in for a lack of a better something else. The *DSM* does not, probably, construct SSD with the hope of diagnosing vast numbers of patients with mental disorders. There is not likely a conspiracy at work. What do we do when we can't find a reason, and therefore a course of treatment, for a distress? Corporeal idioms of distress offer a theoretical framework through which to meditate on that important question. Conflating physiological and psychological symptoms as corporeal idioms of distress do, moreover, obliquely address stigmas associated with psychogenic symptoms; bodies suffer, and minds are not separate or separable from bodies, so suffering in all its forms flattens out.

For women like Lisa Smiril, the ability to convince a physician of the reality of their suffering is indeed a matter of life or death. As rhetoricians of health and medicine continue to define their disciplinary purview, engaging in studies that take up the complexity of the clinical scene in ways that actively reorient health/medical issues toward recognition of the whole body in context, and toward recognition of kinds of suffering that are currently misunderstood, will be crucial.

NOTE

1.   POTS is notoriously difficult to diagnose and often leads to misdiagnosis.

REFERENCES

American Psychiatric Association. n.d. "Somatic Symptoms Disorder Factsheet." Last modified 2013. https://www.psychiatry.org/psychiatrists/practice/dsm/educational -resources/dsm-5-fact-sheets.
American Psychiatric Association. n.d. "Highlights of Changes from DSM-IV-TR to DSM-V." Last modified 2013. https://www.psychiatry.msu.edu/_files/docs/Changes-From -DSM-IV-TR-to-DSM-5.pdf.

American Psychiatric Associaton. n.d. "What is Somatic Symptom Disorder." Last modified 2020. https://www.psychiatry.org/patients-families/somatic-symptom-disorder/what-is -somatic-symptom-disorder.

Barr, Donald A. 2014. *Health Disparities in the United States: Social Class, Race, Ethnicity, and Health.* Baltimore: Johns Hopkins University Press.

Boissoneault, Lorraine. 2015. "My Doctor Told Me It Was All in My Head; I Might Have Died If I'd Believed Him." *Salon*, November 22. https://www.salon.com/2015/11/22 /everything_is_fine_with_your_thyroid_the_doctor_told_me_youre_just_stressed/.

Chapman, Elizabeth N., Anna Kaatz, and Molly Carnes. 2013. "Physicians and Implicit Bias: How Doctors May Unwittingly Perpetuate Health Care Disparities." *Journal of General Internal Medicine* 28 (11): 1504–1510.

Castro, Yessennia, Joyce L. Carbonell, and Joyce C. Anestis. 2012. "The Influence of Gender Role on the Prediction of Antisocial Behaviour and Somatization." *International Journal of Social Psychiatry* 58 (4): 409–16.

Deaton, Emily. 2015. "When Doctors Told Me My Chronic Illness Was All in My Head." The Mighty: We Face Disability, Disease, and Mental Illness Together, August 10. https://themighty.com/2015/08/when-doctors-told-me-my-chronic-illness-was-all-in -my-head/.

de Jong, Joop T., and Ria Reis. 2010. "Iyang-Yang, a West-African Postwar Idiom of Distress." *Cultural Medical Psychiatry* 24 (2): 301–321.

Durà-Vilà, Gloria, and Matthew Hodes. 2012. "Cross-Cultural Study of Idioms of Distress among Spanish Nationals and Hispanic American Migrants: Susto, Nervios and Ataque de Nervios." *Social Psychiatry and Psychiatric Epidemiology* 47 (10): 1627–1637.

Fassler, Joe. 2015. "How Doctors Take Women's Pain Less Seriously." *Atlantic*, October 15. https://www.theatlantic.com/health/archive/2015/10/emergency-room-wait-times -sexism/410515/.

Graham, S. Scott. 2015. *The Politics of Pain Medicine: A Rhetorical-Ontological Inquiry.* Chicago: University of Chicago Press.

Harvard Health Publishing, Harvard Medical School. 2008. "Anxiety and Physical Illness." https://www.health.harvard.edu/staying-healthy/anxiety_and_physical_illness.

Hinton, Devon E., and Roberto Lewis-Fernández. 2010. "Idioms of Distress among Trauma Survivors: Subtypes and Clinical Utility." *Culture, Medicine and Psychiatry* 34 (2): 209–218.

Hoffman, Diane E., and Anita J. Tarzian. 2001. "The Girl Who Cried Pain: A Bias against Women In the Treatment of Pain." *Journal of Law, Medicine and Ethics* 28 (4): 13–27.

Jung, Julie. 2005. "The Perfected Mother: Listening, Ethos, and Identification in Cases of Munchausen by Proxy Syndrome." In *Rhetorical Agendas: Political, Ethical, Spiritual*, edited by Patricia Bizzell, 345–350. Mahwah, NJ: Lawrence Erlbaum.

Katz, Joel, Brittany N. Rosenbloom, and Samantha Fashler. 2015. "Chronic Pain, Psychopathology, and DSM-5 Somatic Symptom Disorder." *Canadian Journal of Psychiatry* 60 (4): 160–167.

Keränen, Lisa. 2012. "'This Weird, Incurable Disease': Competing Diagnoses in the Rhetoric of Morgellons." In *Health Humanities Reader*, edited by Therese Jones, Delese Wear, and Lester D. Friedman, 36–49. New Brunswick, NJ: Rutgers University Press.

Keys, Hunter M., Bonnie N. Kaiser, Brandon A. Kohrt, Nayla M. Khoury, and Aimée R. Brewster. 2012. "Idioms of Distress, Ethnopsychology, and the Clinical Encounter in Haiti's Central Plateau." *Social Science and Medicine* 75 (3): 555–564.

Kleinman, Arthur. 1986. "Social Origins of Distress and Disease: Depression, Neurasthenia, and Pain in Modern China." *Current Anthropology* 27 (5): 499–509.

Kohrt, Brandon A., and Daniel J. Hruschka. 2010. "Nepali Concepts of Psychological Trauma: The Role of Idioms of Distress, Ethnopsychology and Ethnophysiology in Alleviating Suffering and Preventing Stigma." *Culture, Medicine and Psychiatry* 34 (2): 322–352.

Ladwig, Karl-Heinz, Birgitt Marten-Mittag, Natalia Erazo, and Harald Gündel. 2001. "Identifying Somatization Disorder in Population-Based Health Examination Survey: Psychosocial Burden and Gender Differences." *Psychosomatics* 42 (6): 511–518.

Mol, Annemarie. 2003. *The Body Multiple: Ontology in Medical Practice*. Durham, NC: Duke University Press.

Mol, Annemarie, and John Law. 2004. "Embodied Action, Enacted Bodies: The Example of Hypoglycaemia." *Body and Society* 10 (2–3): 43–62.

Morrison Zachary J., David M. Gregory, and Steven Thibodeau. 2011. "It's Not Just about the French Fry: Avoidance as an Idiom of Distress among Overweight and Obese Adolescent Boys." *American Journal of Men's Health* 5 (6): 517–523.

Nations, Marilyn, and Ana Paul S. Gondim. 2013. "'Stuck in the Muck': An Eco-idiom of Distress from Childhood Respiratory Diseases in an Urban Mangrove in Northeast Brazil." *Cadernos de saúde pública* 29 (2): 303–312.

Nicther, Mark. 2010. "Idioms of Distress Revisited." *Culture, Medicine, and Psychiatry* 43 (2): 401–416.

Novella, Steven. 2009. "It's All in Your Head." Science-Based Medicine: Exploring Issues and Controversies in Science and Medicine, November 4. https://sciencebasedmedicine.org/its-all-in-your-head/.

Núñez, Lorena C. 2009. "Is It Possible to Eradicate Poverty without Attending to Mental Health? Listening to Migrant Workers in Chile through Their Idioms of Distress." *Journal of Health Management* 11 (2): 337–354.

Oxford English Dictionary, s.v. "corporeal." Last modified 2000. www.oed.com.

Oxford English Dictionary, s.v. "idiom." Last modified 2010. www.oed.com.

Ratcliffe, Krista. 2005. *Rhetorical Listening: Identification, Gender, Whiteness*. Carbondale: Southern Illinois University Press.

Reynolds, J. Fred. 2008. "The Rhetoric of Mental Healthcare." In *Rhetoric of Healthcare*, edited by Barbara Heifferon and Stuart Brown, 149–157. Cresskill, NJ: Hampton.

Scott, J. Blake, Judy Z. Segal, and Lisa Keränen. 2013. "The Rhetorics of Health and Medicine: Inventional Possibilities for Scholarship and Engaged Practice." *Poroi* 9 (1). https://ir.uiowa.edu/poroi/vol9/iss1/17/.

Skovenborg, Elisabeth L., and Andreas Schröder. 2014. "Is Physical Disease Missed in Patients with Medically Unexplained Symptoms? A Long-Term Follow-Up of 120 Patients Diagnosed with Bodily Distress Syndrome." *General Hospital Psychiatry* 36 (1): 38–45.

Snow, Rachel C., Angela M. Williams, Curtis Collins, Jessica Moorman, Tomas Rangel, Audrey Barick, Crystal Clay, and Armando Matiz Reyes. 2013. "Paying to Listen: Notes from a Survey of Sexual Commerce." *Community Literacy Journal* 8 (1): 53–69.

So, Joseph K. 2008. "Somatization as Cultural Idiom of Distress: Rethinking Mind and Body in a Multicultural Society." *Counselling Psychology Quarterly* 21 (2): 167–174.

Wool, Carol A., and Arthur J. Barsky. 1994. "Do Women Somatize More Than Men? Gender Differences in Somatization." *Psychosomatics* 35 (5): 445–452.

2

ART-I-FACTS
A Methodology for Circulating Infertility Counternarratives

Maria Novotny and Elizabeth Horn-Walker

INTRODUCTION

The year 2013 was a particularly hard one for the two of us. In May, Elizabeth learned she was miscarrying twins. Further complicating this loss was the financial reality that this failed pregnancy was the result of an IVF[1] cycle. That same year, Maria was deciding whether or not to start a PhD program, knowing full well this would postpone any fertility treatment. Despite all the prayers, the tracking of cycles, and the restricted diets, the reality was sinking in for her that a natural pregnancy would never happen. While we each had tried for years to naturally conceive, 2013 was our breaking point—either do anything to get pregnant or take a step back. We both decided, without knowing each other at the time, to do the latter.

Reflecting on this decision, while many of the nuances are a bit blurred, we shared one poignant reason: we no longer recognized ourselves. We had to stop. Our cisgender bodies felt foreign to us. While we looked healthy, young, and emotionally in control, we were living in a shell of ourselves, disguised as a person who truly did not exist. Infertility had changed us. Very few people knew how disoriented we felt, and some had no knowledge we were trying to conceive or the challenges we faced in that process.

We share our own stories to establish personal exigency for this work and contextualize the methodology we built and describe here. After coming to terms with our decisions to take a break, our paths were brought together. In May of 2014, the two of us met at an infertility advocacy event. There, we disclosed versions of the stories above, and a friendship naturally developed as we discussed our feelings of fatigue, noting our embodied frustration in how infertility somehow made us "incomplete." While we could not naturally have children, we knew that we were part of families and that even though we could

DOI: 10.7330/9781607329855.c002

not get naturally pregnant, infertility was not a terminal disease. Our bodies, while unable to get pregnant naturally, were not threatened. We still had the option to not do anything, to take a break. Yet despite this realization, narratives of infertility continue to echo pathological assumptions that an infertile body is an unhealthy, diseased, incomplete body. That was not our story, nor was it the story of many other infertile friends we had come to know. Realizing the need to circulate infertility stories that did not follow such a path, we decided to create an organization to rebuild public perceptions and narratives of infertility. Drawing on our areas of expertise, Elizabeth's with art and photography and Maria's with oral-history methods and cultural narratives, we created The ART of Infertility, and in doing so, developed a methodology to gather counternarratives of infertility.[2]

This chapter unpacks the conflation of infertility, biomedicine, and gender so as to disrupt the pathology that is infertility. Describing our methodology and demonstrating its approach with two of our participants, we discuss the need to make visible narratives that counter pronatalist assumptions that correlate fertility with femininity. We suggest art may serve as a method to support the circulation of narratives that counter the gendered pathologization of infertility and point to a few examples that demonstrate this approach in action. We see art as a particularly useful method for making visible the gendered constructions of biomedicine and (in particular) infertility, which resonates with Leslie Anglesey's discussion of the rhetorical construction of endometriosis found in chapter 3 of this collection. It is our hope that this chapter speaks back to the pathologization of infertility and inspires more critical and compassionate models of public support for those who learn they are one in eight.[3]

INFERTILITY, BIOMEDICINE, AND GENDER

Infertility is a particularly challenging disease to diagnose. For one, it is a disease that does not have easily identifiable biomarkers, which allow for a measurable detection symptomatic of a potential disease. Lack of biomarkers leaves physicians needing to test a variety of factors and conditions in both men and women. Additionally, to receive an official infertility diagnosis, on average an individual must have spent more than six months having unprotected intercourse without resulting in a pregnancy. Frequently then, infertility is not realized until after months, sometimes even years, of trying to conceive. An embodied silence thus lurks in the body when it is infertile, a silence often only detectable once a person struggles in their desire to become pregnant. This silence is coupled with the reality that unlike disease with physical characteristics such as tumors or tremors, infertility can be hidden from others, meaning one's body is not easily *seen* or detected as an infertile body compared to bodies read as pregnant or as having cancer.

Social science scholars have studied how the silence surrounding infertility perpetuates feelings of shame and stigma, especially when gender ideologies are wrapped together with normative notions of reproduction (Allison 2011). For example, Arthur Greil's (2002) work discusses how normative views on gender reinforce feelings of failing gendered expectations amongst infertile women. He explains that "from the vantage point of American infertile women . . . infertility is a major disruption in one's projected life course, a failure to live up to normative notions about what it means to be an adult woman in American society" (101). From a young age then, girls in particular are taught through sociocultural messages that "being a mother is some-thing often central to identity. Thus, [with infertility] a sense of loss of identity and feelings of defectiveness and incompetence are quite often experienced" (Galhardo et al. 2011, 2409).

The integration of gender with reproductive norms reinforces pronatalist attitudes, whereby social value becomes linked to pro-creation (Parry 2005). And while second- and third-wave feminist efforts have attempted to refute and resist pronatalist ideologies, stud-ies continue to indicate motherhood remains a valued and desired identity—particularly biological motherhood (Jordan and Revenson 1999). And while biomedicine has allowed others (such as single parents by choice or LGBTQ persons) who previously could not expe-rience biological motherhood or fatherhood to carry a pregnancy, we remain concerned with how fertility treatment pathologizes bod-ies through normative attitudes towards gender and reproduction. Pathologizing the abnormal, infertile female body within a pronatalist framework makes possible the ability to fix and correct the abnormal body through fertility treatment, thereby perpetuating normative attitudes toward gender and reproduction by emphasizing fertility treatment as the only "resolution to the often life-altering experience of infertility" (Britt 2000, 208). Such a framework acts as a backbone to the most visible narratives of infertility, which are those that contain "success stories," by proliferating language that infertility is a disease that can and must be beaten so as to fulfill one's desire to become a mother/parent.

In what follows, we describe our resistance to these success narratives by offering an arts-based methodology that literally makes visible and calls into question the pathologizing of bodies when ideological norms of reproduction and gender conflict. We elaborate on this by sharing the counternarratives of two cisgender women who donated pieces of art to The ART of Infertility. These pieces of art act as a rewriting of what infertility stories get heard and make space for validating moments of biomedical failure, echoing similar narratives offered by Lori Beth De Hertogh in chapter 10 of this collection. We offer conclusions that explore how art acts as a disruptive discourse expanding cultural assumptions of infertility and consider the role of circulating art in traveling exhibits as a model of public pedagogy, calling attention to the gendered pathology of infertility and reproductive loss.

ART-I-FACTS: A METHODOLOGY TO VIEW INFERTILITY

The ART of Infertility operates on the premise that infertility continues to be stigmatized and experienced in silence/isolation and that—because of the availability of fertility treatments—an embedded cultural narrative persists that an infertile body is an abnormal body, correctable through a variety of medical procedures. We strive to trouble such sociocultural orientations to infertility. Consequently, we use art, a visual representation of infertility, to make clear the everyday challenges and forms of resistance infertile persons confront once given an infertility diagnosis. We see art as a method making infertility visible and facilitating more critical conversations about its experience amongst the greater public. Our hope is that the display of these artistic representations in public spaces (1) allows for a community of support to emerge, meaning individuals no longer see themselves as being alone and realize infertility impacts many and (2) creates awareness among the general public about the everyday challenges infertile persons face, inviting the public to revise practices and policies that fail to account for challenges to living with infertility.

To do this work then, we have established an art-i-facts-based methodology. Three points support our rationale for using art-i-facts. One, this methodology requires participants to bring artifacts, such as art. Two, this methodology is a play on words, drawing on what Kathy Mantas (2016) has called "notions of fact (i.e., scientific facts) and fiction (i.e., artfully crafted forms), especially as they relate to telling and retelling, remembering, and memory" (118). Finally, *art-i-facts*, like The ART of

Infertility, is a play on *assisted reproductive technology*, sometimes referred to as *ART*.

Beyond its name, it should be noted that this methodology is a phased methodology, meaning there are several parts that happen over time. This approach is influenced by Bump Halbritter and Julie Lindquist's (2012) LitCorps project, a literacy sponsorship project in which researchers and participants engaged in moments of *looking, listening*, and *strategically deferring interpretive closure*. Drawing on Halbritter and Lindquist's focus on the reflective learning emerging through a phased-out and scaffolded methodological structure, we sought to mimic its approach so as to enhance moments of reflective learning and factor in a strategy to circulate findings beyond academic bounds. Accordingly, we created a three-phased methodology to gather reflective participant data, assemble and make meaning out of such data, and then circulate and repurpose the data for public consumption.

Phase 1: Preinterview

First, participants are asked to fill out a preinterview form indicating general information about their experiences with infertility. This form serves as an artifact in itself, allowing us as researchers to have a more fully developed sense of what the participant may speak to in regard to infertility. Knowing such details assists us in structuring the conversation and focusing on experiences that counter more dominant narratives of infertility, such as male-factor infertility or failed fertility treatments.

Phase 2: Interview with Artist and Art

After reviewing that form, we arrange face-to-face interviews with participants. During this portion, we invite individuals to select two to four pieces of artwork to bring to the interview. Drawing upon the artwork and the preinterview form, together we interview individuals and develop questions to guide them in a rhetorical analysis of their artwork. Examples of questions include, Can you tell me why you opted to create an oil painting? Why use oil paints? Did that medium allow you to express something in particular about your infertility experience? After conducting the interview, photographs of the pieces of artwork are taken so they can be included in the exhibition of art. At times, participants offer to donate their artwork for exhibition and/or loan it to the project.

Phase 3: (Re)Creating and Circulating

Our final phase is a (re)creation and circulation phase. We transcribe the interview using discourse analysis to (re)create a short narrative from our interview to serve as an artist label for the exhibit. Unlike traditional art exhibitions, this label contains a summarized narrative of the person's infertility story and reflective analysis of their art. With the images and narrative (re)created, we move to circulate the pieces frequently in public spaces, including our website and public art galleries around the country.

In what follows, we share the stories and art of two participants who donated their work to The ART of Infertility. We highlight these two narratives below as they reinforce this edited collection's intention to "reconcile data within the context of embodied experience" (6). While we could have incorporated works and narratives from the over two hundred pieces collected for exhibition, we focus on the stories below, as these are bodies that don't fit certain categories commonly represented when discussing infertility. These stories are counternarratives of infertility. They contest and complicate biomedicine's gendered promise that it can change and fix bodies that cannot conceive into more normalized, feminine bodies.

Too often the success stories of infertility are heard and shared, and they reinforce a cultural norm that infertility can be resolved. These stories fit nicely within a rhetoric of hope that positions biomedicine as a life-changing, and, even perhaps more acutely, a life-creating technology that helps people become parents. Many times, however, patients must undergo several rounds of biomedical treatment, like in vitro fertilization, before even becoming pregnant (Smith et al. 2015). These stories of when fertility treatment does not grant immediate success, we find, are too often erased from fertility conversations and, even more, are underserved in terms of being cared for and listened to. We seek in this piece to begin the process of caring for and listening to these stories. Consequently, in the stories shared below, we follow a feminist rhetorical methodological approach, in line with Maureen Johnson et al.'s (2015) embodied methodological inquiry, which finds value in individuals tacking into their own embodied experiences.

MEG'S AND SARA'S ART-I-FACT NARRATIVES

Meet Meg and Sara. Both women identify primarily as patient artists who turned to art as a method of coping and a need to document their experiences with infertility. We met Meg as a participant in May 2015. We met Sara in October 2015. In the subsection that follows, we demonstrate the application of our phased methodology with Meg and Sara.

Meg

Phase 1

By reviewing the preinterview form, we learned Meg was diagnosed with DOR[4] and ovarian dermoids (mature teratomas).[5] Additionally, she revealed that prior to their relationship, her husband had a vasectomy, which further complicated their fertility. In total, Meg and her husband had three surgeries between the two of them and attempted seven IUIs[6] and nine IVFs—all of which did not succeed. At the time of our interview, she indicated they are now in the process of grappling with the reality that treatment may not work and living child free may be their path of family-building resolution.

Phase 2

During the face-to-face interview, Meg brought us two artifacts. "My Consent" (fig. 2.1) is a piece of blackout poetry she created from a medical release form, an artifact she collected from one of her prior treatments. The poetry reads, "I / perform / observe / authorize / certain risks / I / will be disposed / used for research / no right or entitlement / My consent / not an exact science / no guarantee / all-inclusive." The second artifact is "Bloodlines" (fig. 2.2), an acrylic painting on canvas.

Phase 3

Throughout the interview, Meg shared with us the stories of infertility reflected in her artwork. She reflected in particular on "Bloodlines" during our interview, stating,

> It's a little un-PC, but it is how I feel. It's a base. It's a primal need. My desire to have a child has always been very primal. I want to feel pregnant. I want to give birth and there's something about bloodlines in there and I can't get around it. I'm smart enough to have researched epigenetics, but it just does not cut it for me. It wasn't enough and I do think there's a part around how dysfunctional my family of origin is, and really wanting to change that patterning and I think that that plays into it, the desire that there has to be a genetic link so I can fix the family somehow. It's not logical. I don't necessarily think it's the healthiest, but I know that that's part of it. I don't know if that makes any sense.

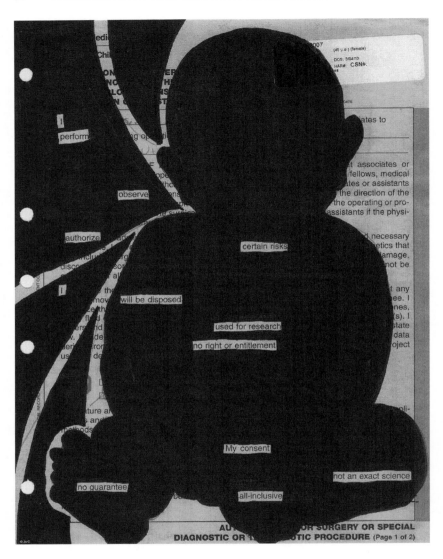

Figure 2.1. "My Consent" by Meg

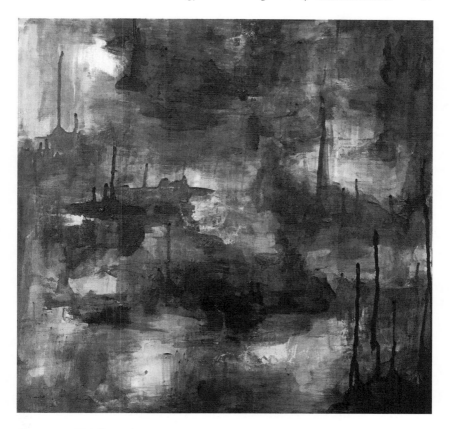

Figure 2.2. "Bloodlines" by Meg

After the interview was transcribed and coded, the following labels were created for an upcoming exhibit.

"MY CONSENT" LABEL FOR ART OF INFERTILITY EXHIBIT
I
perform
observe
authorize
certain risks
I
will be disposed
used for research
no right or entitlement

"BLOODLINES" LABEL FOR ART OF INFERTILITY EXHIBIT

In *Bloodlines* I express the complexity of one's relationship to ancestry when infertility wipes out your descendants. I was also exploring the symbolism of bloodletting in human reproduction: the monthly offering of menstrual blood. This bloodletting is initially seen as a signal of health and fecundity, but quickly becomes a trigger of despair the longer you are unable to conceive. As I embarked on intensive fertility treatments, many more rites of blood offerings followed. While more clinical, they are no less sacred rites of the body:

The almost daily blood draws to monitor hormone levels and follicular growth.

The Beta test to find out if hCG, the pregnancy hormone, coursed through my veins.

The track marks left on my belly, hips, and butt from injections.

The blood red sharp containers filled to the brim with discarded syringes.

My vaginal wall punctured by needle during each egg retrieval.

Sara

Phase 1

Sara, as we learned from her preinterview form, was just preparing to begin her second IVF cycle. She had been diagnosed with infertility at the age of thirty-seven, and a number of factors were complicating her fertility, including possible exposure to diethylstilbestrol (DES)[7] when she was in utero as well as a PCOS diagnosis,[8] which she contests and believes is simply not accurate. Her multiple diagnoses and multiple factors impacting her fertility have led her to consulting (and at times) firing doctors and to leaving her feeling as if she must "fight for [her] healthcare."

Phase 2

For our interview, Sara brought us "Failed IVF #1," (fig. 2.3) a mixed-media piece constructed from a body cast of Sara's stomach and decorated with vials, syringes, and an ultrasound image from an embryo transfer, which was unsuccessful.

Phase 3

During our interview, she was asked "Why a body cast?" In answering this question, Sara explained,

I've always had anger issues towards this ridiculous model that we're supposed to fit as females. We are supposed to be perfectly beautiful, we're

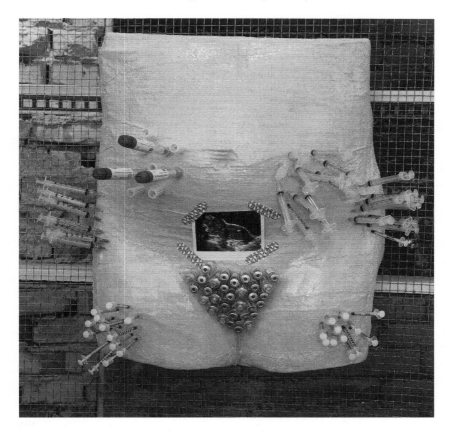

Figure 2.3. "Failed IVF #1" by Sara

never supposed to age. We are supposed to have amazing careers and be fabulous mothers. I am never going to be tall. I apparently am never going to be fit and who knows if I'm going to get to be a mother. I'm going to try, but that may not happen. All of these norms that are set up for women may never fit me. It's really hard too because there is something about kids and this society. Everybody loves children and it is okay in this society for someone you don't know or hardly know to ask you if you have children. As an infertile female, that's such a big question.

After the interview was transcribed and coded, the following labels were created for an upcoming exhibit:

> **"FAILED IVF #1" LABEL FOR ART OF INFERTILITY EXHIBIT**
>
> I knew when I was getting ready to go through the IVF and while I was going through the IVF, I knew that I would do something with all the needles. It's such an overwhelming experience . . . When they [medications] come in the mail, they come packaged in like ice and stuff and it's a huge box full of medicines, syringes, a sharps container, vials, like all this stuff. It is overwhelming looking at it thinking, "I am going to put all this crap in my body. Holy cow." I don't think people get how much goes into an IVF. Anyways, I was trying to figure out what I could do with my syringes. I was just marinating on the idea trying to figure it out and then the idea hit me. I was like, Oh, duh. Just make a cast of yourself and put the needles back in. Duh.
>
> I've always made casts. I have a cast of my entire right side and I turned myself into an island, because no man could be an island, but one woman in our society is absolutely expected to be one. I made myself into an island, why not? That was when I was like, Oh, duh, this is perfect. I should just cast myself. I just wanted some way for people to see how much medicine goes into this. I wanted to show people IVF.

MAKING VISIBLE: INFERTILITY, RISK, AND FAILURE

What emerges through this methodology is that an infertility diagnosis involves the navigation of both medical and sociocultural factors. Both Meg and Sara make claims about the need to make infertility more visible to others. Related to this sense of becoming visible, they recount how sociocultural gender norms, idealizing motherhood, and attaching notions of fertility to femininity make living with infertility a challenge.

Here, we tend to three specific findings that emerged out of participants' art. One, there is a perceived health and sociocultural risk to embodying femaleness and infertility. This means fertility treatment itself positions infertile women in decisions of risk. We situate this with the market model of infertility medicine. Further, to be an infertile woman is to embody a particularly risky subject—challenging larger sociocultural assumptions of femininity. Second, this sense of embodying risk because of one's inability to conceive derives from sociocultural notions of failing to be female. We note how this sense of failing fertility emerges from pronatalist culture. This sense of failure is heightened when fertility treatments fail.

From these two findings emerges our third takeaway. This finding argues that the medical invasiveness of infertility often fails to be visible. Many disregard the medical risk attached to fertility treatments. Meg's and Sara's interviews nod to this when they recount how others, in response to learning of their infertility, say, "Well you can just do IVF" or "You can always just adopt." Fertility treatment, which puts female patients at risk, fails in these larger sociocultural discourses to be recognized as a medical risk. Further, when treatment fails and one must grapple with the reality of living without children, there is an additional component to the invisibility of infertility. Both Meg and Sara talk of this need to make infertility more visible to stakeholders and the general public. They view art as a way to make infertile experiences, the counternarratives of success, more visible to others. This sense of needing art to raise awareness leads us to a discussion about the final phase of our methodology—the circulation of these experiences via art exhibitions.

Risk and Infertility

The artwork created by Meg and Sara does not explicitly comment on the subject of risk. However, we focus on the incorporation of medical art-i-facts in these pieces of artwork. Sara's decision to include syringes and Meg's incorporation of a medical consent form serve as evidence of underlining moments of risk attached to infertility, specifically fertility treatment. This understanding of risk is informed by Tasha Dubriwny's (2013) examination of contemporary women's-health movements. Her work argues that current health-advocacy campaigns construct notions of being a healthy woman through discourses of risk. Her work seeks, through biopolitical advocacy, to disrupt larger sociocultural beliefs that idealize women's health. Dubriwny's work is important to understanding how health becomes a risk, particularly in the context of women and infertility.

Infertility as engaging in risk has been discussed primarily in the context of multiple births (Hall 2015; Shivas and Charles 2005). However, this discussion of infertility and risk is limited and assumes infertility is always accompanied by successful fertility treatment. We complicate this discussion of risk and infertility by drawing upon what we learned from the interviews with Meg and Sara. Specifically, we pay attention to how their artwork visualizes risk more explicitly than their interviews do. For example, Meg's "My Consent" is an artifact signaling a sense of risk attached to fertility treatment. While she does not explicitly talk of the potential side effects of the treatment, she does indicate in her poem the reality that there is "no guarantee" of the treatment's success. Sara's "Failed IVF #1" also does not explicitly speak to becoming a subject of risk. Yet her decision to keep and incorporate the syringes and vials from her failed treatment does indicate the medical invasiveness of such fertility treatments. Together, these two pieces remind viewers that fertility treatment is risky in that (1) there is an injection of hormones and the possibility that the treatment may result in multiple births and (2) that the treatment is a risk, meaning it might not be a success.

Market models of medicine have encouraged medical professionals to actively examine the risk of hormone injections, such as the correlation of fertility hormones with various forms of cancer. More recently, many have advocated for the reduction of the number of embryos transferred in each cycle so as to reduce risks associated with multiple births, preterm delivery, and low birthweights for infants (Sunderan et al. 2014). Yet, market models of medicine have failed to really consider the impact of the second potential risk—treatment not working. While there have been many studies indicating the improving success rates of treatments like in vitro fertilization, the reality remains that treatment may not work. Meg and Sara are examples of treatment failing. They speak to the reality of embodying a new risk—finding happiness in the reality that they may not be mothers or have a biological child. This is a risk to pronatalist culture, as we explain in our next finding.

Failing Fertility; Failing Femininity

This sense that risk emerges through a failed fertility treatment, and the inability to become a mother, can be traced to pronatalism. Carolyn Morell (2000) explains pronatalism through feminist theory and suggests its increasing presence in Western culture is a direct response to second-wave feminists, who "de-emphasize[d] the positive importance of motherhood in women's lives" (315). As a consequence, pronatalism has become more readily adopted in US culture by religious movements that emphasize the identity of a wife as a mother. This conservative ideology, as a result, has adopted a "racist dimension, attacking middle-class and upper middle-class white women who remain childless or postpone childbearing and castigating women of color who have children as single parents in non-optimal circumstances" (315). Pronatalism, then, approaches infertility as an identity in need of correction. This position provides insight into contemporary health discourses that position infertility as something to be "beaten," akin to notions of "beating cancer" and "not letting the disease beat you." Larger cultural ideologies of gender, health, and the neoliberal family are thus embedded in these discourses of health advocacy. But there are moments when one may choose not to undergo fertility treatment or to accept the reality that fertility treatment simply may fail.

Meg's and Sara's interviews and artwork speak to the reality of failure and fertility treatment. Both, as subjects of fertility-treatment failure, comment on the effects of pronatalism and their infertility identity. Sara's piece, "Failed IVF #1," perhaps most directly indicates a sense of failure, and her interview indicates deep frustration with both the promise of medicine to fix her infertility and larger sociocultural beliefs attaching fertility to feminine ideals. In the interview for Meg's piece "Bloodlines," we learned that, while not as explicit as Sara's piece, "Bloodlines" reflects sentiments of failure and the loss of a biological connection with a child. These sentiments of failure, we argue, are directly tied to infertility's connection to pronatalist culture and discourse. Such discourse is further embedded in biomedical practices, aiming to fix culturally deemed nonnormative bodies, such as the infertile female body. Failing fertility treatment indicates then not just a failure of biomedicine but also a failure to conform to larger sociocultural notions of what it means to be a woman.

Infertility and Invisibility

Drawing upon the two findings above, we found that Meg and Sara often feel their infertility is invisible to others. This finding is significant given the invasiveness of an infertility diagnosis. We learned from Meg and Sara that women often experience infertility through a deeply biomedical model of medicine. Such a model poses risks to infertile women, who are often the primary recipients of fertility treatment. Further, this model, when it fails, positions women at risk of being unable to conform to sociocultural ideals of gender and family. This failure to recognize infertility as a medical condition and to recognize the psychological challenges of feeling as if one's identity is always at odds with dominant notions of femininity is challenging and must be noted.

In our interviews, we learned more about how Meg and Sara feel invisible. For example, from Sara we learned how frustrated she felt with the insensitivity of many individuals who did not understand her struggle to conceive. Further, Meg's piece "Bloodlines" serves to speak to the challenges of coming to terms with possibly never having a biological child and never making the continuation of her "bloodline" or DNA visible to others. This is further mirrored in "My Consent" with the image of the black silhouette of a baby—suggestive of an absence that will never be filled.

Social science studies examining this perception of feeling infertile and invisible (Greil and McQuillan 2010; Whiteford and Gonzalez 1995) suggest such an experience has led to a sociocultural stigma of infertility. Attempts to reduce such stigma and silencing around infertility have included national advocacy health events such as April's annual event National Infertility Awareness Week (NIAW), which aims to spread awareness about experiences of infertility, and the creation of several infertility advocacy blogs such as *Our Misconception* or *The Broken Brown Egg*. The central idea behind many of these infertility advocacy campaigns is for the circulation of infertility stories so as to make infertility a more recognized health condition and reduce its sociocultural stigma. While these campaigns focus on written or oral discourse, we argue that our findings suggest that art, too, can be a powerful outlet in which words and images come together to represent the realities of infertility—making infertility more visible. Similarly, art becomes a powerful communicative tool with which patients can represent embodied experiences of pain and medicine to medical professionals. The need to listen to subjective patient experiences is further emphasized in the introduction to this collection.

Feminist art scholar Marissa McClure (2014) elaborates on the need to make more nuanced narratives of infertility, and motherhood, visible. She explains that while feminist artists and art activists have a well-documented and exhibited history of confronting sociocultural attitudes towards motherhood, infertility and infertile bodies "remain largely invisible in both artistic practice and academic discourse" (253). It is through absence that McClure offers the phrase " ," which suggests how art "perpetuates misunderstandings of the complex reality of mothering and parenting experiences in all their expressions" (253). Calling for a more critical feminist take on topics of motherhood represented in art, McClure advocates that art education needs an artistic reorientation to the bodies s/m/othered by the overwhelming dominance of motherhood. This reorientation should include the fostering, through a feminist-arts public pedagogy, of creative practices to make infertility experiences more visible to larger publics. We find that McClure's call to artists and educators for more critical inquiry towards female bodies, along with our findings, surfaces implications for rhetoricians committed to interrogating embodied sites of gender, health, and broader sociocultural identity constructions, such as motherhood.

ART AS PUBLIC PEDAGOGY

2020 marks six years since the two of us met and established The ART of Infertility. Today, we remain on a break for a variety of personal and professional reasons. One main reason has been the reception of and interest in this project, The ART of Infertility. Over the past few years, this project has evolved from a self-funded "pop-up" organization into a sponsor-funded, nonprofit corporation hosting month-long exhibitions across the country. What has emerged in the years of building and learning from this organization is the continual response from the general public of "I had no idea." Art makes the stories of infertility visible, makes the struggles of infertility clearer, and as a result fosters a sense of community compassion and support.

By using a methodology that focuses a viewer's attention on the art-i-facts created by infertile persons, the shame, stigma, and silence so often embedded in these stories—the reasons it is often so difficult for infertile persons to share their stories—gets told in a new medium: through art. Art performs as a discourse-mobilizing action. Barbara Kirshenblatt-Gimblett (1998), in her work facilitating art as public pedagogy, notes art not only shows and speaks "but does." We find then that art as a discourse is embodied—its words are material compositions of bodies, inviting others into the corporeal compositions of their infertile lives. Simultaneously, art also is a method that invites the patient-artist to reflect on their experiences (Hogan 2003). While it can invite outsiders to see moments of personal coping, it also provides the patient-artist opportunities to cope and grieve, needs "often heightened at times of mourning" (Malchiodi 1992, 114). The personal healing that can come from creating art has been rather underexplored by feminist rhetoricians exploring issues of health and medicine and opens up a new space for mapping future research trajectories in rhetorical studies.

Art also allows for a greater circulation of and accessibility to stories. Hosting curated art exhibitions of art gathered from this project allows us to share stories across a broader series of networks. By making visible the gendering of infertility using art-i-facts, we hope the general public may revise common beliefs and become more culturally sensitive to the stigmatization of infertility. Further, we hope the exhibits, taken as an assemblage of stories, provide more inclusive, less prescriptive definitions of infertility success. Viewing, for example, Meg's and Sara's pieces begins to make space for broader, less uniform, and more complex notions of infertility. This, we argue, is significant to disrupting conflated understandings of infertility as a gendered pathology.

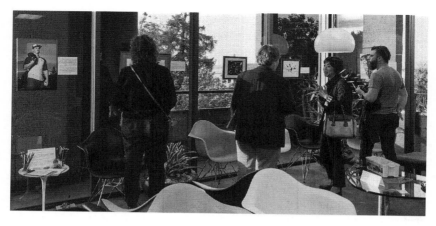

Figure 2.4. Picture Your Fertility: An Interactive Art Event. *Invited by a urology clinic based in California, The ART of Infertility created an exhibit themed around Men's Health Month. Attendees of this exhibit included members of the Association for Reproductive Medicine, including mental health and medical professionals, participants in The ART of Infertility, and individuals broadly interested in the intersection of medicine and art.*

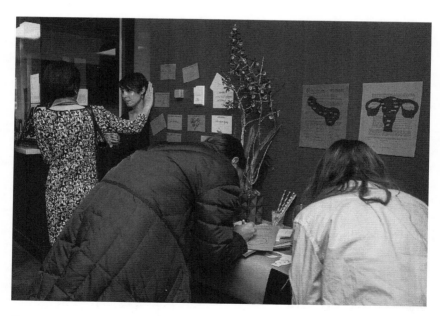

Figure 2.5. Meg's "My Consent" *served as inspiration for individuals to create their own consent art forms using blackout poetry techniques. This activity occurred at the* Picture Your Fertility: An Interactive Arts Event *exhibit. The purpose of interactive art is to invite others to reflect on their own embodied relationships to health and medicine. A similar event was conducted during the Coalition of Feminist Scholars in the History of Rhetoric and Composition (CFSHRC) Action Hour at CCCC in Houston, Texas.*

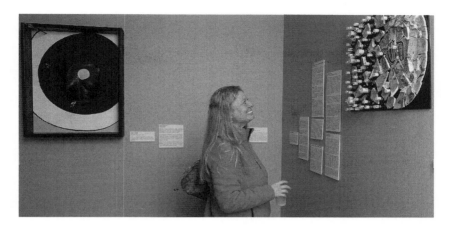

Figure 2.6. This exhibit was hosted at a local fertility clinic in Michigan. Physicians at this clinic wanted to host the exhibit as a way to connect to patients and aid communication between staff and patients about the intense emotions of infertility. Such approaches of attending to patient and staff communication have been documented in improvements needed for fertility patient-centered practice (Dancet et al. 2011).

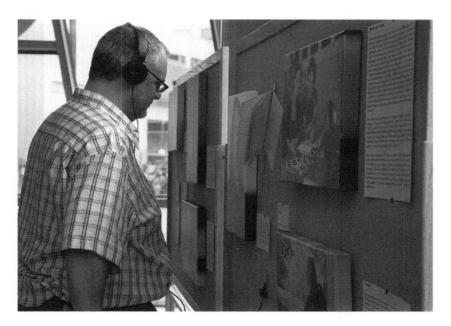

Figure 2.7. This exhibit was displayed at the Examined Life Conference, a medical humanities-based biannual conference hosted by the Roy J. and Lucille A. Carver College of Medicine at the University of Iowa. Here, patient perspectives represented through artwork and creative writing were shared with a range of medical stakeholders, including medical students, medical educators, and physicians and nurses.

Art becomes, then, a method to facilitate interventions in the gendering practices of health and medicine. We share with you the figures in this chapter to illustrate and make visible the variety of spaces and networks the project circulates across so as to illustrate how inhabiting particular spaces—using art as a method—may work to intervene in the sociocultural pathologizing of infertility. We see this work as imperative to engaging in public rhetoric by blurring the lines of who such scholarship is for: academics or communities we work with. We see the need for both and find art is a method to facilitate a reimagining of public rhetorical work.

NOTES

1. In vitro fertilization (IVF) is a process in which egg and sperm are combined outside the body and grown for several days, then the embryo is transferred back to the uterus.
2. To read more about counternarratives of infertility see Maria Novotny (2019).
3. One in eight is a statistic generated by the Centers for Disease Control and Prevention, citing that one in eight couples in the United States report trouble conceiving or maintaining a pregnancy. See *Facts About Infertility* (Resolve n.d.) for more information.
4. DOR is an acronym for the medical diagnosis diminished ovarian reserve.
5. Dermoids (mature teratomas) are dermoid cysts found on the ovary.
6. Intrauterine insemination (IUI) is when "washed" sperm are manually placed inside the uterus in an effort to help more sperm reach the fallopian tubes.
7. DES refers to an estrogen treatment used on women from 1938 to 1971. Its use was stopped once birth defects were linked to DES exposure. One cited birth defect is the development of an anteverted uterus, which tilts the uterus and makes it difficult to conceive.
8. A PCOS diagnosis refers to polycystic ovarian syndrome, which has been linked to infertility.

REFERENCES

Allison, Jill. 2011. "Conceiving Silence: Infertility as Discursive Contradiction in Ireland." *Medical Anthropology Quarterly* 25 (1): 1–21.

Britt, Elizabeth. 2000. "Medical Insurance as Biopower: Law and the Normalization of (In)Fertility." In *Body Talk: Rhetoric, Technology, Reproduction*, edited by Mary Lay, Laura J. Gurak, Clare Gravon, and Cynthia Myntti, 207–222. Madison: University of Wisconsin Press.

Dancet, Eline A., Inge W. Van Empel, Peter Rober, Willianne L. Nelen, Jan A. Kremer, and Thomas M. D'Hooghe. 2011. "Patient-Centred Infertility Care: A Qualitative Study to Listen to the Patient's Voice." *Human Reproduction* 26 (4): 827–833.

Dubriwny, Tasha N. 2012. *The Vulnerable Empowered Woman: Feminism, Postfeminism, and Women's Health*. New Brunswick, NJ: Rutgers University Press.

Galhardo, Ana, Jose Pinto-Gouveia, Marcla Cunha, and Marcia Matos. 2011. "The Impact of Shame and Self-Judgment on Psychopathology in Infertile Patients." *Human Reproduction* 26 (9): 2408–2414.

Greil, Arthur L. 2002. Infertile Bodies: Medicalization, Metaphor, and Agency. In *Infertility around the Globe: New Thinking on Childlessness, Gender, and Reproductive Technologies*, edited by Marcia C. Inhorn and Frank VanBalen, 101–118. Berkley: University of California Press.

Greil, Arthur L., and Julia McQuillan. 2010. "'Trying' Times." *Medical Anthropology Quarterly* 24 (2): 137–156.

Halbritter, Bump, and Julie Lindquist. 2012. "Time, Lives, and Videotape: Operationalizing Discovery in Scenes of Literacy Sponsorship." *College English* 75 (2): 171–198.

Hall, Jennifer G. 2015. *Women's Health Communication: High-Risk Pregnancy and Premature Birth Narratives.* Lanham, MD: Lexington Books.

Johnson, Maureen, Daisy Levy, Katie Manthey, and Maria Novotny. 2015. "Embodiment: Embodying Feminist Rhetorics." *Peitho* 18 (1): 39–44.

Hogan, Susan. 2001. "Approaches to Feminist Art Therapy and Gender Issues in Art Therapy." In *Arts—Therapies—Communication: On the Way to a Communicative European Arts Therapy,* edited by Line Kossolapow and Sarah Scoble, 108–116. Piscataway, NJ: Transaction Publishers.

Jordan, Caren, and Tracey A. Revenson. 1999. "Gender Differences in Coping with Infertility: A Meta-Analysis." *Journal of Behavioral Medicine* 22 (4): 341–358.

Kirshenblatt-Gimblett, Barbara. 1998. *Destination Culture: Tourism, Museums, and Heritage.* Berkeley: University of California Press.

Malchiodi, Cathy. 1992. "Art and Loss." *Art Therapy: Journal of the American Art Therapy Association* 9 (3): 114–118.

Mantas, Kathy. 2016. "ART-i-facts: A Work in Progress." In *On Mothering Multiples: Complexities and Possibilities,* edited by Kathy Mantas. Bradford: Demeter Press.

Martins, Mariana V., Brennan D. Peterson, Patricio Costa, Maria E. Costa, Rikke Lund, and Lone Schmidt. 2013. "Interactive Effects of Social Support and Disclosure on Fertility-Related Stress." *Journal of Social and Personal Relationships* 30 (4): 371–388.

McClure, Marissa. 2014. "S/M/Othering." *Studies in Art Education* 55 (3): 253–257.

Morell, Carolyn. 2000. "Saying No: Women's Experiences with Reproductive Refusal." *Feminism and Psychology* 10 (3): 313–322.

Novotny, Maria. 2019. "Infertility as Counterstory: Assembling a Queer Counterstory Methodology for Bodies of Health and Sexuality." In *Re/Orienting Writing: Queer Methods, Queer Project,* edited by Will Banks, Matthew Cox, and Caroline Dadas. Logan: Utah State University Press.

Parry, Diana C. 2005. "Work, Leisure, and Support Groups: An Examination of the Ways Women with Infertility Respond to Pronatalist Ideology." *Sex Roles* 53 (5–6): 337–346.

RESOLVE: The National Infertility Association. n.d. "Get the Facts." Last modified April 15, 2015. https://resolve.org/infertility-101/what-is-infertility/fast-facts/.

Shivas, Tricha, and Sonya Charles. "Behind Bars or Up on a Pedestal: Motherhood and Fetal Harm." 2005. In *Women and Children First: Feminism, Rhetoric, and Public Policy,* edited by Sharon M. Meagher and Patrice DiQuinzio, 283–201. New York: SUNY Press.

Smith, Andrew D.A.C., Kate Tilling, Scott M. Nelson, and Debbie A. Lawlor. 2015. "Live-Birth Rate Associated with Repeat In Vitro Fertilization Treatment Cycles." *JAMA* 314 (24): 2654–2662.

Sunderam, Saswati, Dmitry M. Kissin, Sara B. Crawford, Suzanne G. Folger, Denise J. Jamieson, Lee Warner, and Wanda D. Barfield. 2014. "Assisted Reproductive Technology Surveillance—United States, 2012." Centers for Disease Control and Prevention. *Morbidity and Mortality Weekly Report Surveillance Summaries* 64: 1–29.

Whiteford, Linda M., and Lois Gonzalez. 1995. "Stigma: The Hidden Burden of Infertility." *Social Science and Medicine* 40 (1): 27–36.

SECTION II

Patienthood and Patient-Provider Communication

3

"WE'RE ALL STRUGGLING TO BE A COMPLETE PERSON"
Listening to Rhetorical Constructions of Endometriosis

Leslie R. Anglesey

Doctor and patient approached each other with an agenda that they wished to articulate in the consultation. The implicit question, "are you listening to me?" turned into a symmetrical struggle for the role of the speaker.

—Dianna T. Kenny

INTRODUCTION

If you were to ask me to describe the pain I experience because of endometriosis in six words, I would say something like this: surprise, wrenching, intense, unbearable, searing, and alone. If you were to look through my chart for the same question, you might find a list with terms like "chronic pelvic pain in female" and "dysmenorrhea."[1] Of course, no healthcare professional has asked me this question, but this simple exercise highlights one of the greatest challenges faced by female patients. While both lists attempt to capture the pain associated with endometriosis, they communicate the experience in vastly different ways because, as the epigraph to this chapter suggests, doctors and patients have their own agendas for each consultation (Kenny 2002, 297). Patient agendas range widely. At times, patients seek validation; other times, patients like Shelley Raymond seek a diagnosis. Raymond revealed that in the moment she was finally diagnosed with the condition, she experienced relief; as she recalled, "The diagnosis didn't heal the pain. But after all these years of living with the unknown, a doctor had finally put a name to what was wrong with my body" (Kirkey, *Ottawan Citizen*, August 7, 1992).

These agendas (always personal, always political) do not, however, always align with the agendas of doctors, which are framed by the doctor's own political and personal experiences, beliefs, and knowledge

DOI: 10.7330/9781607329855.c003

sets. Because these agendas are often at odds with one another, it follows that one party is likely to lose out in controlling what happens when doctors and patients meet. For example, the woman knows she is in pain and, therefore, that something is wrong based on her experience of the pain. However, Western medicine trains doctors to look for the etiological causes of pain: a pinched nerve, internal bleeding, a broken bone, an ectopic pregnancy, and so forth. Even when some doctors "believe" their endometriosis patients' subjective self-reports, their medical training requires them to seek physical evidence.

Endometriosis, as I demonstrate in this chapter, poses significant challenges to medical professionals and patients alike. Because patients and doctors have different beliefs about the nature of a female patient's pelvic pain, it can be difficult for both parties to construct endometriosis-related pain in mutually intelligible ways. Increased attention to medical discourses of endometriosis, and female pelvic pain more broadly, is fraught with social assumptions and consequences. I explore my own experiences as a patient with endometriosis in order to trace how medical discursive practices and assumptions about the pain experienced by women dislocate female patients as authorities over their own bodies. I conclude with a brief exploration of the ways narrative medicine may assist gynecological practices in incorporating the voices of female patients.

CONNECTING EPISTEMOLOGY AND PATHOLOGY

To begin this chapter, I highlight an important tension between female epistemology and pathology by discussing the varying epistemologies of female pelvic pain, or the ways the very nature or existence of such pain is understood. As I argue throughout this chapter, female patients' day-to-day reality is informed by bodily knowledge and their experiences with pain that interferes in their ability to carry out various tasks. To live with chronic pain is to experience pain as a salient factor of daily life. This patient epistemology, rooted in experiential knowledge, sits in opposition to the medical establishment's ontology of chronic female pelvic pain, which is based on an ability to determine a pathogenesis. Pathogenesis in the case of endometriosis is achieved by visualizing lesions and implants, which is currently only accomplished through surgery. Given the high costs of surgery, doctors are not quick to do exploratory surgery to diagnose endometriosis. The delay in diagnosis keeps women's pain pathologically *unreal* and perpetuates, as Margrit Shildrik (1997) suggests, "the standards of an objective, universalized body" (76).

Because of the reliance upon notions of an idealized, "healthy" female body and assumptions about the kinds of pain women are expected to deal with, women are dislocated from their status as authorities about the pain they experience regularly.

Women have trouble discussing pain because their access to tools for reporting their pain (narratives) are coded within mainstream Western medicine *as* feminine practices. Thus, female patients with complaints of chronic pelvic pain are doubly gendered as they use discursive practices coded as feminine to talk about "womanly" pain, which is often received as hysteria (see next section). As the account of Shelley Raymond earlier in this chapter suggests, many doctors are quick to dismiss women's complaints of pelvic pain as illegitimate. She was told there was nothing wrong with her except that she was "'high strung'" (Kirkey, *Ottawan Citizen*, August 7, 1992). But Raymond is not alone. Heather C. Guidone, another woman diagnosed with endometriosis, once explained doctors often told her "'periods are supposed to hurt. It's a woman's lot in life to suffer'" (Glenza, *Guardian*, September 8, 2015). Another woman, who wished to remain anonymous, noted that a doctor dismissed her: "At one point [the doctor] told me I was a little girl who cried wolf, and one day I would be really sick and no one would believe me. And so I just kind of shut up" (Glenza).

These stories demonstrate the object, universalized female body Shildrik (1997) suggests. An objective understanding of the female body requires the regular experience of pelvic pain. It is thus natural and expected that women of childbearing age would experience pain, and because that pain is normalized, their reports of pain are most often filtered through the expectation that what they are experiencing is normal. Cara E. Jones's (2016) discussion of the gendering of endometriosis, its pain, and diagnosis, is telling. She observes that because of the "gendered norms" surrounding women's experience of pelvic pain, which make endometriosis pain "invisible in public discourse," "those with endo symptoms must seek legitimization through diagnosis to achieve what little support is available from friends, family, and social systems" (556). These socially accepted norms force women to seek substantiation through the long and arduous road to diagnosing endometriosis. But even within medical contexts, women's narratives of chronic pain must overcome substantial barriers in order to be listened to seriously.

To fully appreciate how these narratives are dismissed on the basis of a universalized, objective female body that experiences pain regularly, we can compare a woman's report of pelvic pain against a man who might report pelvic pain to his doctor. Because pelvic pain is not read as a regular occurrence of the male body's growth and development, any reports of pelvic pain by a man would be routed as symptomatic of something *wrong* with his body (prostatitis, appendicitis, diverticulitis, bowel obstruction, etc.), not something right (or at least something normal), as it is with women. Reports of pain by women are not dismissed only because of the ways female bodies are expected to experience pain but also because of the longstanding rhetorical figure of the hysterical woman, which is still prevalent in medical discourse today.

METHODOLOGIES

This chapter relies upon accounts of my own experiences with doctors. The decision to use my own experiences is not without political and methodological implications. However, part of my goal is to actively reorient the medical community away from large generalizations toward personal accounts. This reorientation must be done, in part, because the only record I have of most of my interactions with doctors are the copies of my charts provided to me, which by and large do not fully capture our conversations. Without traditional documentation, my experiences stand mostly as anecdotal evidence, which makes such data more difficult to generalize. However, the gaps in the "official" record of my past and ongoing treatments—the fact that I remain as a silent nonparticipant in my own charts, emphasizes the problem I address: namely, that female patients are nonauthorities on their own pain.

To highlight the issue of a woman's silence in her records, I want to draw attention to differences between a woman's absence in her medical records when she complains of chronic pelvic pain and a man's absence in his medical records when also complaining of pelvic pain. While it may be easy to see these absences as equal, they are not. The difference between the records of pathology for the man and the woman is that the man's reality of being in pain or the very reality of his condition is not likely to be challenged, whereas the woman's will likely be. It's not that a man will not use narrative to articulate his pain. The issue arises because a man is likely to be believed to have his condition, in part because his narratives about pain are easily corroborated by diagnostic tools; for a man presenting with pelvic pain, conditions like prostatitis, appendicitis, bowel obstruction, and diverticulitis can be diagnosed through urine samples (diverticulitis, prostatitis), CT scans (diverticulitis, appendicitis), and x-rays (appendicitis, bowel obstruction). His narrative accounts are made visible by diagnostic tools, and thus the absence of his voice does not illegitimate his claims of pain, whereas it can for a woman complaining of pelvic pain. On the other hand, a woman who reports pelvic pain may diagnostically *appear* healthy, which may make her narratives about pain more likely to be dismissed or read as exaggeration of normal female pain. Her absence from the medical records, then, constitutes an epistemological loss.

My attempts to reread my own experiences are examples of what Jacqueline Jones Royster and Gesa Kirsch (2012) have called reflective methodologies. Methods such as critical imagination and strategic contemplation, Royster and Kirsch (2012) argue, are central to feminist research. Critical imagination, for example, is a research tool for taking stock of what has been noticed and what has been unnoticed, a method for exploring why certain things are observed, and a technique for speculating about what could be (20). This research project would be incomplete without the ability to imagine the events of my own treatment and listen (in memory and in my charts) to what occurred and did not occur. To accomplish this task, I have taken care to ground my reflection in both the texts and contexts of the events (21).

As Royster and Kirsch (2012) further suggest, critical imagination is not a stand-alone method, and it is not treated as such in this project. I also employ what they call "strategic contemplation," a process by which a researcher engages their research subjects in dialogue, even if only imaginatively. This engagement allows researchers to recover voices ignored or intentionally silenced and to more critically reflect on what the researchers' own thoughts and interpretations of such silences may be. This process of listening, however, is complicated by the fact that I must alternately take upon myself the roles of researcher and subject. While it may be easy to see this dynamic as problematic, I view it as an opportunity. As Rita Charon (2006) has observed, an "autobiographical gap" is created "any time a person writes about himself or herself" (70). This gap allows the "narrator-who-writes and the protagonist-who-acts" to meet in a "reflective space . . . in a heightened way, revealing fresh knowledge about its coherent existence" (70). In other words, methodologies that meditate upon experiences from multiple (sometimes imagined) standpoints offer researchers opportunities to better understand the critical potential of events and provide subjects the opportunity to make sense of what they have experienced.

ENDOMETRIOSIS: A CASE OF DELAYED DIAGNOSIS

Because of the gendered nature of diagnosis and the pathologizing of women's bodies, delays in diagnosis of multiple conditions have been documented. As Kerri K. Morris's chapter in this collection also demonstrates, the delay of diagnosis can be attributed to the gendered nature of medical diagnosis, even when the condition is common to both men and women, such as bladder cancer. Endometriosis, however, is an example of delayed diagnosis partially because it is a condition specific to female bodies, with only a few cases of endometriosis being documented in men (Jabr and Mani 2014). While not often discussed in popular culture, endometriosis is a serious and persistent chronic pain condition that effects an estimated 6 to 10 percent of women of reproductive age and up to 60 percent of women who suffer with pelvic pain (Giudice 2010, 2389). In addition to the primary symptom of pain, women with endometriosis also experience "immunological and gastrointestinal disorders, chemical sensitivities, and allergies" (Jones 2016, 555). In women with endometriosis, cells containing functional endometrial glands are found outside the uterus, typically within the abdominal cavity. The presence of these cells outside the uterus causes pain because they behave like the endometrial lining within the uterus; as a woman progresses through her monthly menstrual cycle, endometrial cells implant, thicken, and ultimately shed just like the endometrial lining within the uterus, resulting in bleeding and inflammation. Because these cells cannot escape the body after shedding, they develop over time into adhesions (Hogg and Vyas 2015). Endometriosis results in more common menstrual pain (pain before/during menstruation), as well as chronic pelvic pain throughout the month and painful intercourse (Giudice 2010; Hickey et al. 2014). The condition is not only a pain condition; many women with endometriosis also experience subfertility (Giudice 2010) or infertility (Hickey, Ballard, and Farquhar 2014).

The seriousness of endometriosis is compounded by two factors. The first is that the cause of endometriosis is not fully understood (Hickey, Ballard, and Farquhar 2014). Second, the only way to confirm a woman has the condition is through laparoscopic procedures (Giudice 2010, 2389). When a laparotomy is performed, a fiber-optic instrument is surgically inserted into the body through the abdomen, allowing the surgeon to utilize imaging technology to visually confirm the presence of endometrial adhesions and implants. It is only at this point that the surgeon can also evaluate the extent of the spread of endometriosis and rate its severity (Hickey, Ballard, and Farquhar 2014). Since diagnostic laparoscopies are surgical procedures, the cost prohibits most patients from obtaining early diagnosis and thus better treatment. As Susannah Hogg and Sanjay Vyas (2015) observed, patients in the United Kingdom averaged seven and a half years from the onset of symptoms to diagnosis

(134). Crystal Weibe (*Lincoln Journal Star*, May 18, 2003) reports that women in the United States average a nine-year wait for a proper diagnosis. This means a woman must endure years of suffering and multiple treatment attempts without an official diagnosis and better treatment.

Irreconcilable Discourses

At this point I turn my attention to my experiences as a patient with endometriosis to demonstrate how this patient dislocation occurs. The first time I experienced severe pelvic pain, I was about seventeen years old. Up until then, I had experienced what I considered to be "normal" pain associated with my menstrual cycle. For reasons I cannot fully explain, around that time the pain felt different to me: more intense, perhaps. When I tried to describe the pain to others, I often fell back on the same metaphor: "Imagine someone has reached into your gut with their hands and is twisting all your insides around." To some extent, I was experiencing what Elaine Scarry (1985) has called the "unsharability of pain" (4). While Scarry believes the inexpressibility of pain should lead doctors to coax pain into clarity by listening with acuity (6), most people dismissed my characterization of my pain as the kind of melodrama to which young women are supposed to be prone, and I was recommended over-the-counter (OTC) pain relievers, accompanied by faces that expressed displeasure at my fanciful narratives. In retrospect, however, there is a wealth of information about my experiences with my own bodily pain wrapped up in this description.

The autobiographical gap created through this research helps me recognize the horror and violence of my adolescent self's pain. The image conjures up graphic violence of the body being violated by another unknown body. The hand must somehow penetrate the abdomen but without surgical instrumentation, a process that would be crude, painful, and bloody, yet nowhere in my charts does my own anxiety or fear about the pain I was experiencing manifest. Instead, my doctors remark that "the patient has noted increased cramping with menstrual cycles." A year later, at another annual exam, my charts simply state, "She complains of cramping with periods for years." These are not my words, of course, but impressions that reflect a biomedical interpretation of the female body in pain. There is no urgency, no concern, despite repeated visits with increasing pain. I am woman "in otherwise good health," as my doctors observe.

The twisting description is also worth pausing over. In 1975, Ronald Melzack and Warren Torgerson developed an inventory of descriptive pain categories, later known as the McGill Pain Questionnaire (Noble et al. 2005). This scale, now a widely used pain index, has been used for cancer treatment (Ferreira, Pais-Ribeiro, and Jensen 2015), both neuropathic and nonneuropathic pain studies (Dworkin et al. 2009; Lovejoy, Turk, and Murasco 2012), and suggests that one category of pain could be described as "flickering, throbbing" or "pounding," while another type of pain could be "tight, squeezing" or "tearing" (Noble et al. 2005, 17). *Twisting* is not found within the pain scale. Close siblings to *twisting* appear on the questionnaire, such as "squeezing" or "tugging," but neither of these fully encapsulates my experiences. Simply put, the narratives that made sense to me as a female likely experiencing the early symptoms of endometriosis were unrecognizable within the established medical discourse on pain.

Even though my pain does not map neatly onto widely used pain scales, my early narrative of pain does show similarities to reports by others about endometriosis pain. Dr. David Redwine (2009), a noted physician in obstetrics and gynecology specializing in endometriosis, describes the reports of endometriosis-related pain as "'sharp,' 'knife-like,' 'stabbing,' 'like shards of glass'" (22). These reports align with my own on several layers. Each description presents a dimension of pain related to endometriosis that cannot be captured on the McGill pain scale, which is designed to capture several dimensions of pain: sensory (pain location, intensity, quality, and pattern), affective (fear, depression, and anxiety related to pain), cognitive (overall pain appraisal), and behavioral (aggravating and alleviating actions) (Ngamkham et al. 2012, 28). Yet, when looking at my own description of pain, what I see is a dimension of pain related to the body being violated, a biopsychosocial dimension of pain not captured on the McGill pain scale. Other accounts of pain by women with endometriosis, especially within the context of pain experienced during sexual intercourse, reinforce the necessity of understanding endometriosis pain as an experience of bodily violation. Mary Lou Ballweg (1995), former president of the Endometriosis Association, recounts the stories of anonymous women trying to narrate their experiences with endometriosis: "Knifelike pain, right through the rectum, without warning. One moment I'd be standing in line for a movie, talking with a friend, and then I'd be doubled over, trying not to black out. . . . The worst was telling people where the pain was. No one wants to hear about this symptom—believe me—and then they don't want to accept that it's related in some way to bad periods. I don't think there's anything harder than having to live with a symptom nobody is even willing to hear about" (35). Ballweg further reports on the Endometriosis Association's solicitating women to draw what their endometriosis looked like. She reports that the most common depiction of their pain was in the form of a devil or a monster. In some instances, women drew their pain as a powerful or sinister male. In one picture, a male figure with broad shoulders and clenched fists scowls at the viewer with two speech bubbles that say, "'I'll get you' and 'I've got control!'" (350–351). My own experiences, taken together with a collection of other narratives, suggest at least one dimension of endometriosis-related pain the McGill pain scale is simply not designed to account for and often described through women's use of narrative.

For my experiences to be "heard" within the medical discourse, I would learn over time that I needed to adapt my own narratives about my pain to different discursive patterns. My initial description was very rarely given in the doctor's office. The first time I described the reaching-in-and-twisting sensation, my doctor patronizingly smiled at me as if to so say "here we go again." Most doctors' visits, however, never gave me an opportunity to describe in my own words what I was experiencing. I would be asked where I was having pain and to rank the pain on a numerical rating scale. When doctors were interested in what kinds of pain I was experiencing, I was often given a multiple-choice question, such as, "Would you describe your pain as . . ." followed by any number of adjectives: *sharp, aching,* or *cramping,* to name a few.

These seemingly mundane experiences with doctors—the kinds of interactions women have with doctors regularly—disrupt female patients' abilities to narrate their experiences to themselves and to their healthcare providers. The difference between the hand twisting my innards and a chart stating a seventeen-year-old patient "presents with mild to moderate pelvic pain associated with menstruation" or even a diagnosis of "dysmenorrhea" is significant. What does not get captured by my doctor's records, but is implied by my narrative, is my own shock over what was happening. Choosing graphic symbols to describe the experiences could have (or maybe should have) been an indication to my physician that something was amiss. It could also have been easy to establish my own narratives of menstrual pain prior to my first complaint to realize that, however feverish the narrative may appear, I had never used such descriptions before. This could be an indication of a new experience with pain, thus warranting at least a few minutes of discussion. Because my descriptions of pain were often dismissed as exaggerations, as "disordered imaginations," I was treated as an undisciplined patient and therefore denied the legitimacy of being treated as a patient with acknowledged pain. Women are expected to accept menstrual pain without much protest because it is "natural." It seemed as though arguing for the significance of my pain associated with menstruation or the pelvic region was to trespass into hysterical territory.

Rather than listening to how I interpreted my own experiences, for the nine years it took to finally be diagnosed with endometriosis doctors provided me with stock phrases to complete my own picture of my pain. I learned to describe my pain as "dull" or "aching" when referencing pain in my back and "sharp" when describing pain located in my abdomen. From that point on, I was being coached in how to communicate my body.

Coaching Representations of Pain

At the age of twenty-six, I voluntarily enrolled in an experimental research program testing the efficacy of a new drug. The drug being investigated functioned by suppressing sex hormones (like estrogen), which ultimately stops the menstrual cycle, as well as the spread of endometriosis. Because this study involved human subjects, strict IRB protocols were to be observed to produce consistent results among all participants (at the time of my participation, 1,781 women had received at least one dose of the drug). An electronic diary was given to each participant, and for the duration of the trial, subjects were asked to complete series of daily questions related to changes in menstrual cycles (such as the onset and cessation of periods and bleeding not associated with a cycle) and about pain. The diary prompted us to rate how bad our pain was on a scale of zero to three (with zero representing no pain), as well as when we engaged in sexual intercourse. Above the image of each number was a word representing what each "meant:" *no, mild, moderate,* and *severe* (from 0 through 3, respectively). This form of pain scaling combined a numeric pain scale with a visual analog scale (Hawker et al. 2011). After declaring the level of pain experienced, subjects were also asked to report which (if any) of the prescribed "rescue" analgesics were used for the pain (naproxen and hydrocodone with acetaminophen).

While it may be hard to determine whether pain on any given day is a 1 or a 2, the use of both scales together may be intended to prompt a subject to report consistently throughout the study. This was confirmed in my in-person conversations with the research-site director (administrators who met with subjects regularly, even when exams were not scheduled with the physician). During these meetings, I often had to review with the site director my entries in the electronic diary, sometimes because I forgot to complete the diary and my responses needed to be collected. Other times, however, the site director reviewed my responses with me. Sometimes the director simply wanted to "make sure" I did actually have four days of severe pain. On these occasions, the site director often took the opportunity to help me interpret the scale. For example, I was told I should consider entering a 3 if the pain was bad enough that, if I could have stayed home from work because of the pain without repercussions at work, I would have. A 3, it was added, should only be selected on days I stayed home from work if I was scheduled, resulting in some repercussions, such as loss of pay. These descriptions, however, are nowhere to be found in the study materials.

These quiet, off-the-record moments are important to consider when trying to understand how female patients are dislocated as authorities over their own pain. Giving seemingly unauthorized interpretations of what severe pain *should* look like in a patient's life belies the vast lived experiences of sufferers with chronic pain. At that time, I was a contingent faculty member, and the idea of not going to work no matter how intense the pain became was out of the question. Using the baseline of whether I would call in sick from work or not was a poor representation of what severe pain meant to me. At no time I can recall was I asked what I thought it meant to experience severe pain daily. Instead, someone else's measuring stick was exerted over my experiences, coloring the ways I thought about my pain.

I have deliberately used the term *coaching* to describe these interactions with healthcare professionals because, after decades of exchanges with different primary care physicians, OB/GYN specialists, OB/GYN surgeons, clinicians, nurses, and interns, I fully believe these experts in medical discourse thought they were helping me be a better patient, however misguided this pursuit may be. Each interaction taught me how to present my case better than the last time. These discursive interventions—reframing for me and with me—were meant to help me communicate with doctors more efficiently; what they did, however, was mold me into a disciplined patient subjectivity. The patriarchal undertones of being coached by healthcare professionals are important to consider in order to gain a richer understanding of how women are disciplined into being patients.

Producing Pain(ed) Performances

Partway through the study, I met with the site director before a scheduled physical exam with the doctor. In this meeting, she explained to me what the exam would entail, including a full pelvic exam. She then told me the doctor would press on multiple areas of my abdomen and he would ask me about any pain I experienced when he did so. I was reminded of the need to be honest with my reports; however, if I did experience any pain, I needed to make it clear to the doctor. The site director suggested I moan. At the time, this instruction seemed odd and made me uncomfortable. Moaning is not how I usually express pain. I may do it from time to time at home when pain feels unbearable, but never, until then, had I moaned in pain in public, but she insisted that the doctor might not notice I'm expressing pain if I simply wince or "make faces." The sexual dynamic of this scene cannot be underscored enough. When young female patients are told to moan at the touch of a male doctor, those patients are yet again disciplined into marginalized subjectivities. I do not wish to suggest my doctor or the site director thought of me as a sexual object. In fact, that neither of the professionals in the room demonstrated any belief that there might be something wrong with instructing me to moan at the (male) doctor's touch is further evidence of how fossilized these attitudes are in contemporary practices.

In many ways, this encounter is evidence of how little gynecology has improved over the centuries. Julie-Marie Strange (2000) has highlighted the gendered implications of gynecology. As she argues, "Whilst the manifest purpose of gynaecology was to nurture and heal the female generative capacity, women were often sexualised in medical texts in a language of danger, violence, and immorality. Some case reports carried aggressive sexual connotations, such as references to 'plunging' through the hymen or 'thrusting' into the vagina" (610). While these references were written over a hundred years ago, women are often subjected to same kinds of sexualization today by being asked to represent their pain in ways that may be construed as sexual in nature, like moaning.

My encounter raises implications for understanding how pain discourse is negotiated between doctors and patients. It yet again suggests that, as patients being asked to *perform* pain, women are not perceived to be reliable reporters of pain. Rather than listening to how *I* chose to respond to his touch (through guarding, wincing, shortened breath, etc.), I was expected to perform what a doctor supposes pain to be. But my presentation did not end with merely biological indicators of pain; as has been suggested by the biopsychosocial model of medicine, my doctor and the sponsors of the research *could have* chosen to observe the psychological and social signals that I was experiencing pain. My experiences align with the findings of Leandra Hernández and Marleah Dean in this collection, who found that women experienced doctors as "patronizing/belittling" (109), a figure characterized by an unwilling-ness to consider women's experiential knowledge, rejecting it in favor of biomedical knowledge about women's bodies.

I remember getting fidgety during painful examinations and want-ing to get off the table. Knowing this was not good for the trial, I often endured those moments by trying to distract myself. I memorized how many clear jars were on the table (four) and what they contained (cot-ton swabs, cardboard tongue depressors, etc.). The doctor or the site director had pinned a poster to the ceiling of the room just above the head of the table, and many afternoons were spent counting how many blue butterflies and orange butteries and monarch butterflies were on the poster. To distract myself from the pain, I engaged in these kinds of "games" to the point that I did not hear questions the first time they were asked. If the doctor had wanted to listen to my body and me, he could have probed into this distraction—What was bothering me, if I needed a minute to relax or focus, and why? These kinds of interactions, however, never came about. Only my body was communicated with, and so long as I spoke his language, my doctor appeared to be satisfied. In the words of Caitlin Leach (see her chapter in this collection), I had not gained subjecthood. My ongoing compliance with the requested performances of pain, born out the confusion, the humiliation, and the reality of my pain, gained me only patienthood. This patienthood served as a double-edged sword. As Leach observes, it was not personally liberating for me and, in fact, diminished my ability to communicate about my pain and my body in ways meaningful to me. For the study, however, because I operated within the prescribed patienthood, my doctor's interpretation and analysis of pain moved a major pharmaceutical study forward. As of the summer of 2018, the medication had received FDA approval and would shortly be available for consumers in the United States.

CONCLUSION

Throughout this chapter I have tried to utilize my own experiences as a patient with endometriosis as a springboard for understanding the gen-dered nature of pain communication. I argue that female patients are dislocated as authorities about their own experiences with pain through the process of delayed diagnosis and by regular doctors' refusals to lis-ten to female patients' discursive representations of their pain, replac-ing them with coached representations. In doing so, I do not claim to represent the experiences of all women with endometriosis; instead, I hope this work can serve as part of the ongoing conversations about negotiating power and pain between doctors and patients. Rather than seeing medical discourses and personal discourses as incommensurate, I wish to conclude this work by exploring how Charon's (2006) narrative medicine can help doctors and patients listen to one another in order to accomplish both parties' goals.

Doctor-patient interactions are marred in part by issues of power, gender, class, clinical training, and patients' expectations (Charon 2006). Some of these issues could be mitigated by a more holistic approach to treating patients; under the narrative-medicine model, doctors would

> come to understand that patients and caregivers enter whole—with their bodies, lives, families, beliefs, values, histories, hopes for the future—into sickness and healing, and their efforts to get better or to help others get better cannot be fragmented away from the deepest parts of their lives. (12–13)

The task doctors would undertake within narrative medicine would be to listen to the many narratives patients tell—"through the patient's words, silences, gestures, facial expressions, and bodily postures, as well as physical findings, diagnostic images, and laboratory measurements" (132). This would be no easy task for, as Charon acknowledges, these diverse narratives will inevitably tell competing and conflicting stories about the patient. Charon sees listening to these narratives as central to a doctor's job and that the task to "cohere these different and sometimes contradictory sources" into "at least provisional meaning" is the goal of medicine (132).

Narrative medicine poses significant risks to the established norms of Western medical communities, but it also holds vast potential. It would work to do what S. Scott Graham (2015) claims postmodernism never could accomplish—overthrow the dualism between body and mind. If doctors assumed diagnosis requires listening to messy and conflicting reports about the body from multiple authorities, personal discourses and medical discourses would not be inherently at odds with one another. Female patients could be recognized as authoritative reporters about what's happening in, with, and to their bodies.

I am not trying to suggest doctors should immediately look to perform exploratory surgery to diagnose endometriosis at a woman's first complaint of pelvic pain. I am, however, trying to suggest that practices can be improved upon. To give an idea of how this might be accomplished, we can consider those patients' long-neglected narratives of their pain. If these narratives were listened to, written down in charts, and tracked over time, doctors might get a better understanding of how patients are making sense of their experiences. Medical professionals could explore how those narratives change over time and through different treatments. Does a regimen of OTC or prescription-strength pain medication change a patient's narrative? In what ways does their understanding of their own pain evolve over time? If patients persist over time in producing strong reports of pain in narratives, what next steps (including surgical intervention, where appropriate) can be taken? Narrative medicine would help explain and explore "invisible" conditions like endometriosis and authorize new ways of seeing those conditions, perhaps leading to early diagnoses and improved treatments. Through narrative medicine, healthcare could finally begin to embrace some of the methods feminist inquiries have long advocated for—partnerships between researchers and subjects, reflection, and serious listening that might bridge the divide between doctors and patients.

NOTE

1.   The medical term for pain associated with menstruation.

REFERENCES

Ballweg, Mary Lou. 1995. *The Endometriosis Sourcebook*. Chicago: Contemporary Books.

Charon, Rita. 2006. *Narrative Medicine: Honoring the Stories of Illness*. New York: Oxford University Press.

Dworkin, Robert H., Dennis C. Turk, Dennis A. Revicki, Gale Harding, Karin S. Coyne, Sarah Peirce-Sandner, Dileep Bhagwat, Dennis Evertone, Laurie B. Burke, Penney Cowan, John T. Farrar, Sharon Hertz, Mitchell B. Max, Bob A. Rappaport, and Ronald Melzackj. 2009. "Development and Initial Validation of an Expanded and Revised Version of the Short-Form McGill Pain Questionnaire (SF-MPQ-2)." *Pain* 144 (1–2): 35–42.

Ferreira-Valente, Maria Alexandra, José Luís Pais-Ribeiro, and Mark P. Jensen. 2011. "Validity of Four Pain Intensity Rating Scales." *Pain* 152 (10): 2399–2404.

Giudice, Linda C. 2010. "Endometriosis." *New England Journal of Medicine* 362 (25): 2389–2398.

Graham, S. Scott. 2015. *The Politics of Pain Medicine: A Rhetorical-Ontological Inquiry*. Chicago: University of Chicago Press.

Hawker, Gillian A., Samra Mian, Tetyana Kendzerska, and Melissa French. 2011. "Measures of Adult Pain: Visual Analog Scale for Pain (VAS Pain), Numeric Rating Scale for Pain (NRS Pain), Mcgill Pain Questionnaire (MPQ), Short-Form Mcgill Pain Questionnaire (SF-MPQ), Chronic Pain Grade Scale (CPGS), Short Form-36 Bodily Pain Scale (SF-36 BPS), and Measure of Intermittent and Constant Osteoarthritis Pain (ICOAP)." *Arthritis Care and Research* 63 (S11): S240–252.

Hickey, Martha, Karen Ballard, and Cindy Farquhar. 2014. "Endometriosis." *British Medical Journal* 348 (7950): g1752.

Hogg, Susannah, and Sanjay Vyas. 2015. "Endometriosis." *Obstetrics, Gynaecology and Reproductive Medicine* 25 (5): 133–141.

Jabr, Fadi I., and Venk Mani. 2014. "An Unusual Cause of Abdominal Pain in a Male Patient: Endometriosis." *Avicenna Journal of Medicine* 4 (4): 99–101.

Jones, Cara E. 2016. "The Pain of Endo Existence: Toward a Feminist Disability Studies Reading of Endometriosis." *Hypatia* 31 (3): 554–571.

Kenny, Dianna T. 2002. "Constructions of Chronic Pain in Doctor-Patient Relationships: Bridging the Communication Chasm." *Patient Education and Counseling* 52 (3): 297–305.

Lovejoy, Travis I., Dennis C. Turk, and Benjamin J. Morasco. 2012. "Evaluation of the Psychometric Properties of the Revised Short-Form McGill Pain Questionnaire." *Journal of Pain* 13 (12): 1250–1257.

Ngamkham, Srisuda, Catherine Vincent, Lorna Finnegan, Janean E. Holden, Zaijie Jim Wang, and Diana J. Wilkie. 2012. "McGill Pain Questionnaire as a Multidimensional Measure in People with Cancer: An Integrative Review." *Pain Management Nursing* 13 (1): 27–51.

Noble, Bill, David Clark, Marcia Meldrum, Hank ten Have, Jane Seymour, Michelle Winslow, and Silvia Paz. 2005. "The Measurement of Pain, 1945–2000." *Journal of Pain and Symptom Management* 29 (1): 14–21.

Redwine, David B. 2009. 100 *Questions and Answers about Endometriosis.* Sudbury, MA: Jones and Bartlett.

Royster, Jacqueline Jones, and Gesa E. Kirsch. 2012. *Feminist Rhetorical Practices: New Horizons for Rhetoric, Composition, and Literacy.* Carbondale: Southern Illinois Press.

Scarry, Elaine. 1985. *The Body in Pain: The Making and Unmaking of the World.* New York: Oxford University Press.

Shildrik, Margrit. 1997. *Leaky Bodies: Feminism, Postmodernism, and (Bio)Ethics.* New York: Routledge.

Strange, Julie-Marie. 2000. "Menstrual Fictions: Languages of Medicine and Menstruation, c. 1850–1930." *Women's History Review* 9 (3): 607-628.

4

SIMULATING GENDER
Student Learning in Clinical Nursing Simulations

Lillian Campbell

"I love her earrings!" a female nursing student exclaims when she first encounters Josie. "Oh, she's wearing a bra, just noticed that!" comments a male student. Josie, or Joe, is a robotic patient manikin a group of nursing students are meeting for the first time. In addition to earrings and a bra, the white male manikin is wearing a grey wig, and its penis has been replaced with a plastic vagina. This will enable students to practice catheter insertion on their elderly female patient once the simulation begins.

Nursing education has a rich history of incorporating simulated care into student training. Historically, students practiced procedures on models of body parts or worked with volunteers who could provide real-time feedback. However, since manufacturer Laerdal's introduction of the first affordable patient simulator in 2000, SimMan, simulations have included life-sized robotic manikins that can respond to treatment (Rosen 2008, 162). As the title SimMan suggests, physical interactions with simulators have the potential to impact students' understanding of the role of gender in their care of patients. At the same time, the technical skills acquired from physical care in simulations are only one dimension of student learning. Simulations also prompt conversations about the power relationships in clinical settings and promote a view of nurses as patient advocates. At times, conversations explicitly address gender, as students and instructors discuss how to appropriately lift an older female patient's gown or correct a self-assured physician's error. Overall, nursing's feminized nature, as well as its integration into the masculinized world of medicine, makes nursing simulations a site for frequent and often conflicting opportunities for gendered learning.

This chapter uses a material rhetorical lens to build on previous feminist research on patient simulation by studying simulators not just as static objects but also as apparatuses in action (Johnson 2005; Sundén 2010). To account for "gender-and-scientists-in-the-making," to expand

DOI: 10.7330/9781607329855.c004

on Karen Barad's (2007) concept, I argue that research on simulation must capture both the technical learning that occurs at the physical interface between student and machine and the interpersonal lessons that emerge in conversations with the simulated patient. Thus, I draw on field research with third-year nursing students that included observations of over thirty clinical simulations and the activities that surrounded them. I also include excerpts from interviews with five focal students (four female and one male). This range of data offers access to the multitude of ways nursing students are taught to orient to and perform gender in simulations.

Studying gendered lessons in simulations necessitates a heuristic for understanding what we hope students learn about interacting with patients on a gender spectrum. Ultimately, I see this as an opportunity for rhetorical scholars and nursing instructors to collaborate, as I discuss in the conclusion. For my purposes, however, I draw on the work in this volume (informed by both rhetoric of health medicine scholarship and feminist theory) to offer three premises for gendered interactions. First, research shows men's experiences continue to be normalized in medical care and practice. Kerri Morris's analysis in this collection of how bladder cancer is often considered a men's disease and misdiagnosed as UTIs in women provides a compelling example of this normalization. Thus, students should understand how and why their patient care will differ in response to gender. Second, research indicates that even within a single gender, care cannot be generalized because gender interacts with other identity factors including sexuality, class, race, age, and disability (see De Hertogh and Liz in this collection). Thus, students should take an intersectional approach to gendered care that accounts for the influence of different demographic backgrounds and identities. And finally, nurses must understand every patient interaction is different and act responsively to emerging patient needs rather than approaching care statically. Leandra Hernández and Marleah Kruzel's discussion in this collection of how individual experiential knowledge is often discounted during the patient-physician exchange highlights the importance of responsive care. I see such care as deeply rhetorical—immersed in a specific context, tied to a unique individual, and emerging in response to a pressing exigence.

Using these three premises, I discuss a number of overlapping and at times contradictory gendered lessons that emerged for students during their physical and verbal interactions with the patient simulator. First, I argue that the simulator and the simulation coordinator both establish "typical" gender features and expectations for student care. These typifications emphasize how care is different for men and women, but they can also support stereotyping and reliance on shared experience. Perhaps because of the risks of stereotyping, intersectional identities are rarely portrayed when establishing typical gender features, with the exception of age. Thus, students had limited opportunities to address specific strategies for intersectional gendered care.

Second, I demonstrate how the simulator and instructor disrupted student expectations, necessitating that the future nurses learn to act responsively. I use the word *disruption* to describe actions that disturbed, redirected, or overturned the existing simulation scenario. The simulator's disruptions came in the form of its imperfect representations of both a human body and a gendered body, while the instructor's disruptions were often strategically introduced. In both cases, disruptions provided opportunities for students to reflect on how they would modify their care for different kinds of bodies, supporting an awareness of variation and flexibility with interventions. In the conclusion, I elaborate on why these physical and verbal disruptions are so critical to the gendered lessons in clinical simulations. I also discuss the potential for integrating diffractive strategies into debrief conversations to help students think through the challenges of intersectional care.

GENDER AND SIMULATION

Nursing as a field has long been feminized. As Rachel Prentice (2013) explains, "The gendered distinctions that make technical work the physician's province and leave caring work to nurses remain. The work of caring often becomes coded as 'soft' or as 'woman's work'" (226). In contrast, patient simulators have been critiqued for promoting a dehumanized view of the patient that aligns with the "technical work" of physicians (Johnson 2005; Sundén 2010). Thus, research on nursing simulations can consider how gendered learning occurs at the intersection of feminized and masculinized domains. In this section, I briefly overview scholarship on gender and simulation from the fields of nursing and gender studies to set the groundwork for my own investigation.

Nursing scholarship on gendered learning in clinical simulations has focused primarily on differences in how male and female students respond to simulation technology (Grady et al. 2008; Mould, White, and Gallagher 2011). These studies found that male students were more likely to report higher levels of comfort and confidence in high-fidelity environments. Research argues that outside simulation contexts, male nurses must find ways to negotiate often feminized modes of care. For example, Murry Fisher (2009) draws on interviews with twenty-one male nurses to describe how they perform bodywork ("the labour performed on others' bodies . . . , emotional labour, and the effects of work on one's own body" [2669]) that is gendered as female. Fisher finds that male nurses leverage a range of strategies including providing detailed descriptions of upcoming procedures, receiving patient consent before interacting, and avoiding unnecessary bodily exposure or touching. He concludes that "gender implications of bodywork should be included in nursing curricula" (2676). Clinical simulations provide an ideal context to study this embodied gender learning.

Conversely, gender studies scholars have considered how medical simulators perpetuate problematic conceptions of gender for health-care providers. Notably, this research is confined to considering how manikins represent male and female genders, since companies have not yet created manikins with identities outside of this binary. Jenny Sundén (2010) researched Noelle, a simulation manikin made by Gaumard designed to provide students with hands-on practice in supporting labor and delivery. Sundén argues that adding details like hair and breasts but not the fluids, odors, or sounds that accompany birthing represents a "selective bodily awareness" that supports problematic gender conceptions in the medical imagination (107). However, Sundén's analysis is based only on physical simulators and manuals, interviews with design-ers, and promotional materials, not on simulator use in practice. In contrast, Ericka Johnson (2005) draws on ethnographic research on an anesthesia simulator to argue that the simulator's removable plastic pelvis emphasizes reproductive organs as the defining gender feature (156). According to Johnson, these one-sex models position female bodies as less developed versions of male bodies, contributing to the normalization of male medical care. Meanwhile, Johnson (2007) reflects on the difficulty during data collection of reconciling practitioners' general attitudes towards gender ("politically correct, gender sensitive, and pedagogically concerned with integrating female students into their practices" [150]) with their disinterest in gender during simulations. Thus, there is still a need for more attention to how interactions with patient simulators teach students both to orient to differences in gender in their care and to embody gendered professional roles.

FIELD CONTEXT

I took a "rhetorical field methods" approach to this project, which immersed me in many activities surrounding clinical simulations (Endres

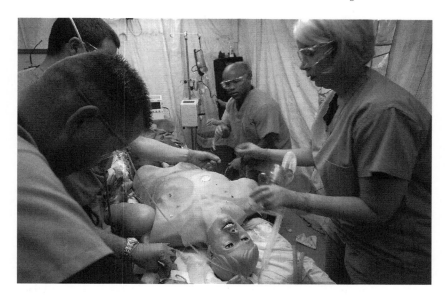

Figure 4.1. Air force medical personnel practice patient care on a male manikin similar to the one used by nursing students in this study.

et al. 2016). Over the course of a year, I followed a group of eighty third-year baccalaureate nursing students through their three different clinical simulations at a midsized private university in the Northwest. The simulations took place in two high-tech simulation suites, which each included a patient manikin—Joe/Josie in the adult suite and Hal in the obstetric/pediatric suite—as well as most supplies needed for care (gloves, oxygen, catheters, telephone to reach other providers, etc.). The simulation coordinator, the students' clinical instructor, and I sat in the simulation control room, which is positioned between the two suites with a large one-sided window looking into each. The simulation coordinator, Maura, operates a computer that controls all the simulator's vital signs and a microphone that connects to its speaker box.

After an orientation to the simulation room, three groups of two to four students are immersed in a narrative set up by Maura. Each group takes a turn caring for the patient for approximately twenty minutes while the patient's condition worsens. During their turn, students practice conversations with one another and with the patient, engage in critical thinking to prioritize problems, and decide on interventions. They also have physical interactions with the simulation environment and the simulator—applying sanitizer, putting on latex gloves, checking a wound, and so forth. While one group provides care, the other two groups sit in a nearby classroom watching a live stream. After each group's turn, the students, clinical instructor, and simulation coordinator reconvene in the classroom for a debrief. This is a formal instructor-facilitated conversation in which students reflect on their experience and receive feedback from their peers and instructors.

Of the simulations I observed, the first involved an elderly female patient, Eliana Ruiz, who was diabetic and experiencing complications after a leg operation. The second was with a young male patient, Jason Lee, who was recovering after a leg surgery caused by a car accident. And the third was caring for a male infant, Eric Joslin, with a respiratory infection. Despite the age and gender differences between Eliana and Jason, the same white male robotic manikin was used for both simulations. My analysis below focuses primarily on these first two simulations, as they offer contrasting case studies of how students were taught to orient towards gender through both physical and verbal patient interactions. Despite the fact that both Eliana and Jason were ethnically marked by their last names and the pictures that accompanied their patient profiles, I found students largely ignored race in interactions. In the conclusion, I consider how diffractive debriefs could be leveraged to support more intersectional learning in simulated contexts.

A MATERIAL RHETORICAL FRAMEWORK

As I turned to a rich data set that included interviews with focal students and observations of over thirty clinical simulations and their surrounding activities, I wanted to analyze patient simulators not as static objects but as active rhetorical agents. Thus, I drew on research in material rhetorics, which considers the persuasive capacities of nonhuman objects and spaces. Barad's (2007) concept of intra-action, specifically, can account for the rhetorical force of the simulator while also addressing power relationships between individuals.

By engaging in a material rhetorical analysis of simulators, my aim is to move beyond a critique of the simulated body on the grounds that it does not accurately represent a human body. As other authors have emphasized, representational accuracy is not the goal for simulation design; fidelity of physiological experience is paramount (Johnson 2010). Both Prentice (2013) and Johnson (2010) turn to Bruno Latour's actor-network theory (ANT), which posits that human and nonhuman "actants" share agency and thus provides a framework for understanding rhetorical action at the interface between bodies and machines. However, feminist scholars have expressed concern that posthuman research like Latour's has the potential to obscure unequal power relations—like gender, race, and class—between human actants (Booher and Jung 2018).

In fact, Barad (2007) argues that overlooking human power relations is a trend in posthuman science studies research: "While [science studies] scholars insist on the importance of tracking 'science-in-the-making' . . . they fail to attend to 'gender-in-the-making'—the production of gender and other social variables as constituted through technoscientific practices" (87). Thus, Barad's theory of "agential realism" synthesizes posthuman work with feminist poststructuralism, like Judith Butler's theory of gender performativity (57). Key to this framework is the notion of "intra-action," which emphasizes how objects and bodies come together to create apparatuses and ultimately phenomena that "matter" in particular moments. In order to demonstrate how intra-action can reorient posthuman scholarship towards power disparities, Barad uses the story of a key discovery in the field of quantum physics—a demonstration of space quantization that depended upon the smoking of a cheap cigar in the lab. She asserts that the cigar is a "'nodal point,' as it were—of the working of other apparatuses, including class, nationalism, economics, and gender" (167). Barad recognizes that attributing causal agency to the cigar is misguided but demonstrates how ignoring the experiment's entanglements in gendered and class-based material practices would create a limited account of "science-in-the-making."

In this way, Barad's agential realism offers a posthuman approach for studying scientific practice with attention to gendered, class-based, and race-based materializations. Thus, recent work in feminist medical rhetoric, like Christa Teston's (2016) research on genetic biomarkers in cancer care, turns to Barad as a theoretical stronghold. This chapter demonstrates how Barad's theories can be mobilized to better understand classroom practices and student learning as well, or "gender-and-scientists-in-the-making." By calling attention to how particular classroom apparatuses like patient simulators teach students to embody gendered roles, this research can offer insights not just into nursing practice but also into nursing training and curriculum.

GENDERED LESSONS IN SIMULATIONS

Across all aspects of the simulation, students were exposed to lessons about how to perform gender as nurses and how to orient to their patient's gender during care. As one example, their clinical instructor reminded them to "get to the point" in a phone call with the physician, describing nurses' tendency to be storytellers as a female trait. However, given my interest in the simulator's rhetorical role, the following analysis focuses specifically on gendered lessons that emerged in physical and verbal intra-actions between students and the patient simulator. Ultimately, I demonstrate how these intra-actions at times created opportunities for students to practice modifying their care to meet men's and women's differential needs and at other moments disrupted students' expectations, teaching them to be responsive providers.

Physical Intra-actions with the Simulator

On the preparation sheet students received prior to their simulation, there was a photo of their elderly patient, Eliana, shown wearing a thick grey sweater, a crimson scarf, and a black hat. Her dress was conservative, cuing students into the fact that modesty should be prioritized. Indeed, part of what students learned in their physical intra-actions with Eliana was how to best maneuver her gown to uncover only the body parts they needed to access—heart, leg wound, or genitals. During one group's simulation, a male student attempted to lift up Eliana's gown to listen to her heart, but another student suggested he reach the stethoscope through the neck-hole of her gown instead. During their debrief, the simulation coordinator encouraged students to check in about a patient's comfort level with nurses of a different gender, remarking, "Don't make a big deal of yourself as a man, but with any patient ask if it's okay."

Practicing lifting a medical gown modestly teaches students to be thoughtful about modifying their care for patients of different genders, as well as individuals whose cultural backgrounds might impact their expectations about privacy. Johnson (2010) argues that simulators do not provide the same feedback as patient actors, who often comment on things like eye contact, tone of conversations, or the temperature of the medical instruments. However, intra-actions with Eliana did provide students with an array of opportunities to consider how their touch could foster comfort or embarrassment. In addition, students were also given hands-on practice with a gender-specific procedure: female catheter insertion. While they had practiced this on a pelvic simulator during skills lab, students had to be more attentive to patient experience during the simulation. For example, my focal student Michelle reflected on her experience of the instructor responding to her touch through the manikin's speaker box, saying, "I forgot to warn the patient that I was going to touch her genitals and she was obviously just like, 'Oh, oh my gosh . . .' so I was just like, 'Whoa, okay, this is real like I need to actually warn her.'"

Nursing students are constantly intra-acting with every inch of the patient's body as they inspect, palpate, listen to, and ultimately feel how the bodies of their patients resist or yield to their aims. Aspects of Eliana's robotic body provided students with cues to practice intra-acting differently with a female body. Her bra was a cue for students to consider how to modestly maneuver her gown, and the removable genitals enabled students to practice a gender-specific procedure. However, physical intra-actions with the simulator patient also disrupted students' expectations for a female human body—which was not quite human and not quite female. In our conversation following her first simulation with Eliana, my focal student Kira reflected, "The first thing I noticed was that my patient was a very big woman." Later, she elaborated, "I don't know how to describe, but she was HUGE. She must have been like seven feet tall. And she's got these man-hands and so I was like struggling to lift up one of her legs . . . I see people as these bendable moveable objects and so when it's just dead weight but it's stiff dead weight it's even worse." According to Kira, Eliana's simulator body represented an imperfect human body, in part because of its stiffness/dead weight. Along similar lines, Ryan, a male focal student who was responsible for performing a catheter insertion during his group's simulation, reflected on the ways the imperfect simulator body disrupted his care: "It doesn't move like a person . . . like putting a catheter in a female, you would have them bend their own legs and spread their legs rather than you adjusting them and you have to be a lot more rough with the manikin."

For both Kira and Ryan, the simulator's lack of fidelity as a human body became apparent in their intra-actions with the machine. As they lifted it, repositioned it, and attempted to orient to it so they could provide care, the machine acted back, resisting these movements. This resistance called attention to its inhumanness, but it also provided students with opportunities to reflect on the differences between their intra-actions with the simulator and with a "regular patient." Ultimately then, the machine fostered meta-awareness for students about how their practice must be responsive to each individual patient's body rather than suggesting certain technical approaches are universal.

However, Eliana's simulator body is not just imperfectly human, it is also not the appropriate size or shape for a female. Gender matters for these nursing students in part because the size of the male patient body significantly impacts their ability to maneuver the patient during care. Thus, Kira described Eliana first euphemistically as "a very big woman"

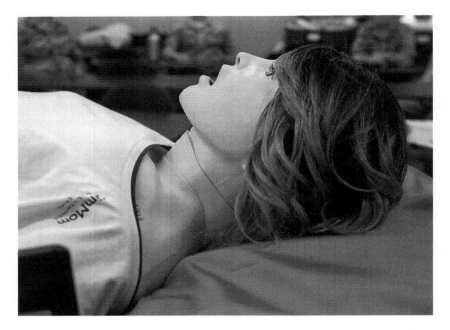

Figure 4.2. Nursing instructors often use wigs to transform a male manikin into a female for the simulation.

but then later emphasized the unbelievable scale of her size: "HUGE . . . like seven feet tall." Kira also observed how Eliana's hands were incongruent with her gender, referring to them explicitly as "man-hands." Though it was offered only as an aside, this comment was important because it was the only instance in which Kira's feedback about the simulator body was an aesthetic critique, not addressing how Eliana's body felt in intra-action. In this way, it resembled a disturbing moment Ben Singer (2013) describes when a group of nursing students laughed after arranging a simulated body so that the top half was male and the bottom half was female. Singer argues, "The laughter of these students, if neither purposeful nor malicious, reveals that trans-specific embodiment is unthinkable, hence invisible, in clinical settings" (250). Along similar lines, Kira's comment articulates intolerance for the incongruity between a female patient and male hands and in doing so undermines the wide range of possibilities for bodily variation. This comment, rather than helping Kira be reflective about how her simulated patient differed from future patients and fostering responsive care, set clear boundaries between categories of bodies and in doing so planted the seeds for derision or, like Singer's example, even mockery.

Overall, then, examining several instances of physical intra-action with Eliana during simulations demonstrates how the patient simulator can directly support physical lessons for students about how to differentially provide care—from the procedure for inserting a female catheter to the proper direction for lifting a dressing gown. Meanwhile, the manikin also frequently disrupts these lessons through its inability to perfectly replicate intra-actions with a human body. The physical distance between intra-acting with a simulator and with a real human body provides students with opportunities to reflect on how they will modify and revise their care for different kinds of bodies, supporting an awareness of variation. Student critiques of the simulator become problematic, however, when they emerge in an attempt to define what constitutes normal. On the other hand, patient feedback, delivered through the instructor's microphone, has a crucial role to play in student learning as well. Eliana gasps when she is touched without warning, groans when a catheter bag pulls on her urethra, and expresses embarrassment when she is left uncovered. Thus, to fully understand how students are learning to orient to gender in their care, it is important to consider the patient's voice as key to the intra-action of machine and student as well.

Verbal Intra-actions with the Simulator

In contrast to Eliana, twenty-year-old male patient Jason presented students with the chance to consider how they would need to adjust their care for a young male. From requesting a hamburger two hours after surgery to asking whether he would have "cool" scars from his operation, simulation coordinator Maura, whose microphone was connected to Jason's voicebox, ensured conversations with Jason would reflect a typical positioning. One of the primary ways Maura represented this perspective was by having Jason ask a male nurse questions about the catheter. For example, during focal-student Ryan's shift, Jason called Ryan over, saying,

> JASON: It's kind of embarrassing. How long do I have to have that tube in my penis . . .
> RYAN: So you're on day one right now. So you'll have it until tomorrow.
> JASON: Okay yeah it's—I didn't want to ask the other nurses . . .
> RYAN: I totally understand . . .

Later on, when Ryan informs Jason that he is going to clean the catheter, Jason responds, "I'm glad it's you." Overall, Ryan discussed these exchanges positively during our interview: "He was like, 'Oh I'm glad that it's you because I don't want that other nurse to look at me' and then, it made sense. Before now I never understood why it would be an issue that I was a male but now I understand when a male's more comfortable with me, that fell into line, which was cool." Thus, for Ryan the exchange with Jason represented a rare instance in which he felt his gendered perspective was uniquely useful. He describes clarity from the exchange about how his gender will sometimes be an asset. Of course, not every male patient feels comfortable with another man talking about or examining his genitals. Ryan will ultimately need to learn to "listen metonymically" to both male and female patients, a key tactic for rhetorical listening that "assumes that a text or person does not share substance with all other members of its/his/her cultural group but, rather, is associated with them" (Ratcliffe 2005, 99). This tactic explicitly addresses the kind of overgeneralization Ryan makes in assuming all male patients will react to his gender in the same way.

At the same time, while Jason's attitude towards male caregivers helped Ryan feel valued in his simulation, identification also comes with risks of "erasure and alienation," as discussed by Kerri Morris (this collection). Indeed, one of my female focal students, Liz, described feeling distanced from the patient: "Allen had to take out the patient's foley [catheter] . . . the patient was definitely more comfortable with a male figure just because he was male so didn't want us to impose as much." If one assumes patient connection is created through shared experiences, when nurses cannot easily identify with patient experience—because of age, gender, race, class, or disability—this can create a barrier to relationship building. This need for identification is why current feminist scholarship is calling for new ways of imagining how connections might be built between individuals to account for and value their different experiences (Hesford 2011; Ratcliffe 2005). For authors coming from a materialist perspective, objects and environments (nonhuman actants) have a role to play in promoting these ethical relationships to others and the world (Bennett 2010).

Ultimately, many students struggled to connect with Jason during his simulation, not only because of differences in gender but also because there were many technical tasks to accomplish. One strategy Maura used to counter students' task-focused care was to make Jason cry. Actual liquid could flow from the simulator's eyes, which often surprised students. As one student explained during debrief, "With anyone else crying you'd see eyes welling up, puffy, but it was like, 'Oh okay, he's crying!'" Even though Jason's tears were not perfectly human, they disrupted student actions and redirected care. For example, in the following exchange, a nursing student is taking Jason's pulses when he suddenly begins to cry.

KYLIE: What's going on? Talk to me.

JASON: I think it's all just starting to hit me. What happened.

KYLIE: [Grabs a tissue and dabs the tears] Yeah? Are you in any pain right now?

JASON: Yeah I'm hurting a little bit, but mostly I'm just starting to worry about everything.

KYLIE: What are you worried about?

JASON: Well you may have heard that when I had the [car] accident I was drinking and I've never even been in trouble. I just haven't been in trouble before and never ever had a problem and I don't know how mad my dad's going to be.

KYLIE: Do you want me to call your dad and we can talk to him? We can have him come in . . .

JASON: [Exhales] I'm just not ready to face [my parents] so no, thank you but not yet.

KYLIE: Of course, is there anyone else you want to talk to?

JASON: I don't know, I just—I don't know if I can go back to school, I just don't know a whole lot of stuff. It's just all hitting me what happened and I just can't [inaudible].

KYLIE: I know. It's okay we're just going to get you well and then you can focus on it once you feel better, okay? Is there something I can do for you right now, though?

JASON: [Exhales] No, just uh—you're right I just have to focus on getting better.

KYLIE: That's okay, do you want to talk about it?

JASON: Well go ahead and do whatever you gotta do and I'll—I'm okay, thanks for listening. I'll be all right.

At the beginning of this conversation, Kylie tries to intervene to "fix" the crying. As a reversed version of the many instances Cathryn Molloy (this collection) describes of providers attributing women's pain to psychological origins, Kylie begins by assuming the crying male patient is suffering from physical pain. Once she discovers the pain is emotional, she makes several offers to contact Jason's parents or others for support. Ultimately, though, Kylie realizes Jason is just looking to talk about his feelings, so her last offer is simply to listen. The exchange between Kylie and Jason is notable because the solution is to set aside instincts for identification or intervention and listen to the patient's experience from their point of view, a mode that closely resembles "standing under," another tactic for rhetorical listening (Ratcliffe 2005).

Ratcliffe (2005) emphasizes that "standing under" necessitates a shift from listening *for* a speaker's intent or our own interests to listening *with.*

In this instance, and undoubtedly many clinical contexts, the provider's automatic response is to listen *for* the problem so they can identify an intervention. However, Maura's disruption necessitates that Kylie listen *with* and let the patient's experiential "discourses wash over, through, and around" (28). A materialist lens also calls attention to the rhetorical role the simulator plays in fostering this exchange. The crying was a catalyst for Kylie's responsive intra-action. The imperfect tears worked in tandem with the coordinator's words to disrupt Kylie's agenda and foster a different kind of listening.

Broadly, then, like the physical intra-actions with Eliana, verbal intra-actions with Jason also provided two kinds of gendered lessons. Some lessons focused on teaching students to orient to "typical" characteristics of a young male patient, emphasizing, for example, the likelihood that a male patient would want to ask a male nurse questions about his catheter. While these intra-actions helped a male student understand how his gender might be an asset, they ran the risk of suggesting all male patients will react similarly. In addition, these exchanges tie empathy for patient experience to assumptions of sameness. In contrast, the simulation coordinator also strategically introduced conversational disruptions to redirect students away from their plans for care and to emphasize patient interaction. Learning to dwell in the uncertainty of such moments helped students navigate between their premeditated, often static plans for a patient and the persons' emergent needs, ultimately gaining the rhetorical skills to be a responsive caregiver.

DISRUPTION AND DEFRACTIVE DEBRIEFING

Fisher's (2009) study emphasized that "the gender performances of male nurses were not fixed dualities . . . but were fluid and tailored to individuals, located in a specific space and in a historical moment" (2672). Ultimately, the simulator and instructor's capacity for disruption become a significant resource in fostering this fluid and responsive orientation to and performance of gender in simulation settings. My analysis throughout this chapter demonstrates that both the simulator and the instructor serve as sources for disrupting students' orientations to gender in their care. The simulator body, in being not perfectly human and not perfectly gendered, disrupts physical intra-actions, while instructors speaking as the patient provide verbal sources of redirection. In both cases, students must act as responsive caregivers, not assuming that what works for one patient will work in all instances.

Thinking back to the three premises for student learning about gender I introduce at the beginning of this chapter, however, it is clear that premise two, taking an intersectional approach to gendered care, is receiving the least attention in simulations. The simulator and the instructors worked together to establish "typical" physical and verbal features that provided students with opportunities to think through how they might differentiate care by gender. At the same time, there were rarely opportunities to address how these practices might be modified for patients from different races, gender identities, cultural backgrounds, and so forth.

In order to establish typical gender features, instructors had to rely on stereotypes and generalizations that would have been more noticeably problematic if modified to suggest, for example, that Black women or homosexual men act in certain ways. This, in part, demonstrates the way gendered stereotypes continue to be normalized in workplace contexts (Frost 2016; White, Rumsey, and Amidon 2016). In addition, the simulation coordinator and clinical instructors may have limited knowledge of the experiences of individuals from different backgrounds. In a rare instance when a student who was familiar with Chinese culture tried to strike up a conversation with Jason about his favorite Chinese New Year food, Maura was at a loss for a response. Finally, recognizing the active role of the physical simulator in gendered learning, physical modifications that might call attention to intersectional differences are more complex than adding a wig or a brassiere. Even when the image of their patient on their preparation sheet indicated a nonwhite cultural background, the manikin students were caring for was still white. As Sundén (2010) discusses in her analysis of birthing simulator Noelle, which is also "routinely portrayed and sold as white," the simulator's whiteness enables students and instructors to efface race in their care (110).

With those limitations in mind, the debriefs that follow clinical simulations offer a rich space for "mak[ing] white strange," as Sundén (2010, 110) describes it, as well as making straight, able-bodied, middle-class, and other normalized identities strange. In order to do so, instructors could shift the conversation away from only reflecting on the simulation interactions to imagining how interactions and care might change for patients from different backgrounds. For example, following Ryan's catheter exchange with Jason, instructors could ask the group to think about how this interaction would change if Jason came from a cultural background that vilified homosexuality, and then how it might change if Jason identified as a trans man but had not had bottom surgery. Rather than putting the onus on a single simulated patient (and thus a single coordinator) to represent a particular identity, debrief conversations could open a space for students and instructors to draw on their own experiences and previous clinical interactions to offer possibilities for responsive care. These questions would be line with the current debrief model, which already tends towards discussing a number of possible approaches rather than a single right answer. It would also shift the conversations from a mode of reflection, which Barad (2007) argues is often self-referential and oriented towards sameness, towards diffraction, which is attuned to differences and the material "effects they have on the world" (72).

Barad (2007) describes the methodology of diffraction as "reading insights through one another in attending to and responding to the details and specificities of relations of difference and how they matter" (71). In this way, diffraction also resonates with Ratcliffe's (2005) call for listening metonymically and being attuned to individuals' material experiences of difference while at the same time not attempting to generalize them. Diffractive debriefing conversations would offer students and instructors opportunities to multiply the strategies for intersectional gendered care while avoiding the challenge of having to represent a single "typical" example of these identities. Working in tandem with both instructor and simulator disruptions during the simulations, diffractive debriefings have the potential to help students think expansively about how they both perform and orient to gender in their care without offering easy answers.

Of course, the effectiveness of diffractive debriefing relies on the ability of instructors to facilitate challenging conversations about the influences of student and patient identity. My analysis throughout this chapter builds on existing calls for more pedagogical collaboration between rhetoricians of health and medicine and health instructors (Campbell 2018). Nurses have developed a number of evaluative tools for simulations that are often attentive to considerations of gender and identity. For example, one checklist for evaluating health communication in an obstetric simulation includes items such as "Touched patient appropriately" and "Avoided stereotyping behaviors (re: teen mom, unwed mother, ethnicity, sexual orientation, gender, or economic diversities, etc.)" (Campbell et al. 2013, e547). Meanwhile, rhetoricians of health and medicine can bring to the table alternative ways of understanding how simulations might foster ethical communication strategies, like this chapter's attentiveness to the role of the physical simulator and the simulation space in gendered learning. These perspectives have the potential to disrupt typical ways of thinking about gendered communication in the nursing field and thus can generate flexible and innovative strategies for simulation pedagogy.

REFERENCES

Barad, Karen. 2007. *Meeting the Universe Halfway: Quantum Physics and the Entanglement of Matter and Meaning.* Durham, NC: Duke University Press.

Bennett, Jane. 2010. *Vibrant Matter: A Political Ecology of Things.* Durham, NC: Duke University Press.

Booher, Amanda K., and Julie Jung, eds. 2018. *Feminist Rhetorical Science Studies: Human Bodies, Posthumanist Worlds.* Carbondale: Southern Illinois University Press.

Campbell, Lillian. 2018. "The Rhetoric of Health and Medicine as a 'Teaching Subject': Lessons from the Medical Humanities and Simulation Pedagogy." *Technical Communication Quarterly* 27 (1): 7–20.

Campbell, Suzanne Hetzel, Michael P. Pagano, Eileen R. O'Shea, Carol Connery, and Colby Caron. 2013. "Development of the Health Communication Assessment Tool: Enhancing Relationships, Empowerment, and Powersharing Skills." *Clinical Simulation in Nursing* 9 (11): e543–e550.

Endres, Danielle, Aaron Hess, Samantha Senda-Cook, and Michael K. Middleton. 2016. "In Situ Rhetoric: Intersections Between Qualitative Inquiry, Fieldwork, and Rhetoric." *Cultural Studies <=> Critical Methodologies* 16 (3): 1–14.

Fisher, Murry J. 2009. "'Being a Chameleon': Labour Processes of Male Nurses Performing Bodywork." *Journal of Advanced Nursing* 65 (12): 2668–2677.

Frost, Erin A. 2016. "Apparent Feminism as a Methodology for Technical Communication and Rhetoric." *Journal of Business and Technical Communication* 30 (1): 3–28.

Grady, Janet L., Rosemary G. Kehrer, Carole E. Trusty, Eileen B. Entin, Elliot E. Entin, and Tad T. Brunye. 2008. "Learning Nursing Procedures: The Influence of Simulator Fidelity and Student Gender on Teaching Effectiveness." *Journal of Nursing Education* 48 (9): 403–408.

Hesford, Wendy. 2011. *Spectacular Rhetorics: Human Rights Visions, Recognitions, Feminisms.* Durham, NC: Duke University Press.

Johnson, Ericka. 2005. "The Ghost of Anatomies Past: Simulating the One-Sex Body in Modern Medical Training." *Feminist Theory* 6 (2): 141–159.

Johnson, Ericka. 2007. "Surgical Simulators and Simulated Surgeons: Reconstituting Medical Practice and Practitioners in Simulations." *Social Studies of Science* 37 (4): 585–608.

Johnson, Ericka. 2010. "Simulating Medical Patients and Practices: Bodies and the Construction of Valid Medical Simulators." In *Technology and Medical Practice: Blood, Guts and Machines,* edited by Ericka Johnson and Boel Berner, 119–144. Surrey: Ashgate.

Mould, Jonathan, Haidee White, and Robyn Gallagher. 2011. "Evaluation of a Critical Care Simulation Series for Undergraduate Nursing Students." *Contemporary Nurse: A Journal for the Australian Nursing Profession* 38 (1–2): 180–190.

Prentice, Rachel. 2013. *Bodies in Formation: An Ethnography of Anatomy and Surgery Education.* Durham, NC: Duke University Press.

Ratcliffe, Krista. 2005. *Rhetorical Listening: Identification, Gender, Whiteness.* Carbondale: Southern Illinois University Press.

Rosen, Kathleen R. 2008. "The History of Medical Simulation." *Journal of Critical Care* 23 (2): 157–166.

Singer, Ben. 2013. "The Human Simulation Lab—Dissecting Sex in the Simulator Lab: The Clinical Lacuna of Transsexed Embodiment." *Journal of Medical Humanities* 34 (2): 249–254.

Sundén, Jenny. 2010. "Blonde Birth Machines: Medical Simulation, Techno-Corporeality and Posthuman Feminism." In *Technology and Medical Practice: Blood, Guts and Machines*, edited by Ericka Johnson and Boel Berner, 97–117. Surrey: Ashgate.

Teston, Christa. 2016. "Biomedical Attunement: A Study of Genetic Biomarkers as Suasive Materials." Paper presented at the biennial conference of the Rhetoric Society of America, Atlanta, GA, May 27–29.

White, Kate, Suzanne Kesler Rumsey, and Stevens Amidon. 2016. "Are We 'There' Yet? The Treatment of Gender and Feminism in Technical, Business, and Workplace Writing Studies." *Journal of Technical Writing and Communication* 46 (1): 27–58.

5

"I FELT VERY DISCOUNTED"
Negotiation of Caucasian and Hispanic/Latina Women's Bodily Ownership and Expertise in Patient-Provider Interactions

Leandra H. Hernández and Marleah Dean

Language, as Freud reminds us, is never innocent.
—Suzanne Fleischman

The patient-provider interaction has generated significant scholarship over the last five decades, focusing on how medically authoritative power and clashes between experiential and biomedical knowledge shape patient-provider encounters. Central to these interactions are medical and scientific discourses that construct women's bodies, pathologies, and experiences in objectifying, negative, and dehumanizing ways (Davis-Floyd 2003; Katz Rothman 1986; Martin 1987). Furthermore, the words physicians use to describe their patients' bodies are also important when examining medical interactions, as they impact patients' self-perceptions powerfully (Barrett 1994; Fleischman 1999; Mintz 1992). Although scholarship has analyzed the construction of women's bodies in gynecological exams (Galasinski and Ziolkowska 2007), the metaphors and meanings associated with menopause (Ferguson and Parry 1998; Murtagh and Hepworth 2005), and the discursive constructions of women's experiences with depression (Burr and Chapman 2004; Egan et al. 2003), little research has explored how women of all ages encounter a broad spectrum of health experiences, their perceptions of the terms their physicians use to describe their bodies, and women's perceptions of their physicians' responses to their experiential knowledge within the medical encounter. Knowledge of these critical topics can speak not only to the ways patient-provider relationships affect women's self-perceptions but can also illuminate the negotiation of biomedical and experiential knowledge and the potential limitations that characterize the relationship between these negotiations and shared decision-making.

DOI: 10.7330/9781607329855.c005

Thus, in this chapter, we analyze (1) women's perceptions of the words their physicians use while describing their bodies and (2) women's perceptions of the role of their experiential knowledge within patient-provider interactions. First, we review existing literature on discursive constructions of women's bodies and the relationship between medical socialization and shared decision-making. Then we discuss our participants' perceptions of their relationships with their physicians and conclude with a discussion of the role of power and language in healthcare interactions.

LITERATURE REVIEW

Historical, Scientific, and Medical Conceptualizations of Women's Bodies

Women's bodies have been constructed historically and medically in several ways, including as less perfect male bodies (Laqueur 1990), machines (Davis-Floyd 2003), sites of (failed) production (Martin 1987), and sites of discipline and control (Bartky 2003; Weitz 2003). Thomas Laqueur (1990) chronicles the historical split from the one-sex/flesh model to the two-sex/flesh model, in which women's bodies went from being a less perfect version of the male body to a completely different sex. This split set the stage for the construction of women's bodies as being in need of (male) expert control and advice. For centuries, women have been inundated with messages and directives from "experts" about how to deal with PMS, how to cope with menopause, what kind of births to have, how to be a good housewife, and how to mother their children, among others (Ehrenreich and English 2005).

In their historical account of experts' advice to women, Barbara Ehrenreich and Dierdre English (2005) discuss two centuries of advice experts have used to control women's health practices and medical experiences. This "scientific advice" answered one fundamentally masculine question of control, the Woman Question: "What is woman's true nature? And what, in an industrial world which no longer honored women's traditional skills, was she to *do*?" (6). This question, this problem of control, focused on how women "had become an issue, a social problem—something to be investigated, analyzed, and solved" (6). Scientific expertise about women's bodies gained momentum as witches, midwives, and healers lost their credibility; once science became the dominant paradigm and the "biological hegemony of the medical profession" (108) took hold, experts constructed femininity as a disease and constructed women as the weaker, more problematic sex. This legacy of scientific expertise has aided in the construction of dominant medical paradigms that shape and influence healthcare providers' perceptions of women's organs and biological processes.

Emily Martin's (1987, 1988) research has also shed light upon the nuanced ways various medical and scientific discourses converge to construct the female body as a (failed) machine. Using the Cartesian model of the body-as-machine, Martin (1987) and Robbie Davis-Floyd (2003) illustrate how the rise of the technocratic model constructed women's bodies as broken machines that need to be fixed by their (male) mechanic/technician physicians. This conceptualization, which informs several modern-day medical procedures, "eventually formed the philosophical foundation of modern obstetrics" (Davis-Floyd 2003, 51), as well as other medical specialties. Moreover, Martin (1987, 1988) conducted feminist textual analyses of medical textbooks to explore medical metaphors that serve as a lens through which healthcare practitioners view women's bodies. Men's bodies are constructed as strong, virile, and healthy, whereas women's bodies are negatively constructed as sites of failed production, waste, and debris. Ultimately, Martin concludes that contemporary medical textbooks denigrate women's bodies and bodily processes, and that these constructions not only have the potential to manifest themselves insidiously within medical interactions but also shape women's perceptions of themselves.

Gender, Patient-Provider Communication, and the Healthcare Encounter

Another factor that contributes to how healthcare providers perceive women and their bodies is their understanding of the role of patients' gender within healthcare encounters. Research has traditionally focused on the role of the *physician's* gender as it influences their medical practice and communication with patients (Roter and Hall 1998, 2004; Street 2002), but little research has explored the role of the *patient's* gender within the medical encounter. Laura L. Ellingson and Patrice M. Buzzanell (1999) note that gender shapes patient-provider communication in numerous ways: (1) it shapes how both parties share their personal information, (2) it shapes the power dynamics that have traditionally privileged physicians within medical encounters, and (3) it shapes how "bodily integrity is questioned and perhaps violated by disease or injury and subsequent treatment" (156). Moreover, building upon work by Stephany Borges and Howard Waitzkin (1995), Ellingson and Buzzanell (1999) argue that in patient-provider communication, "we see the gendered politics of everyday life" (157). By not seeking to critically explore patient-provider communication, scholars fail to understand how medical discourses reinforce traditionally oppressive gender roles within medical encounters (Borges and Waitzkin 1995; Ellingson and Buzzanell 1999).

Research that has explored the relationship between women's gender and patient-provider communication is inconclusive at best. Anne Gabbard-Alley (1995) reviewed literature on patient gender and healthcare encounters and found there is a lack of substantial research regarding the role of gender in health communication, which makes it difficult to draw strong conclusions about the role of gender and patient-provider communication. This leads scholars such as Laura Ellingson (2010) and Mohan Dutta and Heather Zoller (2008) to advocate for more expansive approaches to health-communication scholarship, including critical and feminist perspectives that focus on the role of gender and a disruption of "the 'taken-for-grantedness' of the norms of hierarchy and power that pervade health care, illuminating the complexities of communication, revealing manifestations of power, and offering alternatives to top-down power structures" (Ellingson 2010, 96).

Now, we want to emphasize we are not blaming physicians or constructing a victimized female patient/oppressive male doctor dichotomy—this context and socialization process is indeed multifaceted. Based upon past research that explores the role of cultural competence and patient centeredness in patient-provider interactions, despite physicians' best intentions, patients are still stereotyped based on race, ethnicity, gender, and class, to name a few (Hunt and de Voogd 2005; Napoles-Springer et al. 2005). This stereotyping adversely and negatively affects patients' healthcare outcomes and their experiences with their healthcare providers (Geiger 2001; Kleinman and Benson 2006; Perloff et al. 2006). Thus, the patient-provider interaction is a site where many factors converge, such as cultural beliefs, patient attitudes and values, physician biases, biomedical knowledge, and patients' experiential knowledge, among others. As the introduction to this volume illustrates, science is not neutral, biomedicine is gendered; as a result, women patients' experiences are less likely to be taken seriously, in addition to being misdiagnosed or dismissed. Given the national and international push for patient-centered communication (Barry and Edgman-Levitan 2012; De Boer, Delnoij, and Rademakers 2013), a framework that advocates for shared decision-making, patient autonomy, empathy, and egalitarian interactions, we question how historical constructions of women's bodies might seep into healthcare encounters and the degree to which experiential knowledge is valued in healthcare encounters.

Experiential Knowledge

During the second wave of feminism, the women's-health movement as a political project emphasized the role of agency in women's health when, during a consciousness-raising group, women conceptualized how they could take their health matters into their own hands. From this movement came *Our Bodies, Ourselves,* as well as widespread recognition of the notion of experiential knowledge, which was a valuation of women's health self-knowledge (Hernández and Upton 2018; Nelson 2015; Wells 2010). Women became active participants in their health by leading health-education sessions, opening health clinics, and joining the medical profession (Morgen 2002). This idea of an active healthcare participant has carried on into modern-day medical discourses and movements, especially patient-centered care. Reasons for advocating for active patient participation fall into three main categories: patient participation increases the legitimacy of health research, patients have a moral right to participate in decisions that affect them, and patients can improve health research by providing their experiential knowledge (Caron-Flinterman, Broerse, and Bundres 2005; Entwhistle et al. 1998; Goodare and Lockwood 1999; Popay and Williams 1996).

Experiential knowledge can be defined as "the ultimate source of patient-specific knowledge—the often implicit, lived experiences of individual patients with their bodies and their illnesses as well as with care and cure" (Caron-Flinterman, Broerse, and Bunders 2005, 2576). Theoretically, the combination of patients' experiential knowledge and physicians' biomedical knowledge creates an effective and satisfactory treatment plan for an illness, as both parties in the medical encounter are able to voice their knowledges and preferences in search of a path to better patient health (Abel and Browner 1998). However, little research has explored the role of experiential knowledge in healthcare encounters, given structural and interpersonal obstacles that create barriers to the reception of experiential knowledge. Given the tangled relationships among scientific constructions of women's bodies, experiential knowledge, and language in medical encounters, we asked two research questions:

RQ1: How are women's bodies discursively constructed within patient-provider interactions?

RQ2: What is the role of women's experiential knowledge within patient-provider interactions?

METHODS

The data for this project come from a larger research project in which we explored Hispanic/Latina and Caucasian women's perceptions of their healthcare providers' communication broadly, as we were interested in comparing and contrasting cross-cultural healthcare experiences. We recruited participants through a snowball sample (see table 5.1 for participant demographics). Four research assistants conducted in-depth, semi-structured, face-to-face interviews with fourteen Hispanic/Latina and Caucasian women from various cities in Texas. Interviews lasted forty-five minutes to an hour and were recorded and transcribed.

Data were analyzed using the constant-comparison approach, which involves creating and developing themes from the transcripts (Glaser 1965). After research assistants conducted the first four interviews, we read through the transcripts, exploring the utility of our initial research questions and creating initial themes, categories, and codes. This process continued after each round of interviews. After all interviews were conducted, two major themes emerged, each with two codes within each category, resulting in two themes and four codes total.

RESULTS

Data analysis revealed two connected themes: (1) the (re)construction of the pathologized, neurotic, exaggerating female patient who needs to be "fixed" and (2) the denial of patients' experiential knowledge.

The (Re)Construction of the Pathologized, Neurotic, Exaggerating Female Patient Who Needs to be "Fixed"

The Lying Female Patient

All but one of the participants had at least one experience in which her physician implicitly or explicitly called her a liar or implied she was exaggerating. This occurred across a wide spectrum of illnesses and diseases (Crohn's disease, foot problems, gum bleeding, stomach problems), a wide spectrum of physicians (dermatologists, dentists, gastroenterologists, and primary care physicians), and with both male and female physicians. In these scenarios, a patient would tell her physician about her symptoms and pain, and the physician would respond by saying that the patient's symptoms and pain were "fake," "planned," and "unreal." In fact, a few participants' physicians explicitly called them liars to their faces. For example, Betty, a twenty-one-year-old Caucasian female who started showing symptoms of Crohn's disease when she was about six-teen years old attributed her relational problems with her mother to her physicians' construction of her as a liar and an overreacting, erratic teenager. Betty felt her mother resented her and her health problems because of the trajectory of Betty's medical care when she was younger: "So when she would have the time to take me to the doctor and they were sitting there telling me I was faking it for attention, pulling her out and telling her, 'Oh, she's depressed. She's doing this for all the wrong reasons. We don't see anything wrong.' My mom did believe it because it was coming from a doctor, and she started listening to their expertise instead of listening to her child. Here I am getting told that I'm a liar." Betty later mentioned she felt she could not receive an accurate diag-nosis because physicians "were constantly putting [her] down instead of giving [her] a solution, so that was a major problem that they weren't coming from a caring perspective."

Emma, another twenty-one-year-old Caucasian female, recalled a time during her youth when she had a routine check-up: "The [doc-tor] asked if I was sexually active, and I said no, and then he said, 'If you want me to have your mom step out, I will.' And I said no again, and he made my mom go out. He wouldn't believe I wasn't sexually active! He didn't trust me as a patient. Then I was nervous to open up about any other problems. He made me shut down and feel like a victim." Here, Emma attributes her subsequent lack of communication within and withdrawal from the medical encounter to her physician's pressuring her to admit being sexually active. Being a young female, she noted that this offended her and "made her feel terrible about her-self" because her physician did not believe her, and he was supposed to be someone she could trust.

Claudette—a Caucasian woman between the ages of forty and sixty-five—recalled a time she went to her neurologist for testing because of her severe, short-term memory loss. She experienced difficulty receiv-ing a diagnosis because her physicians could not link her memory loss to other health issues: "He didn't really take me very seriously. And although he still ran the physical tests, he made it very clear in his dis-cussion with me even before we ever tested that he did not think that anything was going on. So he kind of used preexisting judgment on me. Rather than see me as a new patient, he saw me as a colleague's patient and acted like he didn't want to tread on anyone else's territory. I felt very discounted in that position." These three examples are but a few of the many times women recounted when their physicians did not believe or trust them.

Female Bodies as Problematic and Abject Sites

Constructing women as exaggerators was the tip of the physicians' discursive icebergs. Women's bodies were also constructed as problematic and abject sites, either because their illnesses were "undiagnosable" or because their treatments wouldn't work; moreover, participants constantly noted that their physicians offended them by using terms like "chronic," "sick," "suppressed," "gross," "depressed," "anorexic," and "fat." While these terms are indeed taught to physicians as part of a standardized biomedical lexicon, these terms negatively impacted participants' self-perceptions and experiences. Participants felt these terms literally transformed their sense of self, resulting in stress and insecurity. When discussing her life with Crohn's disease, Betty noted,

> These words are pretty negative. There is nothing really good that comes from it, and I think word choice *is* kind of big; it did scare me when some of them didn't sugarcoat it. I guess I respected that they didn't, but at the same time, when I would get in the car with my mom I would ask, "What does that word mean?" She'd say, "Oh, you're going to have it *forever*." I did have a lot of those scares and worries keeping me up at night just feeling like, "Will it ever get better? Is this going to cause something else, because I'm having to take care of this."

Physicians' word choice was important for Betty and several other participants. Rosa, a Hispanic/Latina female between the ages of forty and sixty-five, was offended by her dermatologist: "I never thought I had bad acne or anything of the sort. Well, when I walked into the room of the doctor, the first thing he said was, 'Wow! I can see you have acne from walking in the door! It's really bad. I can help.' He made me feel really insecure. I felt really bad afterwards." Rosa felt her dermatologist said this to "benefit himself, as if all he wanted to do was sell [her] an acne product" and left the encounter dissatisfied and offended.

Thus, the "female body as machine" metaphor did not surface in interviews, but past conceptualizations of the neurotic, hysteric female patient were present. A new metaphor, the "female body as abject site," surfaced as well, as participants recalled the denigrating terms used to describe their bodies. Physicians' language choice was a key factor in another aspect of participants' healthcare encounters: practitioners' rejection of patients' experiential knowledge.

Rejection of Patients' Experiential Knowledge

Participants reported that their physicians patronized them and rejected their experiential knowledge, which led to one of two actions: internalization of the doctors' words or outright resistance.

The Patronizing/Belittling Doctor

All but one of the participants stated their physicians rejected their experiential knowledge and asserted the importance of biomedical knowledge (read: *their* knowledge), resulting in dissatisfaction. Participants resisted by expressing their experiential knowledge and treatment preferences, which was met with rejection. Betty experienced constant power struggles with her physicians and the struggle between her experiential knowledge and their biomedical knowledge: "It's your body, it's all you know. And when you know something's off, you know something's off, and I think I always knew there was something more going on. Not only that, but I had a blood infection on top of having Crohn's. They didn't even go to check certain things—like my gallbladder was malfunctioning, my appendix was rupturing, all these things at the same time, on top of Crohn's, and not once were those ideas when you say you're having pain in your abdominal region. They always thought it was anorexia." Emma had a similar experience when she was trying to figure out why she had chronic back pain.

> When I was about 13 or 14, I went to this orthopedic doctor for my back. I described my back pain, and we were trying to figure out what was wrong with my back. He asked me if I ate a lot, and I said not really. He had me lay down on this table, and he did this weird thing over my stomach to feel how much fat I contained. He said, "Oh, well, your abs aren't very strong, so that's why you don't have a good back." I said, "No, sir, I work out every day and try to eat healthy." My mom also jumped in and said that I did soccer and dance, that there was no way I wasn't in shape. He got my self-esteem down. I wasn't fat, but he made me feel fat. I felt uncomfortable, like he was assuming that he knew what was wrong with me without even knowing my opinion.

Participants mentioned that instead of a dialogue or negotiation between the two differing, yet complementary, knowledges, their experiential knowledge was rejected.

Women's Resistance to their Physicians and the Medical System

Although it may seem as if healthcare providers victimized participants, that is not necessarily the case. Approximately half the participants spoke of the damage their physicians did to their self-concepts, whereas the other half of the participants spoke of how they resisted the biomedical hegemony of the healthcare system in agentic and empowering ways. Ginger, a Caucasian female between the ages of forty and sixty-five, spoke of her "chronic" and "undiagnosable" foot problem. Her foot was swollen "like a volleyball" and then proceeded to develop open wounds. Her physicians told her to wrap the wounds, which should cause the foot to heal, yet the wounds persisted for three months. She pleaded with her physicians to cut off the extra skin that was growing around the wounds, which she felt was stunting the healing process. Physicians rejected her pleas because "it wasn't protocol." Ginger took matters literally into her own hands.

> I finally took the extra skin off with a . . . what do you call it? It wasn't a razor, it was a nail thing, like a cuticle clipper thing, but a little stronger. I took that off and was very careful about it. I prefer not to have done it, but at the same time, I was hooked up to so many things. Once I took the skin off, it has healed so much better because that's dead skin and it's not promoting new skin growth. I took care of myself. So, sometimes listening to your own self and common sense is almost dictating what you should do.

Other participants echoed Ginger's wisdom of listening to one's self and the need for physicians to take a walk in their patients' shoes to see what it is like to live within their bodies and experience their pain and frustration. Other resistance strategies included Claudette "sticking to her guns" and not giving in to her physician's recommended treatment at the expense of her preferences; Sherley's insistence upon receiving certain tests, even as her physicians argued the tests were not necessary; and the participants' "fight" to be treated in a more respectful and egalitarian manner.

DISCUSSION

These findings illuminate the power struggles women encounter navigating the healthcare system and asserting power and autonomy within the patient-provider interaction. Nancy Ainsworth-Vaughn (1998) noted over two decades ago that the patient-provider interaction is a site of constant power negotiation among patients, physicians, and their respective knowledge bases. This study points to the importance of two central facets of patient-provider interactions that lead to disheartening healthcare experiences: the terms physicians use to describe patients' bodies and the role of women's experiential knowledge within a medical system that seemingly endorses patient-centered communicative encounters.

The first theme, which focuses on the denigrating terms physicians use to describe their patients' bodies, illuminates the importance of the necessity for physicians' awareness of the words and metaphors they deploy during interactions and the material effects of these choices on patients' self-perceptions. Participants internalized the words and phrases physicians deployed during the medical encounter. Betty, for example, noted that these terms constructed for her a new sense of self.

I think being young at the time when they were saying these things—the "unhealthy" and "underweight" and "extremely skinny"—I guess when I was sick I didn't look . . . I was always small built, but it's not like when I was sick I'd take the time to go step on a scale. I never had those thoughts. When my physicians start saying, "Oh, you're in the 2 percentile of your weight group" and start laying it out using those words, it does make you go home and [think to yourself], "Wow, I'm gross. Look at me!" People look at me—if my doctor sees me that way, then that's what I must be. It's all a vicious cycle.

Physicians' word choices called new identities into existence for certain participants. That is, the physicians' words introduced to participants a new way of looking at themselves, and it was not positive or healthy. It negatively affected their self-esteem, shut down lines of communication within the medical interaction, and led to distrust of both practitioners and the medical system.

This theme questions the inadequacy of the biomedical language taught to medical students. As Lillian Campbell discusses in chapter 4 of this volume, the feminized nature of nursing combined with the masculinized world of medicine constructs opportunities for gendered learning and gendered language use; this research leads one to wonder about larger medical-school requirements and the role of language in medical-student curricula. While physicians do need a standardized medical terminology to utilize when describing illness and disease, is there a space to generate a discussion in which physicians can consider how this language can be offensive and inadequate in relation to patients' lived experiences? What strategies could be used to remedy this issue? Suzanne Fleishman (1999) argues that the conceptual distinction between illness and disease and biomedical knowledge and experiential knowledge maps out in interesting ways. Medical language is abstract—disease, organs, bodily processes—and as a result of being taught the language of disease, physicians lack the language of the illness experience. Participants in this study were sensitive to physicians' language of disease because, as Fleischman notes, "When the body is seriously out of kilter, particularly if the condition is likely to endure, your sensitivity to the nuances of words used to describe it is inevitably heightened. You become critically aware of the subtle ways in which lexical choices define you as a person" (7). In our study, participants became aware of the transformative power their physicians' language had over their medical experiences and sense of self. As Deborah Lupton (1994) argues, "An understanding of language, as used in both written texts and talk, is the primary site of reproduction of power differentials and the struggle for meaning" (61), which became evident as participants in our study recounted their narratives. Physicians' word choices constructed them as neurotic, lying hypochondriacs, rejected their experiential knowledge, and privileged biomedical knowledge at the expense of the women's experiential knowledge.

The second theme, the rejection of experiential knowledge, points to the difficulties inherent within enacting and performing patient-centered communication, particularly shared decision-making, and the difficulties and limitations associated with physicians' attempts to communicate in a patient-centered manner. Participants noted that physicians did not listen to them; treated their symptoms, not the actual problem; and rejected their experiential knowledge and their treatment preferences. This supports Leandra Hernández's (2016) and William Godolphin's (2009) arguments that patient-centered communication—shared decision-making in particular—"is hard to do" (186). It is also indicative of the clash between the voice of medicine and the voice of the lifeworld, or the clash between the biomedical perspective and the biopsychosocial perspective. One's health can be socially constructed, interpreted, and experienced in several ways, and two frameworks have shaped this as it plays out in the medical encounter: the biomedical perspective and the biopsychosocial perspective (Dean 2016). The biomedical perspective is a westernized view of health in which one's health is viewed solely as the absence of disease. This perspective is a paternalistic and linear model in which individuals in positions of power (i.e., healthcare providers, researchers, medical stakeholders) have the most power in terms of defining what is "healthy" and what is "not healthy," often at the exclusion of disenfranchised groups (Airhihenbuwa 1995; Dutta 2008).

The biopsychosocial perspective, on the other hand, privileges the voices of marginalized individuals in the healthcare encounter and provides a more holistic approach to one's health (Sharf and Street 1997). Barbara Sharf and Marsha Vanderford (2003) describe how Elliot Mishler (1984) makes sense of the differences between the biomedical and biopsychosocial perspective when they note that although patients and healthcare providers might be discussing the same histories and symptoms, two important components of the biomedical perspective, "there is nearly always a contrast, and often outright conflict, between what Mishler calls 'the voice of medicine' and 'the voice of the lifeworld'" (quoted in Sharf and Vanderford 2003, 12). The voice of the lifeworld includes social and cultural factors, including religion, spirituality, family members, and peer groups (see Geist-Martin, Ray, and Sharf 2003; Hernández 2010).

Overall, participants noted that their experiential knowledge, the voice of the lifeworld, was rejected within medical encounters, leading to both disempowerment and resistance. Given that patient-centered communication has been a major medical framework and patient-advocate movement for the past few decades *and* the fact that most physicians take continuing-education courses, why are patients still belittled and dissatisfied with their healthcare? Or, as Caitlin Leach discusses in chapter 7 of this volume, why is biomedical medicine touted as the ultimate solution to one's health problems without a focus on the sexism, racism, classism, and ableism women still experience in healthcare contexts (Dusenbery, *Huffington Post*, March 6, 2018; Hernández and De Los Santos Upton 2018; Wetsman 2018)? Given recent pushes for the utilization of experiential knowledge, patient empowerment, and participation within patient-provider interactions, why is women's experiential knowledge still downplayed or rejected? Although this study does not necessarily answer these questions, it *is* a call for medical programs, medical students, and healthcare providers to become aware of the words they use during medical encounters and the implications of the discursive constructions of women's bodies on their self-concepts, identities, and health outcomes. This lack of awareness points to the limitations of medical language and the incompatibilities that lie between the voices of medicine and the voices of the lifeworld. Moreover, it is a call for physicians to think about how they receive and utilize their patients' experiential knowledge within the healthcare encounter—experiential knowledge is not a supplementary knowledge to biomedical knowledge; rather, it is a complementary knowledge that should be utilized so patients can have the best treatment and health outcomes possible.

LIMITATIONS AND FUTURE DIRECTIONS

This study has two limitations that should be addressed. First, the analysis is based upon data from a small sample size, which included the perceptions and experiences of only Caucasian and Hispanic/Latina women. Although this analysis is important and worthwhile because it points to many limitations and flaws that lie inherently within medical encounters, it cannot be generalized to all women. Second, this analysis does not include an important set of voices and perceptions: those of the healthcare providers. As we mentioned earlier, we do not intend to create a victimized female patient/oppressive physician dichotomy, and due to time restraints and access limitations, we were not able to interview physicians about their perceptions of the role of their language

Table 5.1. Participant Demographics

Name*	Race/Ethnicity	Age
Emma Stone	Caucasian	18–30 years old
Becky	Caucasian	18–30 years old
Betty Crocker	Caucasian	18–30 years old
Marie Celero	Hispanic/Latina/Mexican	18–30 years old
Yessica Ayala	Hispanic	18–30 years old
Sasha Jones	Hispanic	18–30 years old
Jennifer Lopez	Hispanic	18–30 years old
Ginger	Caucasian	40–65 years old
Sherley	Caucasian	40–65 years old
Claudette	Caucasian	40–65 years old
Marina	Hispanic/Latina	40–65 years old
Rosa	Hispanic/Latina	40–65 years old

Participants chose their own pseudonyms. Some participants were more comfortable giving an age range, as opposed to their specific age.

choices and the role of experiential knowledge in the healthcare interaction. Future research should include providers' perceptions and observe interactions between long-term patient-provider dyads to provide a more nuanced analysis of the ways patients and providers together navigate and negotiate power within the healthcare encounter.

In short, this study explores women's perceptions of how their bodies are discursively constructed during patient-provider encounters and the ways their physicians react to their experiential knowledge. A thematic analysis of interviews reveals women were often constructed as exaggerating and lying hypochondriacs, women's bodies were constructed as problematic and abject sites, and women's experiential knowledge was devalued and rejected. These experiences occurred across a spectrum of illnesses, symptoms, types of physicians, and ages, and participants reported that both male *and* female physicians practiced medicine in this manner. Historical conceptualizations of the role of women within healthcare encounters still certainly appear in contemporary healthcare experiences, and women responded to this in two ways: they internalized physicians' discursive constructions, resulting in a shattering of their self-concepts and identities, or they resisted the "biological hegemony of the medical profession" (Ehrenreich and English 2005, 108) and took matters into their own hands by cutting their skin, asserting power within the medical encounter, and, at the end of the day, locating new physicians who would treat them better.

REFERENCES

Abel, Emily K., and Carole H. Browner. 1998. "Selective Compliance with Biomedical Authority and the Uses of Experiential Knowledge." In *Pragmatic Women and Body Politics*, edited by Margaret Lock and Patricia Kaufert, 310–326. New York: Cambridge University Press.

Ainsworth-Vaughn, Nancy. 1998. *Claiming Power in Doctor-Patient Talk.* New York: Oxford University Press.

Airhihenbuwa, Collins. 1995. *Health and Culture: Beyond the Western Paradigm.* Thousand Oaks, CA: SAGE.

Barrett, Anna. 1994. "Our Language, Ourselves." *Journal of Medical Humanities* 15 (1): 31–49.

Barry, Michael J., and Susan Edgman-Levitan. 2012. "Shared Decision-Making—The Pinnacle of Patient-Centered Care." *New England Journal of Medicine* 366 (9): 780–781.

Bartky, Sandra Lee. 2003. "Foucault, Femininity, and the Modernization of Patriarchal Power." In *The Politics of Women's Bodies: Sexuality, Appearance, and Behavior*, edited by Rose Weitz, 25–45. New York: Oxford University Press.

Borges, Stephany, and Howard Waitzkin. 1995. "Women's Narratives in Primary Medical Care Encounters." *Women and Health* 23 (1): 29–56.

Burr, Jennifer, and Tom Chapman. 2004. "Contextualising Experiences of Depression in Women from South Asian Communities: A Discursive Approach." *Sociology of Health and Illness* 26 (4): 433–452.

Caron-Flinterman, J. Francisca, Jacqueline E. W. Broerse, and Joske F. Bunders. 2005. "The Experiential Knowledge of Patients: A New Resource for Biomedical Research?" *Social Science and Medicine* 60 (11): 2575–2584.

Davis-Floyd, Robbie E. 2003. *Birth as an American Rite of Passage.* Berkeley: University of California Press.

Dean, Marleah. 2016. "Patient-Provider Communication." In *Storied Health And Illness: Communicating Health: Personal, Cultural, and Political Complexities*, 2nd ed., edited by Jill Yamasaki, Patricia Geist-Martin, and Barbara F. Sharf, 53–78. Long Grove, IL: Waveland.

De Boer, Dolf, Diana Delnoij, and Jany Rademakers. 2013. "The Importance of Patient-Centered Care for Various Patient Groups." *Patient Education and Counseling* 90 (3): 405–410.

Dutta, Mohan J. 2008. "The Culture-Centered Approach to Health Communication." In *Communicating Health: A Culture-Centered Approach*, edited by Mohan J. Dutta, 44–68. Cambridge: Polity.

Dutta, Mohan J., and Heather M. Zoller. 2008. Introduction to *Emerging Perspectives in Health Communication: Meaning, Culture, and Power*, edited by Heather M. Zoller and Mohan J. Dutta, 30–38. New York: Routledge.

Egan, Ronnie, Heather Gridley, Bernadette Hood, and Christine Brew. 2003. "Communication and Control in the Co-Construction of Depression: Women's Accounts of their Interactions with Health Practitioners." *Australian Journal of Primary Health* 9 (1): 26–38.

Ehrenreich, Barbara, and Deirdre English. 2005. *For Her Own Good: Two Centuries of the Experts' Advice to Women.* New York: Second Anchor Books.

Ellingson, Laura L., and Patrice M. Buzzanell. 1999. "Listening to Women's Narratives of Breast Cancer Treatment: A Feminist Approach to Patient Satisfaction with Physician-Patient Communication." *Health Communication* 11 (2): 153–183.

Ellingson, Laura L. 2010. "A Feminist Forecast for Health Communication Research in 2010." *Women and Language* 33 (2): 95–98.

Entwistle, Vikki A., Mary J. Renfrew, Steven Yearley, John Forrester, and Tara Lamont. 1998. "Lay Perspectives: Advantages for Health Research." *British Medical Journal* 316 (7129): 463–466.

Ferguson, Susan J., and Carla Parry. 1998. "Rewriting Menopause: Challenging the Medical Paradigm to Reflect Menopausal Women's Experiences." *Frontiers: A Journal of Women's Studies* 19 (1): 20–41.

Fleischman, Suzanne. 1999. "I am . . . , I have . . . , I suffer from . . . : A Linguist Reflects on the Language of Illness and Disease." *Journal of Medical Humanities* 20 (1): 3–32.

Gabbard-Alley, Anne S. 1995. "Health Communication and Gender: A Review and Critique." *Health Communication* 7 (1): 35–54.

Galasinski, Dariusz, and Justyna Ziolkowska. 2007. "Gender and the Gynecological Examination: Women's Identities in Doctors' Narratives." *Qualitative Health Research* 17 (4): 477–488.

Geiger, H. Jack. 2001. "Racial Stereotyping and Medicine: The Need for Cultural Competence." *Canadian Medical Association Journal* 162 (12): 1699–1700.

Geist-Martin, Patricia, Eileen Berlin Ray, and Barbara F. Sharf. 2013. *Communicating Health: Personal, Cultural, and Political Complexities*. Belmont, CA: Wadsworth.

Glaser, Barney G. 1965. "The Constant Comparative Method of Qualitative Analysis." *Social Problems* 12 (4): 436–44.

Godolphin, W. 2009. "Shared Decision-Making." *Healthcare Quarterly* 124 (4): e186–e190.

Goodare, Heather, and Sue Lockwood. 1999. "Involving Patients in Clinical Research Improves the Quality of Research." *British Medical Journal* 319 (7212): 724–725.

Hernández, Leandra H. 2010. "Are You a Good Person? That's What Makes You Beautiful: A Thematic Analysis of the Sources of Meaning Shaping Female Graduate Students' Social Constructions of Health." Master's thesis, University of Houston.

Hernández, Leandra H. 2016. "'My Doctor Ruined My Entire Birthing Experience': A Qualitative Analysis of Mexican-American Women's Birth Struggles with Healthcare Providers." In *Contexts of the Dark Side of Communication*, edited by Eletra S. Gilchrist-Petty and Shawn D. Long, 151–162. New York: Peter Lang.

Hernández, Leandra Hinojosa, and Sara De Los Santos Upton. 2018. *Challenging Reproductive Control and Gendered Violence in the Americas: Intersectionality, Power, and Struggles for Rights*. Lanham, MD: Lexington Books.

Hunt, Linda M., and Katherine B. de Voogd. 2005. "Clinical Myths of the Cultural 'Other': Implications for Latino Patient Care." *Academic Medicine* 80 (10): 918–924.

Katz Rothman, Barbara. 1986. *The Tentative Pregnancy: Amniocentesis and the Sexual Politics of Motherhood*. London: Pandora.

Kleinman, Arthur, and Peter Benson. 2006. "Anthropology in the Clinic: The Problem of Cultural Competency and How to Fix It." *PLoS Med* 3 (10): e294.

Laqueur, Thomas.1990. *Making Sex: Body and Gender from the Greeks to Freud*. Cambridge, MA: Harvard University Press.

Lupton, Deborah. 1994. "Toward the Development of Critical Health Communication Praxis." *Health Communication* 6 (1): 55–67.

Martin, Emily. 1987. *The Woman in the Body: A Cultural Analysis of Reproduction*. Boston: Beacon.

Martin, Emily. 1988. "Medical Metaphors of Women's Bodies: Menstruation and Menopause." *International Journal of Health Services* 18 (2): 237–254.

Mintz, David. 1992. "What's in a Word: The Distancing Function of Language in Medicine." *Journal of Medical Humanities* 13 (4): 223–233.

Mishler, Elliot George. 1984. *The Discourse of Medicine: Dialectics of Medical Interviews*. Vol. 3. Westport, CT: Greenwood Publishing Group.

Morgen, Sandra. 2002. *Into Our Own Hands: The Women's Health Movement in the United States, 1969–1990.* New Brunswick, NJ: Rutgers University Press.

Murtagh, Madeleine J., and Julie Hepworth. 2005. "Narrative Review of Changing Medical and Feminist Perspectives on Menopause: From Femininity and Ageing to Risk and Choice." *Psychology, Health and Medicine* 10 (3): 276–290.

Nápoles-Springer, Anna M., Jasmine Santoyo, Kathryn Houston, Eliseo J. Pérez Stable, and Anita L. Stewart. 2005. "Patients' Perceptions of Cultural Factors Affecting the Quality of Their Medical Encounters." *Health Expectations* 8 (1): 4–17.

Nelson, Jennifer. 2015. *More Than Medicine: A History of the Feminist Women's Health Movement.* New York: New York University Press.

Perloff, Richard M., Bette Bonder, George B. Ray, Eileen Berlin Ray, and Laura A. Siminoff. 2006. "Doctor-patient Communication, Cultural Competence, and Minority Health: Theoretical and Empirical Perspectives." *American Behavioral Scientist* 49 (6): 835–852.

Popay, Jennie, and Gareth Williams. 1996. "Public Health Research and Lay Knowledge." *Social Science and Medicine* 42 (5): 759–768.

Roter, Debra L., and Judith A. Hall. 1998. "Why Physician Gender Matters in Shaping the Physician-Patient Relationship." *Journal of Women's Health* 7 (9): 1093–1097.

Roter, Debra L., and Judith Hall. 2004. "Physician Gender and Patient-Centered Communication: A Critical Review of Empirical Research." *Annual Review of Public Health* 25: 497–519.

Sharf, Barbara F., and Richard L. Street Jr. 1997. "The Patient as a Central Construct: Shifting the Emphasis." *Health Communication* 7 (1): 1–12.

Sharf, Barbara F., and Marsha L. Vanderford. 2003. "Illness Narratives and the Social Construction of Health." In *Handbook of Health Communication,* edited by T. L. Thompson, A. M. Dorsey, K. I. Miller, and R. Parrott, 9–34. Mahwah, NJ: Lawrence Erlbaum.

Street, Richard L. Jr. 2002. "Gender Differences in Health Care Provider-Patient Communication: Are They Due to Style, Stereotypes, or Accommodation?" *Patient Education and Counseling* 48 (3): 201–206.

Weitz, Rose, ed. 2003. *The Politics of Women's Bodies: Sexuality, Appearance, and Behavior.* New York: Oxford University Press.

Wells, Susan. 2010. *Our Bodies, Ourselves, and the Work of Writing.* Palo Alto, CA: Stanford University Press.

Wetsman, Nicole. 2018. "Doctors Learn to be Sexist in Med School, and Female Patients Pay." *Vice,* February 23. https://www.vice.com/en_us/article/vbpppj/doctors-learn-to-be-sexist-in-med-school-and-female-patients-pay.

SECTION III

Social Construction of Illness /
Biomedicalization of Bodies

6

ORGASMIC INEQUALITIES AND PATHOLOGIES OF PLEASURE

Colleen A. Reilly

In popular culture and even some medical literature, the vaginal orgasm is touted as a superior experience to orgasms produced through the external stimulation of a woman's clitoris. Investigating this issue reveals the medical, cultural, historical, and personal complexities that have contributed to ranking the sexual experiences of women in this manner. Constructing female sexual anatomies and activities—particularly those outside penetration—as pathological and in need of intervention has been a boon to some medical professionals in the past and present. As Carlo Bonomi (2009) argues, in the second half of the nineteenth century, women could be diagnosed with hysteria for a lack of sexual response as well as an excessive interest in sex, especially outside the androcentric paradigm involving heterosexual penetrative sex, ideally with their husbands. During this period, for example, masturbation or suspected masturbation by women was viewed as deviant; medical professionals proposed cures including the "amputation or scarification of the clitoris, . . . the cauterization of the labia, and circumcision" (557–558). Despite the modernization of medicine, the medical literature continues to perpetuate this model of sexuality by privileging vaginal orgasms, which scholars such as Vincenzo Puppo and Giulia Puppo (2015) claim are physiologically unlikely. This results in women seeking unproven and expensive treatments, such as enhancements and injections to the ill-defined G-spot, which is proposed as the trigger area for these elusive orgasmic experiences.

In order to outline the physiological mechanisms for female orgasms, this chapter begins by examining the debates in the medical literature responsible for orgasmic inequalities, including the controversies over the role of the clitoris in female pleasure, the physiological mechanisms of female orgasm, the privileging of vaginal orgasms, and the resulting search for the G-spot. These debates in the medical literature reflect

DOI: 10.7330/9781607329855.c006

that the lack of clear information and disinterested research allows some medical professionals to profit from pathologizing the inability of women to experience satisfaction from androcentric sexual activities alone. After mapping this discussion in the medical scholarship, this chapter then illustrates the inadequacy of the information about female pleasure that reaches publics who frequent medical websites, such as WebMD and the Mayo Clinic site. These sites list symptoms for ailments, including female sexual dysfunction (FSD), linked to orgasmic inequalities and suggest treatments that create more patients in need of counseling, procedures, and medications. The chapter argues that until medical literature and popular media present women and men with physiologically accurate descriptions of the various mechanisms leading to female sexual pleasure, the range of possible sexual responses, and the inadequacies of our historical androcentric constructs, the completely typical experiences of women will continue to be treated as pathological, resulting in unnecessary expenditures of funds and psychological trauma.

ORGASMIC INEQUALITIES

The androcentric construction of sex has historically identified penetration and male orgasm as central to the sexual act, specifically between heterosexual male and female partners (Maines 1999, 5). The clitoris is situated outside the site of pleasure posited by this androcentric paradigm and has been both understudied and inconsistently represented in medical literature. Notably, in chapter 7 of this collection, Caitlin Leach also emphasizes the lack of definitive information in the medical literature concerning the physiological mechanisms of female sexual response. Those who posit the existence of the G-spot claim to empower women by locating a site of female pleasure within the androcentric paradigm; however, this move is troubling, as it is often concomitant with a hierarchy of orgasms that labels vaginal orgasms as superior, resulting in perceptions of inferiority in many women. Identifying the G-spot as a source of female sexual pleasure, and privileging vaginal orgasms in the process, has provided an opening for medical providers to further pathologize women's bodies and pleasure and develop treatments to capitalize upon that pathologization.

In the current medical literature, researchers and physicians generally agree that the clitoris plays a role, and for many, *the* central role in stimulating female bodies to orgasm (Mazloomdoost and Pauls 2015; Pauls 2015; Puppo and Puppo 2015). Fascinating for those of us in rhetoric, current debates in this field focus on the language and visual representations of clitoral anatomy and the physiological processes leading to female orgasms (Mazloomdoost and Pauls 2015, 251; Pauls 2015, 377). As T. Kenny Fountain (2014) argues, "Participants in scientific, medical, and technical contexts accomplish their work and produce relevant phenomena through processes of verbal and visual inscription. . . . In no small part, these displays constitute scientific knowledge by making it visible" (3). In chapters 3 and 14 of this text, Leslie Anglesey and Sage Beaumont Perdue also highlight the role language and visualization play in constructing acceptable bodies and validating medical conditions. Specifically, Anglesey argues that legitimacy is afforded to conditions and anatomical constructs that can be expressed through terminologies authorized by medical professionals; likewise unvalidated conditions may be ignored or dismissed and, in women, attributed to amorphous diagnoses akin to hysteria. The validation of anatomies and conditions takes place in sites designated for professional debate, namely the medical literature, where researchers grapple with ideas, identify areas of agreement, and refute assertions using established scientific conventions, including in-text citations and dueling letters of commentary (Latour and Woolgar 1979).

Representations of the clitoris in medical literature exemplify the power of labels and visual representations to construct female anatomy and provide physicians and the public with definitive albeit simplistic answers about the morphology of female genitalia and sources of sexual pleasure. Even twentieth-century representations of the clitoris vary considerably. In the influential *Gray's Anatomy*, the clitoris appears in diagrams of female bodies in 1901 but is absent by 1948 (Moore and Clarke 1995, 271; Pauls 2015, 376). The situation persists after the 1950s; Lisa Jean Moore and Adele Clarke (1995) found that eight central medical texts published between the 1950s and early 1970s discuss and visually represent the penis while omitting the clitoris entirely or representing it in diagrams while failing to label it or discuss its function (274–275). Freud's influence is cited as central to downplaying the importance of the clitoris and privileging vaginal orgasms. As highlighted by Donna Mazloomdoost and Rachel Pauls (2015), "Freud claimed that the ability to achieve vaginally activated orgasms (VAOs) was central to a woman's psychological development" (246).

According to the androcentric model, female pleasure should derive from penetration resulting in the VAO. The construction of VAOs as superior and the women who experience them as more evolved in seemingly unrelated ways surfaces in current medical scholarship. This

literature presents the G-spot as a site of female sexual pleasure leading to the VAO, empowering women by showing them a pathway to
improved sexual satisfaction (Jannini, Buisson, and Rubio-Casillas 2014,
534). These researchers posit distinct types of female orgasms, a clito-
rally activated orgasm (CAO) and a VAO, defined as "the orgasm experienced after direct stimulation of the anterior vaginal wall by penetration,
without concomitant stimulation of the external clitoris" (Gravina et al.
2008, 612). While offering little empirical support, Emmenuele Jannini,
Odile Buisson, and Alberto Rubio-Casillas (2014) claim that each type of
orgasmic experience results from a different neural pathway: "If several
neural pathways are activated during CUV [clitourethrovaginal] complex stimulation (the pelvic, hypogastric, and vagus nerves) [sources of
the VAO], whereas during clitoral stimulation, only the pudendal nerve
is directly stimulated, this could, at least partially, explain perception
differences between CAO and VAO" (535). Identifying different types
of orgasms leads inevitably to prioritizing the experiences, holding the
VAO as superior. As Jannini, Buisson, and Rubio-Casillas (2014) report,
"For example, orgasms attained through direct clitoral stimulation have
been reported to be sharp, bursting, short-lasting, superficial, and more
localized, being confined only to the pubic area. By contrast, the VAO
has been described as more diffuse, 'whole body' radiating, psychologically more satisfying, and longer-lasting" (534).

Researchers who dispute the existence of these two distinct types of
orgasms in women are vexed by the way women who experience VAOs
are identified as superior in other ways, both psychological and physical
(Pauls 2015). For example, Stuart Brody and Rui Miguel Costa (2011)
link the experience of VAOs with a woman's ability to avoid "immature
defense mechanisms (including somatization, dissociation, displacement, autistic fantasy, isolation of affect)" (2794). While they admit
these mechanisms may "psychologically block the woman from allowing
herself to have a vaginal orgasm, it is also possible that the experience
of specifically vaginal orgasm facilitates emotional growth (thereby
decreasing the use of immature defenses)" (2794). Such assertions har-
ken back to Freud's connection of the absence of VAOs with emotional
immaturity (Puppo and Puppo 2015).

Not surprisingly, Brody and Costa (2011) also highlight physical attributes of women who experience VAOs, such as a "greater likelihood
of a fluid graceful gait, free of blocked or distorted pelvic rotation, as
compared with vaginally anorgasmic women. The disturbance of pelvic
motion and gait could be a psychosomatic symptom coincident with lack
of vaginal orgasm and/or part of a mechanism for inhibiting vaginal

orgasm" (2794; see also Nicholas et al. 2008). As Puppo and Puppo (2015) and others warn, such associations cause distress to women. This is especially troubling because as Giovanni Luca Gravina et al. (2008), whose research supports VAOs, note, research studies derive their evidence about women's experience of VAOs from self-reporting (616); as the researchers explain, while "formal demonstration of the orgasm is theoretically possible . . . the majority of the studies are based on the administration of inventories and questionnaires" (616).

THE SEARCH FOR THE G-SPOT

If VAOs do exist as distinct experiences produced by independent physiological mechanisms, researchers need to posit an anatomical location and process for their production, which is where the G-spot comes in. Despite their support for VAOs as distinct, Jannini, Buisson, and Rubio-Casillas (2014) admit that the pathway giving rise to them has not been established (531) and that research has yet to uncover a physiological link between the clitoris and vagina, the degree to which the vagina has sufficient innervation to give rise to orgasmic pleasure, and the location of a discrete place in the vagina called the Gräfenberg spot (G-spot) (531). Ernst Gräfenberg, writing in 1950 and for whom the G-spot is named, did not identify a specific anatomical structure or provide any scientific support for the G-spot's function; instead, he posits the existence of an unnamed vaginal location based largely on anecdotal evidence: "An erotic zone . . . on the anterior wall of the vagina along the course of the urethra . . . swells out greatly at the end of orgasm . . . after . . . orgasm . . . a complete relaxation of the anterior wall sets in" (quoted in Pauls 2015, 382; see also Hines 2001, 360; Puppo and Puppo 2015). To find the G-spot, empirical studies in the 1980s used palpation of the vagina in small numbers of subjects; Daniel Goldberg et al. (1983) palpated eleven women, four of whom were determined to have G-spots. Such limited research has been dismissed by subsequent scholars because, as Terence Hines (2001) explains, "Almost any gentle, manual stimulation of any part of the vagina can, under the right circumstances, be sexually arousing, even to the level of orgasm" (359).

More recently, panels of scholars were assembled by the *Journal of Sexual Medicine* in both 2010 and 2012 to evaluate dozens of research papers supporting the G-spot and "discounted them" (Schwartz and Kemper 2015, 25). As Amichai Kilchevsky et al. (2012) assert, "Reports in the public media would lead one to believe the G-spot is a well-characterized entity capable of providing extreme sexual stimulation, yet this is far from the truth" (719). Prompted by the lack of documentation of the G-spot's location in the scientific literature he surveyed from 1900 to May 2010, Adam Ostrzenski (2012) developed a unique approach to locating it through fresh-cadaver research, dissecting the vaginal wall to reveal a "distinguishable anatomic structure that is located on the dorsal perineal membrane, 16.5 mm from the upper part of the urethral meatus, and creates a 35° angle with the lateral border of the urethra" (1355). Scholars skeptical of cadaver research, such as Rachel Pauls (2015), have remarked somewhat humorously that "these cadaver specimens were not queried regarding their sensation in relation to orgasm, so labeling this structure the G-spot could be erroneous" (383; for a technical critique of Ostrzenski's research, see Iglesia, Yuteri-Kaplan, and Alinsod 2007, 2013; Puppo and Puppo 2015, 296).

This lack of evidence for a discrete anatomical location for the G-spot has prompted researchers who support the VAO to propose the existence of a complex, the "clitourethrovaginal complex" (CUV) (Jannini, Buisson, and Rubio-Casillas 2014), which then is associated with the G-spot. As Gravina et al. (2008) explain, the resultant CUV could give rise to VAOs: "The close physical proximity of the urethra and the clitoris to the anterior vaginal wall suggests an association between these anatomical structures and sexual function. In fact, the anterior vaginal wall is an active organ, transmitting, during intercourse, the effect of penile thrusting in the vagina to the clitoris, by stretching the two ligaments that insert around its base" (611). Notably, the language here becomes very imprecise, as several researchers first propose the CUV as a replacement for the phantom G-spot and then subsequently conflate the two: "The measurement of the space within the anterior vaginal wall by ultrasonography is a simple tool to explore anatomical variability of the human *clitorisurethrovaginal complex, also known as the G-spot* [emphasis added], which can be correlated to the ability to experience the vaginally activated orgasm" (Gravina et al. 2008, 610; see also Jannini, Buisson, and Rubio-Casillas 2014; Mazloomdoost and Pauls 2015, 252). This sort of slippage in terminology and highlighting of conclusions while eliding the contingencies that produced them recalls the work of Bruno Latour and Steve Woolgar (1979), in which they highlight the tendency of scientists to allow inscriptions to become confirmations, hiding the indeterminate processes that produce them (63).

Researchers who highlight the dearth of evidence for an anatomical location provoking VAOs question the terminology and understanding of anatomy used to posit the CUV. These scholars attribute all female orgasms to clitoral stimulation and point to new information about the anatomy of the clitoris that demonstrates how external and internal stimulation of this organ is possible and could provoke orgasms. The clitoris is now conceptualized as a multiplanar structure "consisting of a glans, prepuce, body (or corpora), crura, bulbs, suspensory ligaments, and root" (Mazloomdoost and Pauls 2015, 246). Pauls (2015) describes the clitoris as having a "boomerang or wishbone shape" whose roots lie "below the vestibular skin and abutting the distal lateral vaginal walls" (377). The shape and position of the roots are significant because they are potentially responsible for orgasms arising from penetration alone, should women experience them, because there is little evidence that the vaginal wall contains innervation capable of producing orgasms (Mazloomdoost and Pauls 2015, 252; Pauls 2015, 382).

While many of the differences highlighted above may seem academic and of little consequence for women's sexual experiences and lives, the search for the G-spot and the corresponding pathologization and medicalization of women's sexual experiences have proven to be psychologically damaging and physically destructive. As noted above, the popular media, including both *Women's Health* (Rimm and Barnes 2019) and *Men's Health* (Editors of *Men's Health* and Zane 2019), continue to promote the existence of the G-spot and to equate heterosexual sex with penetrative intercourse (Braun 2010, 1402). Hines (2001) asserts that "women who fail to 'find' their G-spot, because they fail to respond to stimulation as the G-spot myth suggests that they should, may end up feeling inadequate or abnormal" (361). This perception of abnormality opens women to diagnoses of sexual dysfunction when they seek medical treatment for perceived conditions, such as the inability to experience VAOs. As Puppo and Puppo (2015) bluntly explain, "Female sexual dysfunctions are popular because they are based on something that does not exist, i.e., the vaginal orgasm" (302). Pepper Schwartz and Martha Kemper (2015) concur: "Furthermore, like some of the scientists who have failed to find the G-spot . . . we are worried that women who cannot find it (perhaps because it doesn't exist) will now feel they are sexually deficient in yet another way!" (25).

Unfortunately, the perception of abnormality among some women may be fostered by the medical community. According to Vincenzo Puppo (2015), female sexual dysfunction (FSD) is often measured using a survey: the Female Sexual Function Index (FSFI). Puppo (2015) and Miriam Forbes, Andrew Baille, and Carolyn Schniering (2014) question the validity of the FSFI and critique its apparent focus on penetrative vaginal sex; out of nineteen questions, four address lubrication or lack thereof and three address pain during vaginal intercourse (for support of the FSFI, see Rosen, Revicki, and Sand 2014). The questionnaire is also quite heteronormative, despite using the word "partner." Furthermore, the FSFI was developed with support of drug companies that market treatments for FSD (Puppo 2015, 1419). More disturbingly, FSD related to dissatisfaction with the ability to achieve VAOs is not only treated with medications but also with invasive procedures including injections and surgeries designed to enhance the illusive G-spot. Such interventions are categorized as female genital cosmetic surgery (FGCS), and the procedures are controversial and potentially dangerous. As Virginia Braun (2010) highlights, women are not encouraged to embrace their unique bodies and sexual responses but to seek procedures, which include labiaplasty, vaginoplasty, and G-spot amplification, to reshape their anatomies to some ideal standard (1401). Such a move perpetuates the medicalization of female bodies: "Arguably, the practice and promotion of FGCS render women's genitalia surgical, reinforcing a model of women's genitalia as in need of surgery and women's genital concerns as fixable through surgery" (1403). Because women who do not experience VAOs can be erroneously diagnosed with FSD (Puppo 2015, 1419), they may seek often untested surgical procedures and/or unnecessary medications. Disturbingly, as Cheryl Iglesia, Ladin Yuteri-Kaplan, and Red Alinsod (2013) document, of 238 women surveyed who underwent FGCS procedures, 78 percent did so to enhance their partners' sexual experiences. The androcentric model continues to wield significant power.

G-SPOT AMPLIFICATION AND THE MEDICALIZATION OF FEMALE PLEASURE

While scientific literature presents a detailed debate about the existence of the G-spot and VAOs as well as vaginal rejuvenation, G-spot amplification, and other procedures designed to enhance female bodies' sexual experiences, the popular media does not cover these topics with the same nuance and skepticism. As a result, since the 1982 publication of *The G Spot and Other Recent Discoveries about Human Sexuality* by Alice Kahn Ladas, Beverly Whipple, and John Perry, the existence of the G-spot has been treated as established fact in the public imagination through influence of the media (Hines 2001; Jannini, Buisson, and Rubio-Casillas 2014; Kilchevsky et al. 2012). The G-spot's existence is also assumed in educational texts, including Robert Crooks and Karla Baur's (2014) *Our Sexuality*, which is in its thirteenth edition and is described on Cengage's website as the most influential college human-sexuality textbook. While

Crooks and Baur (2014) warn readers about surgical enhancements to the G-spot, their text provides detailed instructions for finding the G-spot, accompanied by anatomical diagrams (168–169). Such information presents a confused message to readers by codifying the G-spot as fact while simultaneously discounting procedures to enhance it for women who fail to locate this source of pleasure despite adhering to the instructions. As Fountain (2014, 20) explains, visual depictions, such as the diagram of the G-spot included in Crooks and Baur's (2014) influential text, reinscribe the anatomical structure's existence in the minds of readers—and in this case educators—and provide support for activities surrounding it, such as the medicalization of women's sexual experiences.

FGCS is a rapidly evolving field, and new interventions seem to arise each time a web search is conducted. Braun (2010) provides a fairly exhaustive list: "It includes labia minora reductions, vaginal tightening ('rejuvenation'), labia majora 'augmentations,' pubic liposuction (mons pubis, labia majora), clitoral hood reductions, hymen 'reconstruction,' perineum 'rejuvenation, and 'G-spot amplification'" (1393; see also Cain et al. 2013, 170). Braun also points to the complications caused by the proprietary terms used to name some procedures; for example, both a G-Shot and an O-Shot are marketed to women to treat sexual dysfunction without surgical interventions. Potential patients would need to read the online information carefully to determine the differences between the two procedures.

Physician researchers who support the existence of the G-spot and the CUV often run clinics and/or invent procedures to enhance women's abilities to have VAOs—a reality that should prompt skepticism around the science. For example, Ostrzenski (2012), who claimed to locate the G-spot in a cadaver, runs a clinic where he performs a host of FGCS procedures including G-Spotplasty (Ostrzenski n.d.). As Puppo and Puppo (2015) highlight, Ostrzenski does not declare the connection between his business and his discovery of the G-spot in his research article (299); notably, at the conclusion of his article, Ostrzenski (2012) lists his conflicts of interest as "none" (1359). Additionally, Ostrzenski critiques other procedures, such as G-spot amplification, on his website while providing few details about what his G-Spotplasty procedure entails. G-spot amplification, associated commercially with the G-Shot, is defined by Iglesia, Yuteri-Kaplan, and Alinsod (2013) as "a trademarked non-invasive technique intended to amplify the small anatomical region known as the Gräfenberg spot, or G-spot, to increase sexual stimulation during friction with intercourse" (2007) and has become "the center of a multimillion dollar business" (Puppo and Puppo 2015, 299).

The legitimate safety and ethical concerns surrounding procedures such as G-spot amplification have led medical associations to recommend against the procedures and question the ethics of performing them. The American College of Obstetricians and Gynecologists (2020) explains that the procedures are "not medically indicated, pose substantial risk, and their safety and effectiveness have not been established" and warns that "women should be informed about the lack of high-quality data that support the effectiveness of genital cosmetic procedures and counseled about their potential complications, including pain, bleeding, infection, scarring, adhesions, altered sensation, dyspareunia, and need for reoperation." The lack of data is compounded by the secretive nature of the technologies, which make conducting valid research about their efficacy difficult. Despite the admonitions of the medical community, physicians continue to trademark their techniques, market them online, and sell training programs to other physicians (Braun 2010, 1401).

That these procedures are done on female patients who are anatomically typical further calls these physicians' ethics into question (Cain et al. 2013, 169). As the research reflects, many women may only experience CAOs and may be dissatisfied sexually because they do not experience adequate stimulation of their clitoris during sexual encounters. As Puppo (2015) stresses, "If a woman has an orgasm through clitoral stimulation, but not during intercourse, [the absence of the VAO] does not meet the criteria for a clinical diagnosis of female orgasmic disorder" (1419). From this perspective, many of the FGCS procedures designed to treat the absence of VAOs are not medically indicated and should be viewed as unethical (Braun 2010, 1401; Cain et al. 2013, 169; Iglesia, Yuteri-Kaplan, and Alinsod 2013, 2007–2008). The procedures, often performed by plastic surgeons without training in gynecology, confuse the categories of cosmetic and medical surgeries (Iglesia, Yuteri-Kaplan, and Alinsod 2013, 2007)—an elision promoted by the diagnosis of the women with the "disease" of FSD. The American College of Obstetricians and Gynecologists (2020) also warns that the procedures do not offer anything new to patients and that "advertisements in any media must be accurate and not misleading or deceptive. 'Rebranding' existing surgical procedures . . . and marketing them as new cosmetic vaginal procedures is misleading."

ONLINE HEALTH INFORMATION, FEMALE SEXUAL DYSFUNCTION, AND THE G-SPOT

The public often turns to medical websites, such as WebMD and the Mayo Clinic, for health information. Troublingly, individuals who access these sites do not find definitive information that would aid them in avoiding the perception cultivated in the media that the G-spot exists and that VAOs are possible, perhaps even normal. I selected WebMD and the Mayo Clinic websites to examine for this study because eBizMBA Rank (eBizMBA n.d.) lists them as the first and fourth most popular health websites as of December 2016. In contrast to the second and third most popular sites, NIH and Yahoo! Health, which function as aggregators of information from a variety of other organizations, WebMD and the Mayo Clinic provide detailed health information composed by staff writers.

Tellingly, both WebMD and the Mayo Clinic websites address female pleasure in the context of addressing FSD and other sexual problems. When covering FSD, WebMD ("Female," n.d.) explains that physical and psychological causes can be the culprits. Interestingly, the first example provided for psychological causes is "work-related stress and anxiety." WebMD also presents four categories of problems linked to sexual dysfunction, including "inhibited sexual desire," "inability to become aroused," "lack of orgasm," and "painful intercourse." While WebMD presents inhibited desire as potentially stemming from a number of medical problems, such as medical conditions or pregnancy, some of the sources of the other difficulties relate more directly to the andro-centric model. For example, WebMD asserts, somewhat strangely, that "for women, the inability to become aroused during sexual activity often involves insufficient vaginal lubrication." Inadequate stimulation is presented as a less established cause. Similarly, the writers attribute the lack of orgasm to causes associated with the woman's psychology or disposition, including sexual inhibition or inexperience. Again, "insufficient stimulation" is mentioned secondarily. In contrast, the Mayo Clinic ("Female," Symptoms, n.d.) website covers FSD in more general terms. The Mayo Clinic staff writers provide three categories of potential causes for FSD: physical, hormonal, and psychological and social. Notably, the focus on hormonal causes provides an opening for medical interventions. Both sites provide heteronormative constructs of sexual activity and FSD.

The treatments for FSD proposed by WebMD ("Female," n.d.) are vague; the writers emphasize the importance of using a team approach and treating the medical and psychological causes—although the methods recommended for this approach are not detailed. However, they do discuss what they characterize as "other treatment strategies" in more detail. To "enhance stimulation," they recommend using "erotic materials . . . , masturbation, and changes in sexual routines." Two of the other categories seem to repeat these suggestions, including using distraction through videos or reading material and engaging in "non-coital behavior," which might include masturbation. Because the Mayo Clinic is a medical facility, not surprisingly, much of the information it provides about FSD treatments centers around preparing patients for medical appointments; however, it does address some nonmedical interventions, such as communicating with partners, seeking counseling, using lubricant, or introducing a device like a vibrator. The pharmaceutical interventions the Mayo Clinic lists include hormones (estrogen and testosterone), antidepressants, steroids, phosphodiesterase inhibitors, and Viagra. The Mayo Clinic points to the risks related to the use of pharmaceuticals to treat FSD; for example, the clinic warns that "androgen therapy for sexual dysfunction is controversial" and explains that the results are inconclusive and the risks significant, including "heart and blood vessel disease and cancer." The Mayo Clinic also mentions the antidepressant flibanserin (Addyi), which the FDA approved in 2015, and acknowledges its side effects and risks. Interestingly, the remaining information from the Mayo Clinic covers treating FSD through lifestyle changes, home remedies, alternative medicine, and coping and support from partners and medical personnel.

WebMD's medical reference information says little about the G-spot. G-spot amplification is addressed quite generally and with almost no editorializing by the WebMD staff writers. In an article on vaginoplasty and labiaplasty ("Vaginoplasty," n.d.), they describe the procedure as follows: "G-spot amplification. The front wall of the vagina, some experts believe, holds the highly erotic G-spot, an especially sensitive stimulation site for female arousal and orgasm. The G-spot amplification procedure involves injecting collagen into the front wall of the vagina, theoretically to increase pleasure." Although WebMD couches this discussion in supposition, "some experts believe," the writers do not directly warn readers away from this procedure or explain potential dangers in any detail. The writers present potential complications of all procedures at once and in very general terms: "infection, permanent changes in sensation, ongoing pain, scarring." The procedures are not directly linked to specific symptoms.

WebMD also publishes its own health news, and this portion of information from the site does address Ostrzenski's (2012) publication in which he claims to locate the G-spot in the cadaver of an eighty-three-year-old woman (DeNoon 2012). Daniel DeNoon (2012) presents Ostrzenski's work in detail, giving a complete report about his dissection and theory of the G-spot's role in producing sexual pleasure in women. DeNoon quotes two experts, a physician and a sex therapist, who both dismiss Ostrzenski's findings as suspect because they are based on one sample from a deceased person. However, much of the article covers Ostrzenski's justification for his work. On a positive note, when DeNoon mentions FGCS, he points out that "there is no scientific evidence that any gynecologic procedure can enhance a woman's G-spot sensitivity." However, he does not indicate that medical associations oppose these procedures, nor does he indicate that the procedures are considered by researchers to be cosmetic instead of medical (gynecologic).

The Mayo Clinic website does not directly discuss the G-spot or any of the procedures designed to enhance it, possibly because as a world-class medical facility, doctors there would not perform such procedures. The Mayo Clinic staff's discussion of anorgasmia covers much of the same information as their discussion of FSD ("Anorgasmia," Symptoms, Diagnosis, n.d.; "Female," Symptoms, Diagnosis, n.d.). In terms of treatments, they recommend medical interventions that overlap largely with those proposed for FSD, such as hormone treatments, but also emphasize nonmedical approaches including sex therapy and counseling. In defining the condition of anorgasmia, the Mayo Clinic staff writers assert, "In fact, most women don't consistently have orgasms with vaginal penetration alone." While this statement is helpful in calling into question the perception that experiencing VAOs is typical, the statement does not go quite far enough to reassure women who are faced with self-doubt based on their inabilities to have VAOs. On the page that describes how anorgasmia is diagnosed and treated ("Anorgasmia," Diagnosis, n.d.), the staff explain that "most women need direct or indirect stimulation of the clitoris in order to orgasm, but not all women realize this." Although the Mayo Clinic staff make this assertion regarding the importance of clitoral stimulation, they later return to the goal of achieving VAOs in their discussion of sex therapy, where they assert women and their partners "may learn how to combine a situation in which [women] reach orgasm—such as clitoral stimulation—with a situation in which [the women] desire to reach orgasm, such as vaginal penetration." Even the punctuation of this statement is telling in its marginalization of CAOs by placing the mention of clitoral stimulation within em dashes.

The Mayo Clinic staff are frank about the prospect of treating anorgasmia using hormone therapies; they indicate that estrogen may be useful, but testosterone has many potential dangers and is not approved by the FDA. They also address the reality of unrealistic expectations related to orgasms and sexual encounters, possibly engendered through visual media and pornography, and end their discussion of anorgasmia as follows: "Most couples aren't experiencing the headboard-banging, earth-shaking sex that appears on TV and in the movies. So try and reframe your expectations. Focus on mutual pleasure, instead of orgasm. You may find that a sustained pleasure plateau is just as satisfying as orgasm" ("Anorgasmia," Diagnosis, n.d.). Such admonitions could be reassuring although they also could be read as somewhat defeatist, especially as this information is targeted to women. This advice and the entire discussion of FSD contrast revealingly with the discussion of anorgasmia in men, which is addressed only briefly in a discussion of penis health (Mayo Clinic Staff, "Penis," n.d.). Medications are recommended for male anorgasmia by the Mayo Clinic staff. A more complete discussion of male sexual problems is provided through a discussion of erectile dysfunction, which the medical community has tellingly not termed *male sexual dysfunction*. This difference in terminology reflects the disparate approaches to sexual problems in females and males that find the source of the problem in inherent female abnormalities, often psychological in nature, while attributing male difficulties to bodily illness situated in an organ, the penis, not in their entire persons.

In chapter 9 of this collection, Miriam Mara points to similar differences in how the Mayo Clinic site addresses cancer in men and women, legitimizing men's emotions as authoritative while recommending women rely on medical professionals' assessments over their own instincts. As Annie Potts (2000) insightfully explains, "Female 'sexual dysfunctions' become associated with mental illness—madness—and are stigmatized accordingly. Male 'sexual dysfunctions' demand a certain respect that stems from their more or less recognized affiliation with bodily illness" (91). In the "Coping and Support" section of the discussion of erectile dysfunction (Mayo Clinic Staff, Diagnosis, n.d.), the Mayo Clinic staff do not admonish the men to lower their expectations and accept "a sustained pleasure plateau" in place of orgasms but present strategies and encourage continued contact with the medical community.

FEMALE SEXUAL DYSFUNCTION AS THE NEW HYSTERIA

Neither popular health-information websites, including WebMD and the Mayo Clinic, nor popular media represent the nuances of the scientific literature regarding the existence of the G-spot, FSD, and the recommended treatments. The advice women are given on medical websites and in popular media often serves to perpetuate the androcentric model of sexuality and provide the impetus for women to seek medical treatment for ailments that are ill-defined and not correlated definitively with physiological processes. As was the case with hysteria in previous centuries (Bonomi 2009; Maines 1999), FSD is often defined in ways that further medicalize typical female sexual experiences and healthy bodies and, as discussed above, offer opportunities for some in the medical community to profit from their pathologization. While women can locate scientifically sound information in the medical literature if they know where to seek it and have access to it, the information they can find most easily presents the more destructive messages. For example, in searching the web for *G-spot* using the search engine DuckDuckGo, only one result out of the top twenty, published in the *Huffington Post* (Adams, October 14, 2014), connects women to the research by Puppo and Puppo that debunks the G-spot's existence. The remaining nineteen assume the G-spot can be found. The measured but general information on WebMD and the Mayo Clinic sites competes poorly with articles in *Shape* and *Cosmopolitan* that direct women to Dr. Matlock's G-Shot site, where they can gain access to a procedure that according to the doctor's site has helped "87% of women surveyed" gain enhanced sexual arousal/gratification (TheG-Shot.com 2015). The technical medical information discussed above has difficulty inducing skepticism about these promises of improved sexual experience through easy medical treatments. Such treatments exploit the dominance of the androcentric model of sex to benefit some medical providers while causing women greater anxiety and encouraging their perceptions that what is normal for them is actually dysfunctional.

REFERENCES

American College of Obstetricians and Gynecologists. 2020. "ACOG Committee Opinion No. 795: Elective Female Genital Cosmetic Surgery." *American College of Obstetricians and Gynecologists: Clinical Guidance*, January 2020. https://www.acog.org/clinical/clinical-guidance/committee-opinion/articles/2020/01/elective-female-genital-cosmetic-surgery.

Bonomi, Carlo. 2009. "The Relevance of Castration and Circumcision to the Origins of Psychoanalysis: 1. The Medical Context." *International Journal of Psychoanalysis* 90 (3): 551–580.

Braun, Virginia. 2010. "Female Genital Cosmetic Surgery: A Critical Review of Current Knowledge and Contemporary Debates." *Journal of Women's Health* 19 (7): 1393–1407.

Brody, Stuart, and Rui Miguel Costa. 2011. "Vaginal Orgasm Is More Prevalent among Women with a Prominent Tubercle of the Upper Lip." *Journal of Sexual Medicine* 8 (10): 2793–2799.

Cain, Joanna M., Cheryl B. Iglesia, Bernard Dickens, and Owen Montgomery. 2013. "Body Enhancement through Female Genital Cosmetic Surgery Creates Ethical and Rights Dilemmas." *International Journal of Gynecology and Obstetrics* 122 (2): 169–172.

Crooks, Robert L., and Karla Baur. 2014. *Our Sexuality*. 12th ed. Belmont, CA: Wadsworth, Cengage Learning.

DeNoon, Daniel J. 2012. "G-Spot Found? Vaginal Dissection Reveals Elusive G-spot, Surgeon Says." WebMD. http://www.webmd.com/sex-relationships/news/20120425/g-spot-found.

eBizMBA. n.d. "Top 15 Most Popular Health Websites." Last modified January 2019. http://www.ebizmba.com/articles/health-websites.

Editors of *Men's Health*, and Zachary Zane. 2019. "A Step-by-Step Guide to Finding the Female G-spot." *Men's Health*, July 26, 2019. https://www.menshealth.com/sex-women/a19536271/find-g-spot/.

Forbes, Miriam K., Andrew J. Baillie, and Carolyn A. Schniering. 2014. "Critical Flaws in the Female Sexual Function Index and the International Index of Erectile Function." *Journal of Sex Research* 51 (5): 485–491.

Fountain, T. Kenny. 2014. *Rhetoric in the Flesh: Trained Vision, Technical Expertise, and the Gross Anatomy Lab*. New York: Taylor and Francis.

Goldberg, Daniel C., Beverly Whipple, Ralph E. Fishkin, Howard Waxman, Paul J. Fink, and Martin Weisberg. 1983. "The Gräfenberg Spot and Female Ejaculation: A Review of Initial Hypotheses." *Journal of Sex and Marital Therapy* 9 (1): 27–37.

Gravina, Giovanni Luca, Fulvia Brandetti, Paolo Martini, Eleonora Carosa, Savino M. Di Stasi, Susanna Morano, Andrea Lenzi, and Emmanuele A. Jannini. 2008. "Measurement of the Thickness of the Urethrovaginal Space in Women with or without Vaginal Orgasm." *Journal of Sexual Medicine* 5 (3): 610–618.

Hines, Terence M. 2001. "The G-spot: A Modern Gynecologic Myth." *American Journal of Obstetrics and Gynecology* 185 (2): 359–362.

Iglesia, Cheryl B., Ladin Yuteri-Kaplan, and Red Alinsod. 2013. "Female Genital Cosmetic Surgery: A Review of Techniques." *International Urogynecological Journal* 24 (12): 1997–2009.

Jannini, Emmanuele A., Odile Buisson, and Alberto Rubio-Casillas. 2014. "Beyond the G-spot: Clitourethrovaginal Complex Anatomy in Female Orgasm." *Nature Reviews Urology* 11 (9): 531–538.

Kilchevsky, Amichai, Yoram Vardi, Lior Lowenstein, and Ilan Gruenwald. 2012. "Is the Female G-spot Truly a Distinct Anatomic Entity?" *Journal of Sexual Medicine* 9 (3): 719–726.

Ladas, Alice Kahn, Beverly Whipple, and John D. Perry. 1982. *The G spot and Other Recent Discoveries about Human Sexuality*. New York: Holt, Rinehart, and Winston.

Latour, Bruno, and Steve Woolgar. 1979. *Laboratory Life: The Social Construction of Scientific Facts*. Beverly Hills: SAGE.

Maines, Rachel P. 1999. *The Technology of Orgasm: "Hysteria," the Vibrator, and Women's Sexual Satisfaction*. Baltimore: Johns Hopkins University Press.

Mayo Clinic Staff. n.d. "Penis Health: Identify and Prevent Problems." https://www.mayoclinic.org/healthy-lifestyle/mens-health/in-depth/penis-health/art-20046175.

Mayo Clinic Staff. n.d. "Anorgasmia in Women." Diagnosis and Treatment. https://www.mayoclinic.org/diseases-conditions/anorgasmia/diagnosis-treatment/drc-20369428.

Mayo Clinic Staff. n.d. "Coping and Support." Erectile Dysfunction: Diagnosis and Treatment. https://www.mayoclinic.org/diseases-conditions/erectile-dysfunction/diagnosis-treatment/drc-20355782.

Mayo Clinic Staff. n.d. "Female Sexual Dysfunction." Diagnosis and Treatment. https://www.mayoclinic.org/diseases-conditions/female-sexual-dysfunction/diagnosis-treatment/drc-20372556.

Mayo Clinic Staff. n.d. "Female Sexual Dysfunction." Symptoms and Causes. https://www.mayoclinic.org/diseases-conditions/female-sexual-dysfunction/symptoms-causes/syc-20372549.

Mazloomdoost, Donna, and Rachel N. Pauls. 2015. "A Comprehensive Review of the Clitoris and Its Role in Female Sexual Function." *Sexual Medicine Reviews* 3 (4): 245–263.

Moore, Lisa Jean, and Adele E. Clarke. 1995. "Clitoral Conventions and Transgressions: Graphic Representations in Anatomy Texts, c1900–1991." *Feminist Studies* 21 (2): 255–301.

Nicholas, Aurelie, Stuart Brody, Pascal de Sutter, and Francois de Carufel. 2008. "A Woman's History of Vaginal Orgasm Is Discernible from Her Walk." *Journal of Sexual Medicine* 5 (9): 2119–2124.

Ostrzenski, Adam. 2012. "G-spot Anatomy: A New Discovery." *Journal of Sexual Medicine* 9 (5): 1355–1359.

Ostrzenski, Adam. n.d. "Cosmetic-Plastic Gynecology." Last modified October 7, 2017. http://cosmetic-gyn.com/.

Pauls, Rachel N. 2015. "Anatomy of the Clitoris and the Female Sexual Response." *Clinical Anatomy* 28 (3): 376–384.

Potts, Annie. 2000. "The Essence of the Hard On: Hegemonic Masculinity and the Cultural Construction of 'Erectile Dysfunction.'" *Men and Masculinities* 3 (1): 85–103.

Puppo, Vincenzo. 2015. "Female Sexual Dysfunction Is an Artificial Concept Driven by Commercial Interests." *BJOG: An International Journal of Obstetrics and Gynaecology* 122 (10): 1419.

Puppo, Vincenzo, and Giulia Puppo. 2015. "Anatomy of Sex: Revision of the New Anatomical Terms Used for the Clitoris and the Female Orgasm by Sexologists." *Clinical Anatomy* 28 (3): 293–304.

Rimm, Hannah, and Zahra Barnes. 2019. "How to Find Your G-Spot So You Can Have the Strongest Orgasms Ever." *Women's Health*, March 5, 2019. https://www.womenshealthmag.com/sex-and-love/a19927155/how-to-find-your-own-g-spot/.

Rosen, Raymond C., Dennis A. Revicki, and Michael Sand. 2014. "Commentary on 'Critical Flaws in the FSFI and IIEF.'" *Journal of Sex Research* 51 (5): 492–497.

Schwartz, Pepper, and Martha Kemper. 2015. *50 Great Myths of Human Sexuality*. West Sussex, UK: Wiley-Blackwell.

TheG-Shot.com. "G-Spot Amplification." Last modified 2015. http://thegshot.com/physicians/.

WebMD. n.d. "Female Sexual Dysfunction." Last modified 2019. https://www.webmd.com/women/guide/sexual-dysfunction-women#1.

WebMD. n.d. "Vaginoplasty and Labiaplasty." Last modified 2019. https://www.webmd.com/women/guide/vaginoplasty-and-labiaplasty-procedures#1.

7

FROM THE MARGINS TO THE BASEMENT
The Intersections of Biomedical Patienthood

Caitlin Leach

Intersectionality is an analytical framework that takes into consideration the various axes of oppression that give rise to marginalization and subordination. In her 1989 explanation of intersectionality, Kimberlé Crenshaw uses two important metaphors. The first, and most widely utilized, involves a traffic accident that occurs at the intersections of oppressive axes. Black women navigating thoroughfares at the intersections of power are positioned to suffer injury from the traffic flowing from the roads of race, gender, and class simultaneously. Thus, the dangers of these intersections are complex, as multiple axes often overlap and converge to perpetrate injury. Crenshaw's second metaphor invokes hierarchical imagery and places subordinated identities at the bottom of a basement. Stacked with feet standing on shoulders, people occupy the basement according to structural subjugation, with those most disadvantaged at the bottom, furthest from the hatch above through which they may escape. Essentially, the metaphors work together to illustrate the dynamic, multidimensional nature of systemic oppression. As Anna Carastathis (2013) argues in her essay "Basements and Intersections," Crenshaw's intersection metaphor alone flattens the oppressive geography and visually suggests all identities exist along the same plane. Incorporating the basement metaphor in feminist analysis is essential in illustrating the multidimensional nature of power distribution. Indeed, it appears that while we may move from the margins to the center, our centeredness exists in the basement.

In this chapter, I trace how the rhetoric of gender and health in US cardiovascular disease and sexual dysfunction research has evolved by placing women at the center of medical discourse. This discourse problematically implies biomedicine alone can overcome the institutional structures of racism, sexism, cissexism, classism, and ableism as they intersect to impact

DOI: 10.7330/9781607329855.c007

women's cardiovascular and sexual health. I also illustrate the process by which clinical research perpetuates normative gender-binary categories, renders racialized gender invisible, and ultimately excludes genderqueer and transgender people of color. While the obvious solution to exclusion seems to be inclusion, I argue that increased representational visibility can be problematic within unjust institutions. The US medical system is one such institution that promotes hierarchical power relations between the health professional (authority) and the patient (subordinate). The rhetoric of noncompliance, which reveals, constructs, and reinforces power dynamics through language, effectively expresses this hierarchy in which patients are expected to *comply* with a doctor's recommendation. Much of noncompliance rhetoric assumes the superiority of the proposed regimen and the necessary obedience of its object—the patient. This hierarchy relegates patients to a subordinated position within the health-care hierarchy despite their newfound centeredness.

Thus, we can conceptualize patient centeredness not as a liberating subjecthood but as a visible intersection being studied and pathologized through the hatch, from above. While some intersectionality theorists have argued for an intersectional approach to health research and practice in order to remedy these inequities, application remains limited. Study subjects have not gained subjecthood; they have gained patienthood. This patienthood has moved from the margins to the center, and this center exists within the basement of biomedicine.

GO RED FOR (WHITE) WOMEN CAMPAIGN

Recent advances in women's health and research have led to important discoveries in the sex-based differences of disease prevalence and clinical presentation between cisgender women and cisgender men. For example, cardiovascular disease is a major health threat to US women, and female presentation differs from the symptoms typically exhibited by men. Prior to 1993, many of the large trials evaluating the impact and clinical presentation of cardiovascular disease (CVD) excluded women from participation (Hennekens and Eberlein 1985). These results were then extrapolated to represent all bodily experiences of cardiovascular disease, and only when women were dying disproportionately from CVD complications did researchers consider that (cisgender) women may experience disease differently.

Since these discoveries, some women have been increasingly included as study subjects in various clinical trials, but others remain largely underrepresented. The American Heart Association's annual "Go

Red for Women" journal issue demonstrates this evolution but also exemplifies the exclusionary practices of clinical research mentioned above—perpetuating normative gender-binary categories, rendering racialized gender invisible, and excluding genderqueer and transgender people of color. Go Red researchers have called for more trials using a sex-based analysis of data and have noted that, furthermore, "Even beyond sex-based analyses, there may be subgroups of women that warrant particular attention. Although women, as a whole, are often considered to be a subgroup in clinical research, they represent a diverse and heterogeneous population" (Bucholz and Krumholz 2015, S1). The researchers proceed to explain how this diverse nature of women is exemplified by biological life events, with "menopause and pregnancy" as two such events. While the recognition of women as a diverse, heterogeneous group is a welcome initiative, current women's-health researchers promote sex and gender as the only differences worth investigating. Essentially, within the limited framework of these research initiatives, women's destiny and diversity are biology.

Investigating diversity as difference in medical research reinforces difference as rooted in biology rather than in society (Epstein 2007). With its second annual issue published in February 2016, the majority of the "Go Red" articles focus explicitly on sex differences in cardiovascular disease that reify the origins of diversity in biology. The two articles including race in their analysis either fail to explicitly incorporate intersectional identities, indicating in the subheadings that patients experience disease as either a "woman" or "Black" but never both simultaneously (Li et al. 2016), or neglect to address the racial populations most affected by cardiovascular disease (Izadnegahdar et al. 2016). While the former article addresses intersectional identities in an adjusted sensitivity analysis, the majority of the results are reported separately, structured under subheadings of "Disparities According to Sex," "Disparities According to Race/Ethnicity," and "Disparities According to Region" (Li et al. 2016).

Promoting sex and gender as singular and separate factors influencing cardiovascular disease ignores other social dynamics that uniquely and simultaneously, not additively, influence the health of sexed and gendered bodies, including race, ethnicity, socioeconomic status, nationality and sexuality. Women in the women's-health movement and subsequent health policies have historically represented white, wealthy, cisgender, and heterosexual women. The continued categorization of woman as a raceless, classless, opposite sex inadvertently endorses the invisibility of whiteness, wealth, (cis)gender identity, and other identities that affect health and policy. Such practices dangerously reinforce the normativity of certain bodies, enabling representational visibility for some while marginalizing others. Olena Hankivsky (2012) warns of this approach, explaining, "Research on cardiovascular disease (CVD) shows that focusing on sex and gender often obscures the fact that CVD is disproportionately experienced by racial ethnic and low-income groups whose lives are shaped by intersecting processes of differentiation along the lines of age, sex, ethnic group affiliation, socioeconomic class, and geography" (1713). Even in instances in which sex and gender are presumably justified as the focus of research and policy, criteria of who is included in these projects reveal limited conceptualizations of which bodies constitute the categories of men and women.

THE GENDER BINARY AND HEALTH

These limited conceptualizations of gender embodiment that focus on women's health as the alternative to men's health is problematic for addressing the needs of those marginalized by the gender binary. Raewyn Connell (2012) warns of this dichotomous approach, emphasizing that policy "interest centres on the disparities between women as a group and men as a group. Policy documents about gender usually take 'women' and 'men' as fixed, unproblematic categories" (1675). The acknowledgement of gender fluidity is a common omission in the conversation of women's health and gender-based research.

. This omission is challenged by an article recently published in the *Journal of the American Medical Association*, which is boldly entitled "Transgender Care Moves into the Mainstream." Laura Buchholz (2015) writes, "Despite the paucity of research on transgender health issues, physicians seeking education about treating transgender patients now have a number of resources to consult, including several published guidelines," but these guidelines "are not based on long-term prospective randomized trials" (1786), and they rely predominately on physician consensus and expert opinion. Furthermore, the trials available and cited in such guidelines are limited in scope and inadvertently reify the gender binary. Transgender care is taken to be synonymous with hormonal transition and gender-affirming surgery in which patients transition from one sex to the other, excluding consideration of the gender spectrum on which many transgender and genderqueer individuals identify. The male-to-female and female-to-male rhetoric reinforces natal sex categories as binary opposites rather than as extremes along a spectrum.

While incorporating transgender identities within patient-centered medical discourse may seem beneficial, the diagnostic criteria for

gender dysphoria reveals troubling assumptions about gender performativity and embodiment within biomedicine. While some improvements in language were offered by the *Diagnostic and Statistical Manual*
update in 2013, such as the recognition of more than two genders, the
Endocrine Society Guidelines cite the tenth revision of the International
Statistical Classification of Diseases and Related Health Problems (ICD-
10) criteria, implemented in the United States in 2015, for diagnosing "transsexualism," which includes that a boy must assert "his penis
or testes are disgusting or will disappear" and that a girl must assert
"she has or will grow a penis" (Hembree et al. 2009, 9). According to
these criteria, gender is defined by the presence or the lack of a penis.
Anatomizing gender implies gender is rooted in the body—that to be
gender dysphoric is to be body dysphoric. This raises questions about
the access of transition therapy for transgender patients who do not
experience body dysphoria but nonetheless identify as another gender.
The ICD-10 also establishes normative criteria for gender performance,
and patients may be considered dysphoric if they prefer the clothing
and activities exhibited by the "opposite" gender. Finally, one of the
most disturbing aspects of the ICD-10 is the perpetuation of phallocentric rhetoric in biomedicine, which calls into question the notion of
progress in gendered health discourse altogether. It is within this binary
conception of gender and health that the Go Red campaign operates.

Research specifically designed to promote transgender health reveals
exclusive tendencies similar to those offered by Go Red. In an observational, cross-sectional study conducted by Katrien Wierckx et al. (2012),
investigators found cardiovascular morbidity is higher in those trying
to feminize, especially those aged fifty years or older, with at least one
cardiovascular risk factor. In another observational study conducted by
Henk Asscheman et al. (2011), investigators found that the use of ethinyl
estradiol is associated with an increase in thromboembolic events. These
adverse events are attributed to smoking status, concurrent hormone
use, and other cardiovascular risk factors such as hypercholesterolemia
and hypertension. Wierckx et al. (2012) explain, "In our clinical experience, it remains difficult to convince transsexual women to discontinue
smoking but also to adopt a healthier lifestyle" (2647). And Asscheman
et al. (2011) conclude, "Lifestyle behaviors, which include healthy diets,
smoking cessation, and regular exercise, may help to reduce cardiovascular risk especially in the group of MtF" (164). There is no discussion
of social dynamics that may influence and confound these behaviors.
Additionally, the demographics neglect to report race, which promotes
the invisibility of whiteness and ignores the health needs specific to

transgender people of color. The National Transgender Discrimination Survey reveals that while the overall sample of transgender people surveyed report smoking rates 50 percent higher than the general population, Black transgender people smoke at rates 150 percent higher than the general population (Scout 2015). Clinicians should be compelled by these statistics not to increase smoking-cessation initiatives or to modify the behavior of Black bodies but to interrogate the social power dynamics that prevent lifestyle change and make it so "difficult to convince transsexual women" to be compliant patients.

It is further problematic that within the biomedical health system, modifiable risk factors such as smoking are framed as individual problems rather than social ones. Alexandra Choby and Alexander Clark (2014) explain, "Disease is most often understood as an individual problem, with 'health solutions' being targeted to individual bodies and behaviors. This approach overlooks the complex relationship between individuals and social worlds" (89). Increasing the representational visibility of marginalized people in the biomedical health system may result, then, in the increased pathologization of their behavior rather than an interrogation of their marginalized status. This conception of health as an individual responsibility frames remedies as the modification of behaviors and lifestyles. These health interventions are designed despite the fact that many structural factors limit the autonomy and agency of patients. Moreover, this assumption of universalized patient agency is problematic given that these factors operate differently for patients living at multiple intersections of structural oppression. While practitioners encourage patient responsibility under the guise of "patient-empowerment" rhetoric, this rhetoric ignores the systemic oppressions that disempower and disable. As Mary Assad illustrates in chapter 11 of this collection, the Go Red campaign also effaces these structural determinants.

Healthcare professionals' complacency with interventions aimed at the individual level may be elucidated by Choby and Clark's (2014) assessment that liberal values are enmeshed in biomedical institutions and that "furthermore, this insight also reflects the fact that interventions that target power relations may require political action, which may be beyond the scope of what nurses or similar health workers typically identify as their work" (92). Acknowledging that marginalization rather than behavior modification is often the etiology of disease may drastically broaden the scope of health interventions and guidelines. While a provider discharges a patient on antihypertensive therapy, the nurse assesses a blood pressure less than 140/90 mmHg, and the pharmacist counsels on the side effects of calcium channel blockers, no one is challenging the structure of the healthcare system or other institutions that may contribute to hypertension. Rather, patients simply need to exercise, decrease salt intake, and comply with their medication regimens.

In the case of transgender patients, particularly trans women of color, the poor health induced by systemic discrimination is not remedied by the adoption of a "healthy lifestyle." The Transgender Discrimination Survey reveals that 25 percent of transgender respondents report misusing drugs specifically to cope with discrimination, and 41 percent report attempting suicide—compared to 1.6 percent in the general population (Grant et al. 2011). Perhaps this is why smoking-cessation counseling is such an ineffective intervention for this patient population. While some practitioners acknowledge the importance of the social determinants of health, the biomedical guidelines of evidence-based medicine often fail to address these determinants. Additionally, as exemplified by the "Go Red" journal issue, the research from which these guidelines are derived perpetuates the exclusion of genderqueer and trans people of color.

These exclusionary practices are not unique to cardiovascular disease and are exemplified by recent scholarship in female sexual dysfunction and the drug approvals of flibanserin and prasterone. While the intention of this scholarship is to aid those experiencing sexual distress, the rhetoric surrounding sexual interest/arousal disorder and its requisite pharmacologic treatments reveal limited conceptions of female sexual experience and embodiment. Furthermore, they obscure the process by which pharmaceuticalized sexuality is rhetorically constructed.

RHETORICAL CONSTRUCTIONS OF FEMALE SEXUAL HEALTH

The clinical trials leading to the Food and Drug Administration (FDA) approvals of flibanserin and prasterone reveal biomedicine's limited conceptualizations of female sexuality and embodiment. The inclusion criteria of these trials again construct women's sexuality and embodiment as white, cisgender, heterosexual, monogamous, and abled. Similar to how systemic issues in cardiovascular disease are reduced to individual responsibility, the pharmacologic mechanisms of these pharmaceutical agents reduce sexual phenomena to issues of neurochemistry and physiology, ignoring institutional structures that impact sexuality and the significations of embodiment in erotic encounters. These clinical trials exemplify how medical facts become rhetorically constructed and how this construction is ultimately obscured by pharmacology.

Flibanserin was approved by the FDA in August 2015 for hypoactive sexual desire disorder—updated in the most recent revision of the

Diagnostic and Statistical Manual for Mental Disorders (*DSM-5*) (American Psychological 2013) as sexual interest/arousal disorder. Originally investigated as an antidepressant, flibanserin exerts its pharmacologic action as a serotonin and dopamine modulator. Denied by the FDA for a depression indication, investigators later sought approval for its purported effect on the female libido. Denied by the FDA twice more due to lack of safety and efficacy in remedying female sexual dysfunction, flibanserin was finally approved in August 2015. Physicians, bioethicists, and feminist scholars alike have attributed this final approval to the politicization of flibanserin and the use of pseudofeminist rhetoric in the media campaign Even the Score (Chańska and Grunt-Mejer 2016; Jaspers et al. 2016; Segal 2015). Essentially, the campaign contended that sexism was preventing flibanserin's approval rather than the lack of data establishing safety and efficacy. Erroneously claiming men have twenty-six medications to treat erectile dysfunction while women have none, the Even the Score campaign coopted feminist and ethical rhetoric and disseminated misinformation in order to pressure the FDA for approval. This is problematic given that flibanserin provides on average 0.5–1 additional sexually satisfying events per month despite its daily dose, risk of syncope, and interaction with alcohol.

The female sexual-response cycle, including the etiology of sexual interest/arousal disorder, is highly contested in biomedicine (Spurgas 2013). The package insert for flibanserin explicitly states that its mechanism in treating hypoactive sexuality is unknown. Yet, despite its controversial approval history and unknown mechanism, later studies conducted to assess female sexual dysfunction take imbalanced neurotransmission as a given. Bruno Latour and Steve Woolgar (1986) warn of this process whereby data are used to construct problematic causal links that stabilize as facts. These constructions fundamentally appear unconstructed, products of rhetorical persuasions in which no one acknowledges they have been persuaded. The circumstances of these constructions, such as the Even the Score campaign and the business interests of Sprout Pharmaceuticals, vanish from accounts of the drug's approval. Instead, the narrative provided to healthcare professionals and beneficiaries is one in which female sexual interest and desire appear related to imbalanced neurotransmitter functioning. As these constructions stabilize, a shift in understanding about female sexuality takes place (Latour and Woolgar 1986). Flibanserin is no longer viewed as constructing female sexuality as a lack of balanced neurotransmission; instead it merely articulates how female sexuality has been operating all along. This inversion, in which statements about objects become the reality of objects themselves, is evidenced by the clinical trials investigating prasterone, an intravaginal dehydroepiandrosterone (DHEA) suppository indicated to treat dyspareunia in postmenopausal women.

Prasterone is an intravaginal suppository that exerts local action to import "beneficial effects on sexual function in women without systemic action on the brain and other extravaginal tissues" (Labrie et al. 2015). Extrapolated from research in rats, prasterone is hypothesized to provide this effect by increasing the surface area of nerve fibers in the vagina. While the benefit provided by prasterone is a statistically significant increase of 2.59 units on the Female Sexual Function Index (FSFI) score, the clinical significance of this result remains contestable. In claiming prasterone improves female sexual functioning without extravaginal effects, these trials reduce female sexuality to vaginal nerve-fiber density, obscuring the lived experiences of women as sexually raced, classed, queered, and disabled. Sexual relationships do not occur in the absence of institutional influences, and these influences impact women differently based on their sexual identity within intersections of oppressive axes. Reducing these complex relations to atrophied vaginal mucosa effaces the existence and impact of these axes, enabling the biomedical community to address sexual distress without acknowledging the underlying, structural determinants of women's sexual health.

Flibanserin and prasterone provide the newest examples of the pharmaceuticalization of female sexuality—the defining of diverse sexual expressions as a medical condition requiring pharmacologic treatment. But the pathologization of female sexuality is not a new phenomenon and has its origins in the analyses of Freud, Kinsey, and Masters and Johnson. While the sexologists of the twentieth century aided in reconstructing female agency in sexual expression, they relegated this expression to marital fidelity, effectively rendering nonheterosexual, nonmonogamous sexuality invisible (Marshall 2002, 134–135). Essentially, female sexual agency was valued insofar as it reinforced the stability of domesticity and the marital unit. This stability was predicated upon the sexuality of a particularly gendered body: the young, cisgender, feminine, and white sexual woman. The construction of a recognizable and permissible female body also reinforces the stability of binary gender presentation, and the clinical trials used to evaluate the safety and efficacy of flibanserin and prasterone provide another example of this problematic practice applied to women's sexuality.

The demographics of the participants in the three landmark trials leading to the approval of flibanserin reveal the construction of female sexuality as heterosexual, monogamous, youthful, cisgender, and white.

All participants were in monogamous, heterosexual relationships with a mean duration of eleven years, and the mean age of study participants was thirty-six years. Eighty-nine percent of participants were white while only 8 percent were Black, 1 percent Asian, and less than 1 percent American Indian or Alaska Native, Native Hawaiian, or other Pacific Islander (Flibanserin 2015, 11). Despite providing a subgroup analysis for race, given that the overwhelming majority of participants were white, flibanserin can be considered another example of extrapolating white women's experiences to represent the experiences of all women of color. The consequences of these demographics representing the diverse, heterogeneous social category of women include reinforcing normative stereotypes of female sexuality and erasing the lived experiences of nonnormative sexualities. Apparently, sexual interest and arousal disorder, which is purportedly a serious obstacle to female sexual satisfaction, is only worth treating if a woman is white, heterosexual, monogamous, cisgender, and premenopausal.

That postmenopausal women are included in treatment with the approval of prasterone is not a straightforward victory, however. The demographics of the two landmark clinical trials leading to prasterone's approval mimic the exclusionary practices evidenced by flibanserin. Of the 554 participants, 90 percent were white, 7 percent were Black, 1 percent were Asian, while 0 percent were American Indian or Alaska Native, Native Hawaiian, or other Pacific Islander (Labrie et al. 2015, 2404; Labrie et al. 2016, 249). Participants' relationship statuses are not disclosed. While this could be considered an improvement to flibanserin's explicit exclusionary practices, prasterone's may simply be operating implicitly.

The rhetorical construction of female sexuality as imbalanced neurotransmission and inadequate vaginal nerve-fiber density universalizes sexual distress despite the varying significations of embodiment as raced, classed, gendered, queered, and abled. The explanations provided by biomedicine are not exhaustive in terms of women's sexuality and their experiences of sexual distress. Instead, these limited biomedical conceptions compel us to interrogate the institutional structures that intersect to impact women's sexual health.

EMBODIED INTERSECTIONS AND SEXUAL HEALTH

Even if clinicians accept the proposed hypothesis of neurotransmission and vaginal nerve fibers despite the debates on the etiology of sexual distress, it does not stand to reason that rebalancing serotonin and increasing vaginal nerve fibers can alone overcome the institutional structures of racism, sexism, cissexism, classism, and ableism as they intersect to impact women's sexual experiences. Before we can articulate a remedy for female sexual dysfunction, we must analyze these structures and their relationship to sexual distress.

Institutional structures regulate the possible sexualities available to members of oppressed groups. Black women, for example, are historically constructed as hypersexual, deviant, and immoral. Their sexuality is overdetermined by the normative world in which they engage. Black feminist scholars have reacted to this construction with a "politics of silence," which Evelyn Hammonds (1999) critiques as enabling such tropes to persist unchallenged. She explains, "The most enduring and problematic aspect of this 'politics of silence' is that in choosing silence, Black women have also lost the ability to articulate any conception of their sexuality" (97). In the absence of such an articulation, the pathologization of Black women's sexuality through the pharmacologic mechanisms of flibanserin and prasterone is all the more dangerous and, quite literally, prescriptive. The results of a "politics of silence" coupled with the universalization of sexuality as neurotransmission and vaginal nerve-fiber density erases the historical, cultural, and clinical oppression of Black women's sexuality and the impact of these experiences on sexual distress.

Joan Morgan (2015) advocates for a "politics of articulation" and traces how Black feminist scholarship began to engage with counternarratives of Black women's sexuality. The alternatives offered by Black feminists, however, were overwhelmingly heteronormative, "dedicating little attention to issues of pleasure, sexual agency, or queerness" (37). She argues that "the hegemonic narrative of black female sexuality which dominates Black feminist thought in the United States not only erases queer and transgender subjects but also ignores Black multi-ethnicity and the diverse cultural influences currently operating in the world US women occupy" (39). Black women's sexuality as able bodied is also presupposed in many of these conceptions, rendering diverse identities erotically invisible not only in mainstream feminist critiques but also in universalized biomedical approaches to sexual arousal and interest. The structure of racial oppression in the absence of an inclusive articulation of Black women's sexuality is particularly problematic because Black women's sexuality is already prescribed as pathological due to the gendered and raced intersections of their embodiment.

That women's sexual experiences are constructed as heteronormative perpetuates sexual behaviors as phallocentric, measured by the (in)frequency of penile-vaginal penetration. This conflation of the term *sex* with *penile-vaginal penetration* rhetorically forecloses the scope of sexual research, and as Colleen A. Reilly argues in chapter 6 of this book, these standards pathologize women dissatisfied with androcentric sexual activities alone. Jacqueline Cohen and Sandra Byers (2014) explain, "Researchers have found that the term having sex is phallocentric, in that most people do not include genital touching or oral-genital activity, let alone nongenital sexual activities, in their definition" (894). This construction of sex as penetration fails to recognize the diversity of women's sexuality and prescribes how women should perform, measure, and assess the "health" of their sexual engagements. Researchers must recognize that this exclusion of queer sexualities excludes queerness that is simultaneously raced, classed, and gendered. Black queer women, for example, are affected by structures that condition their sexual expression based upon both racial and sexual embodiments.

The cisnormativity of biomedical conceptions of women's sexual health marginalizes the sexual experiences of transgender people. Prasterone's assumption that all women may benefit from alterations to the vaginal mucosa fail to account for the diverse embodiments of women's sexual engagements. Additionally, flibanserin's effects in improving transgender individuals' sexual interest/arousal are unknown given its inclusion only of cisgender women in clinical trials. The inclusion criteria of these trials and the conflation of women with cisgender women undermines the legitimacy of sexual distress experienced by transgender people. While biomedical efforts to remedy women's health issues are welcome initiatives, examples of cardiovascular disease and sexual dysfunction research reveal troubling exclusionary practices. Exclusion from considerations in women's health and from the United States healthcare system as a whole, however, is only disadvantageous if the system actually benefits patients.

THE BIOMEDICAL BASEMENT

Despite its good intentions, the United States biomedical institution, as the privatization of public health resources, operates as a neoliberal project that subordinates patients as objects of the clinical, and increasingly molecular (Clarke et al. 2010), gaze while operating behind the guise of providing patient benefit. Jodi Melamed (2014) explains how neoliberal enterprises work to promote the illusion of social justice for diversified bodies in order to better mask a profit and exploitation-driven system while providing minimal benefit for those exploited. The inclusion of women in cardiovascular disease and sexual dysfunction research can be considered a form of neoliberal multigenderism that sutures feminist rhetoric to health policy in a way that prevents the interrogation of the biomedical institution and its production of privileged and pathologized bodies. It deploys a normative cultural model of gender: the binary of cisgender females and males who perform femininity and masculinity, respectively. This gender is also racialized as invisibly white and, occasionally, visibly colored. And so now that women have entered the realm of patienthood, and that sometimes these women include women of color, biomedicine can assert itself as both a postracist and postfeminist institution.

Biomedical neoliberalism is certainly neither postracist nor postfeminist and often operates paternalistically to modify patient behavior. Patients are positioned to receive instructions from medical authority and comply accordingly. This positioning is not a gained subjectivity but a prescribed patienthood. In the framework of biomedical neoliberalism, the model of the rational, autonomous patient displaces reference to intersectional identities operating within circumstance. Advocacy for inclusion in clinical trials, health antidiscrimination clauses, cultural-competency curriculums, and patient-centered care masks the vertical axes of the physician-patient hierarchy. As Judy Segal (2005) explains, the recent shift to patient-centered medical discourse has done little to deconstruct the relationships that encourage noncompliance rhetoric.

While the attempt of the rhetorical shift—from patient *compliance* to patient *concordance*—seems to work along an inclusive trajectory, it's actually working along other vertical lines to produce the effects of biomedical neoliberalism, such as the reified, rational, and gendered patient. Simply, rhetorical shifts do not prove this hierarchy is no longer operative.

Modifying the rhetoric of biomedical discourse to one of concordance and patient centeredness does not transform the healthcare hierarchy but instead masks the point of vertical intersection that occurs with the centered patient in the biomedical basement. Segal (2005) warns, "What seems to be a challenge to paternalism may be a new cagey version of it. That is, in shared-responsibility medicine, patients have a voice because they are *granted* a voice" (35). The biomedical institution persistently, though perhaps unintentionally, nurtures hierarchical relationships despite changes in noncompliance and medical decision-making rhetoric. The new cagey versions of biomedical inclusion offered by cardiovascular disease and sexual dysfunction research reveal an underlying paradigmatic problem persistent within the institution itself. Intersectionality, as an alternative medicine, offers remedy to the biomedical approach.

INTERSECTIONALITY AS REMEDY

Many intersectional theorists posit that incorporating intersectionality into the biomedical paradigm will ameliorate health inequity and marginalization. However, whether current applications of intersectionality transform the healthcare hierarchy or simply diversifies the patient population within the biomedical basement remains to be established. As illustrated by medicine's noncompliance rhetoric, the biomedical system operates to shape and reinforce social constructions and gradations of appropriate health behavior and embodiment. Behavior modification for cardiovascular disease disciplines compliant patients as adherent to prescribed fitness and diet regimens and medication protocols despite structural barriers that prevent the realization of this idealized, disciplined patient. Additionally, compliance with daily doses of flibanserin and prasterone discipline women as appropriately sexualized irrespective of intersectional axes of oppression that necessarily impact sexual behavior and embodiment. The institution intersectionality seeks to remedy from within actively produces oppressive power dynamics and the categories that reinforce them. As Lynn Weber (2006) explains in *Reconstructing the Landscape of Health Disparities Research*, "From delineating every possible bodily difference between black slaves and whites in the nineteenth century to excluding women from clinical trials because of 'hormonal interferences' for most of the twentieth, physician scientists have played key roles in producing race, class, and gender hierarchies by 'seeing' differences in the bodies of presumably inferior groups" (28). The privileging of medical knowledge often assumes healthcare professionals are objective, rational agents that act as conduits of natural facts rather than as producers of oppression and pathologized, inferior identities. Biomedicine effectively perpetuates this narrative by establishing the etiology of illness within the patient rather than within the biomedical institution. Weber explains that distributional approaches, as adopted by biomedical research, "conceive of these hierarchies as differences that are primarily centered not in their relationships to oppositional groups but rather in women's and men's bodies, in their social roles, in their material resources, and in their various cultural traditions . . . in the things that people are, have, believe, and do" (37). Simply, if only transgender women would stop smoking, their health would improve. The cure to disease lies in behavior and belief modification, material acquisition, and a closer alignment with the mythical norm. Interrogating these structured power dynamics and their relation to health inequity, as intersectional feminism demands, seems necessary in order to provide a more holistic remedy for the multifarious, structural determinants of health.

Intersectionality as a research approach has been applied most often in the social sciences. These works reveal an interrogation of the causes of the causes—the structural origin of the social determinants of health. Recommendations from these studies include policy changes, economic equity, increased education access, and other interventions targeted at institutions, other than biomedicine, that determine health. The application of intersectionality to the biomedical institution remains understudied.

Intersectional approaches to biomedicine not only require analyzing health outcomes according to varying identities such as those provided by an intercategorical analysis according to race and sex, for example, but also require us to consider intracategorical analyses that account for racialized gender and the simultaneity of intersecting axes of identity. Furthermore, significant differences in health outcomes must be attributed not only to biological or behavioral factors but also to structural inequalities and social power dynamics. Intersectionality also requires that the hierarchical relationship between the researchers and researched must be addressed, compelling biomedical researchers to reconceive of themselves as situated knowers rather than as objective observers.

In a recent article addressing the "odd couple" that is biomedicine and intersectionality, Olena Hankivsky et al. (2017) explore how an intersectional approach to biomedical research might manifest. Biomedicine and intersectionality initially seem at odds with each other, the former using predominantly quantitative and physiologically reductionist approaches and the latter using qualitative methods with a focus on social context. But the potential benefits of applying intersectionality to biomedicine—such as addressing multiple systems of inequality at multiple levels of analysis simultaneously, positioning researchers as situated knowers in a particular time and place, and a commitment to social justice—make this odd couple worth weaving together.

Applied to cardiovascular disease research, intersectionality has the capacity to enrich our understandings of disease etiology and progression. While biomedical approaches analyze cardiovascular outcomes according to pieces of individual-level demographic information often in isolation from each other, interviews with people living with heart disease reveal the complexity and simultaneity of identity and structural inequalities that impact their experience of disease (Hankivsky et al. 2017). After conducting in-depth interviews with people of color diagnosed with hypertension or coronary heart disease, Janet Shim (2014) found that lay people attribute their condition to intersecting dynamics of race, gender, and class that impact their risk for and experience of cardiovascular disease. One woman in the study directly attributed her risk for cardiovascular disease to gendered and racialized hiring practices that led her to a lifetime working in physically challenging, low-wage, and low-skilled jobs she felt contributed to her hypertension. While utilizing an intersectional approach to biomedicine can take many forms, this example highlights the capacity of intersectionality to provide a more nuanced understanding of disease that incorporates structural inequality and the simultaneity of intersecting axes of identity. Unfortunately, despite the researchers' promising findings in this example and other concrete examples in HIV, posttraumatic stress disorder, and female genital circumcision/mutilation/cutting (Hankivsky et al. 2017), intersectional approaches in biomedicine remain underutilized.

Current approaches to cardiovascular disease and sexual dysfunction research and its inclusion of women exemplify the narrow scope of gendered biomedical research. Hankivsky (2012) warns against this limited framework, explaining, "Within the confines of such discourses, there appears little space either conceptually or practically for moving beyond two definable sexes and genders, even though intersex and transgendered [*sic*] persons and practices directly destabilize such binary classifications" (1714). She emphasizes that intersectionality is a potential solution to this problem because it recognizes multiple groups of beneficiaries. However, the potential misapplication of intersectionality—that is, horizontally oriented intersectionality—may reinforce biomedical neoliberalism and exacerbate the displacement of subjecthood for patienthood. Essentially, the diversification of beneficiaries offers progress only along a flattened, horizontal geography and ignores the vertical axes operative in the United States healthcare hierarchy.

As Carastathis (2013) argues in "Basements and Intersections," the vertical axis of Crenshaw's basement metaphor remains underutilized. She explains, "The intersection is a flat space where collisions between categorically defined forms of discrimination occur. The point is that the law is not interested in redressing power imbalances and transcending oppressive or exploitive social relations; it seeks to reproduce and legitimate them" (712). The biomedical institution is also interested not in redressing power imbalances but in categorizing nonnormative bodies as unhealthy and noncompliant. Interventions aimed at the individual reproduce and legitimate disease as a consequence of poor health performativity rather than structural oppression. Moving from the margins to the center produces a pathologized patienthood—rather than a liberatory subjecthood—perfectly positioned in the biomedical basement to be the object of the clinical gaze.

We must question the benefit provided to patients rendered visible within the biomedical institution. Intersectionality offers a promising approach to address the hierarchy embedded within neoliberal healthcare insofar as practitioners interrogate vertical orientations as well as horizontal ones. While progress has been made in addressing the researcher-researched relationship through the intersectional framework, the patient-physician relationship remains uninvestigated. The attempted rhetorical shifts in medical practice aimed at empowering patients have not taken an intersectional approach and have not effectively empowered patients as "concordant" with doctors' orders. While visibility within the institution may be problematic, invisibility is certainly not a sustainable position. Health justice within the current biomedical framework can benefit from an intersectional approach that provides improved, inclusive healthcare for marginalized people. Through this approach, we may begin to broaden our conception of health interventions, including remedies aimed at overcoming the institutional structures of racism, sexism, cissexism, classism, and ableism, as they intersect to impact women's health. These interventions must ultimately transform these institutions, including the institution of biomedicine, because gaining patienthood rather than subjecthood cannot be a long-term solution.

REFERENCES

Asscheman, Henk, Erik J. Giltay, Jos A.J. Megens, W. (Pim) de Ronde, Michael A.A. van Trotsenburg, and Louis J.G. Gooren. 2011. "A Long-Term Follow-Up Study of Mortality in Transsexuals Receiving Treatment with Cross-Sex Hormones." *European Journal of Endocrinology* 164 (4): 635–42.

American Psychiatric Association. 2013. *Diagnostic and Statistical Manual of Mental Disorders (DSM-5)*. Arlington, VA: American Psychiatric Publishing.

Bucholz, Emily M., and Harlan M. Krumholz. 2015. "Women in Clinical Research: What We Need for Progress." *Circulation: Cardiovascular Quality and Outcomes* 8: S1–S3.

Buchholz, Laura. 2015. "Transgender Care Moves into the Mainstream." *JAMA* 314 (17): 1785–1787.

Carastathis, Anna. 2013. "Basements and Intersections." *Hypatia: A Journal of Feminist Philosophy* 28 (4): 698–715.

Chańska, Weronika, and Katarzyna Grunt-Mejer. 2016. "The Unethical Use of Ethical Rhetoric: The Tase of Flibanserin and Pharmacologisation of Female Sexual Desire." *Journal of Medical Ethics* 42 (11): 701-704.

Choby, Alexandra A., and Alexander M. Clark. 2014. "Improving Health: Structure and Agency in Health Interventions." *Nursing Philosophy* 15 (2): 89–101.

Clarke, Adele E., Laura Mamo, Jennifer Ruth Fosket, Jennifer R. Fishman, and Janet K. Shim, eds. 2010. *Biomedicalization: Technoscience, Health and Illness in the U.S.* Durham, NC: Duke University Press.

Cohen, Jacqueline N., and Sandra E. Byers. 2014. "Beyond Lesbian Bed Death: Enhancing Our Understanding of Sexual-Minority Women in Relationships." *Journal of Sex Research* 51 (8): 893–903.

Connell, Raewyn. 2012. "Gender, Health and Theory: Conceptualizing the Issue, in Local and World Perspective." *Social Science and Medicine* 74 (11): 1675–1683.

Crenshaw, Kimberlé. 1989. "Demarginalizing the Intersection of Race and Sex: A Black Feminist Critique of Antidiscrimination Doctrine, Feminist Theory and Antiracist Politics." *University of Chicago Legal Forum* 1989 (1): 139–167.

Epstein, Steven. 2007. *Inclusion: The Politics of Difference in Medical Research.* Chicago: University of Chicago Press.

Flibanserin [package insert]. 2015. Raleigh, NC: Sprout Pharmaceuticals.

Grant, Jaime M., Lisa A. Mottet, Justin Tanis, Jack Harrison, Jody L. Herman, and Mara Keisling. 2011. *Injustice at Every Turn: A Report of the National Transgender Discrimination Survey.* Washington, DC: National Center for Transgender Equality and National Gay and Lesbian Task Force.

Hammonds, Evelyn M. 1999. "Toward a Genealogy of Black Female Sexuality: The Problematic of Science." In *Feminist Theory and the Body: A Reader*, edited by Janet Price and Margrit Shildrick, 93–104. New York: Routledge.

Hankivsky, Olena. 2012. "Women's Health, Men's Health, and Gender and Health: Implications of Intersectionality." *Social Science and Medicine* 74 (11): 1712–1720.

Hankivsky, Olena, Lesley Doyal, Gillian Einstein, Ursula Kelly, Janet Shim, Lynn Weber, and Robin Repta. 2017. "The Odd Couple: Using Biomedical and Intersectional Approaches to Address Health Inequities." *Global Heath Action* 10 (sup 2): 73–86.

Hembree, Wylie C., Peggy Cohen-Kettenis, Henriette A. Delemarre-van de Waal, Louis J. Gooren, Walter J. Meyer III, Norman P. Spack, Vin Tangpricha, and Victor M. Montori. 2009. "Endocrine Treatment of Transsexual Persons: An Endocrine Society Clinical Practice Guideline." *Journal of Clinical Endocrinology and Metabolism* 94 (9): 3132–3154.

Hennekens, Charles, and Kimberly Eberlein. 1985. "A Randomized Trial of Aspirin and Beta-carotene among US Physicians." *Preventive Medicine* 14 (2): 165–168.

Izadnegahdar, Mona, Martha Mackay, May K. Lee, Tara L. Sedlak, Min Gao, C. Noel Bairey Merz, and Karin H. Humphries. 2016. "Sex and Ethnic Differences in Outcomes of Acute Coronary Syndrome and Stable Angina Patients with Obstructive Coronary Artery Disease." *Circulation: Cardiovascular Quality and Outcomes* 9 (2_suppl_1): S26–S35.

Jaspers, Loes, Frederik Feys, Wichor Bramer, Oscar H. Franco, Peter Leusink, and Ellen T.M. Laan. 2016. "Efficacy and Safety of Flibanserin for the Treatment of Hypoactive Sexual Desire Disorder in Women: A Systematic Review and Meta-analysis." *JAMA Internal Medicine* 176 (4): 453–462.

Labrie, Fernand, David Archer, William Koltun, Andrée Vachon, Douglas Young, Louise Frenette, David Portman, Marlene Montesino, Isabelle Côté, Julie Parent, Lyne Lavoie, Adam Beauregard, Céline Martel, Mario Vaillancourt, John Balser, and Érick Moyneur. 2016. "Efficacy of Intravaginal Dehydroepiandrosterone (DHEA) on Moderate to Severe Dyspareunia and Vaginal Dryness, Symptoms of Vulvovaginal Atrophy, and of the Genitourinary Syndrome of Menopause." *Menopause: The Journal of the North American Menopause Society* 23 (3): 243–256.

Labrie, Fernand, Leonard Derogatis, David F. Archer, William Koltun, Andrée Vachon, Douglas Young, Louise Frenette, David Portman, Marlene Montesino, Isabelle Côté, Julie Parent, Lyne Lavoie, Adam Beauregard, Céline Martel, Mario Vaillancourt, John Balser, and Érick Moyneur. 2015. "Effect of Intravaginal Prasterone on Sexual Dysfunction in Postmenopausal Women with Vulvovaginal Atrophy." *Journal of Sexual Medicine* 12 (12): 2401–2412.

Latour, Bruno, and Steve Woolgar. 1986. *Laboratory Life: The Construction of Scientific Facts.* 2nd ed. Princeton, NJ: Princeton University Press.

Li, Shanshan, Gregg C. Fonarow, Kenneth J. Mukamal, Li Liang, Phillip J. Schulte, Eric E. Smith, Adam DeVore, Adrian F. Hernandez, Eric D. Peterson, and Deepak L. Bhatt. 2016. "Sex and Race/Ethnicity-Related Disparities in Care and Outcomes after Hospitalization for Coronary Artery Disease among Older Adults." *Circulation: Cardiovascular Quality and Outcomes* 9 (2_suppl_1): S36–S44.

Marshall, Barbara. 2002. "'Hard Science': Gendered Constructions of Sexual Dysfunction in the 'Viagra Age.'" *Sexualities* 5 (2): 131–158.

Melamed, Jodi. 2014. "The Spirit of Neoliberalism." In *Intersectionality: A Foundations and Frontiers Reader*, edited by Patrick Grzanka, 237–241. Boulder, CO: Westview.

Morgan, Joan. 2015. "Why We Get Off: Moving Towards a Black Feminist Politics of Pleasure." *Black Scholar* 45 (4): 36–46.

Scout. 2015. "Trans Smoking." In *Trans Bodies, Trans Selves: A Resource for the Transgender Community*, edited by Laura Erickson-Schroth, 224. New York: Oxford University Press.

Segal, Judy Z. 2005. *Health and the Rhetoric of Medicine.* Carbondale: Southern Illinois University Press.

Segal, Judy Z. 2015. "The Rhetoric of Female Sexual Dysfunction: Faux Feminism and the FDA." *Canadian Medical Association Journal* 187 (12): 915–916.

Shim, Janet. 2014. *Heart-Sick: The Politics of Risk, Inequality, and Heart Disease.* New York: NYU Press.

Spurgas. Alyson K. 2013. "Interest, Arousal, and Shifting Diagnoses of Female Sexual Dysfunction, or: How Women Learn about Desire." *Studies in Gender and Sexuality* 14 (3): 187–205.

Weber, Lynn. 2006. "Reconstructing the Landscape of Health Disparities Research: Promoting Dialogue and Collaboration between Feminist Intersectional and Biomedical Paradigms." In *Race, Class, and Health: Intersectional Approaches*, edited by Amy J. Schultz and Leith Mullings, 21–59. San Francisco: Jossey-Bass.

Wierckx, Katrien, Sven Mueller, Steven Weyers, Eva Van Caenegem, Greet Roef, Gunter Heylens, and Guy T'Sjoen. 2012. "Long-Term Evaluation of Cross-Sex Hormone Treatment in Transsexual Persons." *Journal of Sexual Medicine* 9 (10): 2641–2651.

8

WOMEN AND BLADDER CANCER
Listening Rhetorically to Healthcare Disparities

Kerri K. Morris

Men are three times more likely to be diagnosed with bladder cancer than are women. However, when women are diagnosed, they generally have a worse prognosis, are more likely to be at an advanced stage, and have a higher mortality rate. Finding reasons for this health disparity is complex, making solutions difficult. Despite awareness of the problem for more than twenty-five years, the statistics haven't changed. We know women and their doctors make different treatment choices than men and their doctors do, opting less frequently for bladder removal. Researchers also suspect bladder cancer in women may be biologically different than it is for men (Katz and Steinberg 2009, 12). There may be, in fact, several kinds of bladder cancers, and women may be biologically susceptible to a more aggressive type. However, the most significant research shows women face a diagnostic lag because primary physicians fail to make urological referrals in a timely fashion. In this chapter I explore the delays in referral as a rhetorical problem that requires a rhetorical intervention, arguing that treatment of bladder cancer is complicated by troubled gender identifications, both because it is considered a disease of men and because of the metaphors that frame conversations about women's healthcare.

My interest in bladder cancer and its gendered nature originated in the personal. I was diagnosed with the disease in 2012, and following two surgeries and six weeks of treatment that year, I have been in remission. I was diagnosed after being sent to the ER and admitted to the hospital, where I met the doctor who became my urologist. During my testing and procedures while in the hospital, I had no particular sense of bladder cancer being gender specific, no sense that it was considered a disease of older men. In fact, my experience in the hospital erased my sense of being an individual almost entirely. Everything about the experience was alienating. I was a sick person separated from the healthy, a patient under the care and control of nurses and doctors. People tower over

DOI: 10.7330/9781607329855.c008

patients, and, literally, look down on us. Doctors and nurses are fully clothed, their positions of authority clearly expressed in their uniforms. Patients are covered but not clothed, and we are tethered to the hospital itself by tubes and machines. The color of our socks indicates our fall risk. Through these practices, hospitals strip identification from patients and cast us into an amorphous group of other sick people wearing the same gowns and identification bracelets with barcodes. I knew nothing about bladder cancer when I was in the hospital, and it never occurred to me that my gender was a relevant aspect of my disease. It wasn't until I was in the waiting room during my initial visit to my urologist's office after leaving the hospital that I realized the profound role of gender. In addition to being the only female patient in the waiting room that day, once I was in the examination room, my doctor turned to show me a chart of the urinary system, and it was of male anatomy. From that moment I began thinking of myself as a woman with a man's disease, despite the fact that the bladder isn't a gendered organ. In addition, I would discover my diagnosis was delayed by nine months because my primary care physician interpreted my symptoms as a urinary tract infection and because I considered my symptoms as part of menopause. Both of us misinterpreted symptoms inside a rhetorical space created by social and cultural understandings of women's bodies.

Discourse, such as algorithms for diagnosis and conversations between patient and doctor about symptoms, helps construct this healthcare disparity because of the powerful metaphorical frames we use to talk about women's health. Lisa Meloncon and Erin Frost (2015) urge us to pay closer attention to this kind of discourse in health and medicine, arguing that the "everydayness" of patient interactions with doctors and other members of the health community is often overlooked, yet is "one of the most important dimensions of health and medicine" (7). Using Krista Ratcliffe's concepts in *Rhetorical Listening* (2005), I will describe how everyday discourse obscures a diagnosis of bladder cancer through "identification" and "disidentification" by identifying women as sexually active and viewing them through a lens that magnifies their reproductive potential, inviting both primary care physicians and women themselves to dismiss key symptoms. I first provide background about bladder cancer and delayed diagnosis in women in order to demonstrate the scope of the problem. I then introduce Ratcliffe's theory of rhetorical listening, employing her understanding of identification, disidentification, and metaphor to establish delayed diagnosis as a rhetorical problem embedded in physician and patient discourse. The act of listening rhetorically is a rhetorical *techne*, in the words of J. Blake Scott, Judy

Segal, and Lisa Keranen (2013), that can intervene in and improve the diagnostic process, which I discuss in the conclusion (2).

BACKGROUND ON BLADDER CANCER

The bladder is part of the urinary tract and serves, in part, to filter toxins from the body. Kidneys filter blood, removing toxins stored in the bladder as urine until they are eliminated from the body. The bladder is particularly vulnerable to toxins from smoking and other chemicals because urine sits in the organ for long periods of time, giving ample contact between toxin and cells. People are most often diagnosed with bladder cancer because of gross hematuria, visible blood in the urine. Typically, there is no pain associated with the blood; however, some people present with symptoms that mirror additional symptoms of urinary tract infection, including pain and urgency related to urination.

According to data published in 2016, the National Cancer Institute's Surveillance, Epidemiology, and End Results (SEER) Program estimated 76,960 new cases of bladder cancer in 2016, about 58,950 in men and 18,010 in women. In addition, SEER estimated 16,390 deaths from bladder cancer, about 11,820 men and 4,570 women. It is the fourth and seventh most prevalent cancer in the United States for men and women, respectively; in 2013, an estimated 587,426 people were living with the disease. White people are twice as likely as African Americans to develop bladder cancer, and three times as many men as women are diagnosed. The median age at diagnosis is seventy-three; more than 70 percent are diagnosed between the ages of sixty-five and eighty-four.

Bladder cancer is usually diagnosed at an early stage, but even then it has the highest recurrence rate of any cancer, between 50 and 80 percent. After being diagnosed, people with bladder cancer are monitored closely, from three-month to one-year intervals for the rest of their lives. The gold standard for surveillance is a cystoscopy, during which a scope is inserted into the urethra to examine the bladder internally. Frequent urinalysis and occasional CT scans are also part of surveillance. As a result of the high recurrence rate and the invasiveness of surveillance, bladder cancer is the most expensive cancer per capita to treat.

Despite bladder cancer's prevalence and severity, research is woefully underfunded. In 2012, breast cancer was the fourth most common cancer in the United States, and bladder cancer was the seventh most common in women. However, the United States spent $602 million on breast cancer research and only $23 million on research about bladder cancer (SEER). While breast cancer deaths have decreased about 2 percent each of the last ten years, bladder cancer deaths have remained stable. Until early 2016, there had been no new treatments for bladder cancer in thirty years. With the discovery and federal approval of immunotherapies, we now have a significant new treatment for those with stage-four bladder cancer that is adding many months to the lifespan.

WOMEN AND DELAYED DIAGNOSIS

Even though women are much less likely to develop bladder cancer, they are diagnosed at more advanced stages and are disproportionately more likely to die because of it, with men claiming a five-year survival advantage (Mungan et al. 2000, 877). In contrast, women are significantly more likely to survive cancers of the head and neck, stomach, liver, and pancreas (Cohn et al. 2014, 555). Anyone with unexplained blood in the urine should be immediately referred to a urologist. However, with female patients, research shows a significant delay between the finding of blood in the urine and a referral to a urologist who can provide an accurate diagnosis. In fact, with a clinical finding of blood in the urine, men are 65 percent more likely to be referred to a specialist (Katz and Steinberg 2009, 12). The research of Joshua Cohn et al. (2014) clearly demonstrates that delays in diagnosis negatively affect survival. A six- to nine-month delay creates a 1.19 mortality-hazard ratio, and a delay of more than nine months causes a 1.29 mortality-hazard ratio. Both men and women, especially in younger age groups, face these delays, but the delay is more common and longer for women. One study showed women were more than twice as likely to have had *three or more* visits to a primary care physician with an unexplained finding of blood in the urine before being referred to a urologist. In fact, being treated for a urinary tract infection (UTI) after a finding of blood in the urine was the "single strongest independent predictor of delay in diagnosis of bladder cancer," doubling the risk of delay (Cohn et al. 2014, 560). This finding suggests primary care physicians are treating blood in the urine as a UTI despite the lack of evidence of infection. Even in the case of infection, persistent blood in the urine should raise the alarm and indicate the need to be seen by a specialist, yet women are making three visits to a primary care physician before being referred.

TROUBLED IDENTIFICATIONS AND DIAGNOSIS

In this section, I discuss identification, explaining how it prevents effective diagnosis of bladder cancer in women through current diagnostic protocols and cultural understandings of women, both driven by the power of metaphor. From the physician-researcher's perspective, Mark Katz and Gary Steinberg (2009) identify the standard medical curriculum and the clinical practice of general practitioners as central to the diagnostic lag. However, framing these as sites for everyday discourse allows us to conceptualize the diagnostic delay from a rhetorical perspective. When physicians see hematuria in women as indicative only of a UTI, they are working within a framework powerful enough to direct them away from an accurate diagnosis through a process of identification that is, in Ratcliffe's understanding, coercive.

Identification was originally meant to be an antidote to miscommunication, from Kenneth Burke's view. Burkean identification springs from an understanding that human beings are fundamentally defined by division, an untenable state that must be remedied if we are to live in the world (Ratcliffe 2005, 53). In Burke's conception, identification creates overlaps and bridges by which human beings can connect, find meaning, and coordinate their behaviors through shared language, attitudes, and ideas. Without identification, Burke argues, communication simply isn't possible. Put differently, communication itself creates identification. Language brings along the consubstantial state in which identification is made.

Troubled identifications result from common approaches to medical diagnosis, especially the evidence-based model prominent in our era. James Groopman (2007) explains, "To establish a more organized structure, medical students and residents are being taught to follow preset algorithms and practice guidelines in the form of decision trees" (5). Patterns of symptoms connect one patient to another, clarifying for doctors and patients alike the nature of the patients' disease and, consequently, the approach to their treatment. Medical school prepares general practitioners (GPs) to filter in this way, and without these patterns, it would be difficult to prescribe medications and procedures effectively. As Groopman (2007) argues, clinical algorithms are empowering, enabling consistent diagnoses, but they also prevent doctors from being creative and independent when they need to be. They forget statistics describe large populations but serve to mask individuals, which enhances the process of identification and obscures critical differences. Groopman (2007) describes these troubled identifications in terms of cognitive traps called "anchoring and diagnosis by prototype" (65). He notes that experienced clinicians need only twenty seconds to reach a diagnosis because they see patterns in symptoms and quickly anchor them in a template (34). When physicians use prototypes, they ignore symptoms that contradict the template guiding their diagnosis (44). As Cathryn Molloy argues in this volume, these approaches to diagnosis and a general failure to listen to patients prevent a "full-bodied" understanding of symptoms.

Matching a patient's symptoms to an algorithm produces troubled identifications, but identification creates much more complex problems. Symptoms, patients, and doctors exist inside cultural contexts, the ground upon which identification is built, creating structures that hide difference. With regard to delayed diagnosis of bladder cancer for women, statistics and disease patterns collaborate with our cultural tendency to conflate women with heterosexual, reproductive beings from child-bearing age through menopause. While bladder cancer in women is relatively rare, UTI in women is relatively common. More than 50 percent of women will be diagnosed with a UTI in their lifetimes. Risk factors include using birth-control pills and some other forms of birth control, frequent intercourse, and multiple sexual partners. Thus, hematuria as a symptom in women is seen differently from hematuria in men because women and doctors are under the sway of identification, which obscures the complexity of individual women by encouraging practitioners to see only the commonalities among many female patients across a practice over many years and in their cultural stereotypes. As Leandra Hernández and Marleah Dean explain in this volume, physicians can bring identities into existence through their word choice. If the word *woman* means a heterosexual, fertile female, many women and diagnoses are excluded.

Medical training, disease statistics, and cultural perspectives of women work together to create what Ratcliffe (2005) calls a "troubled identification" (47). In the case of bladder cancer, when a primary care physician sees an individual patient only to the extent that she is like other sexually active women with the same symptoms, "the coercive force of common ground" (47) may lead to misdiagnosis. Common ground draws attention away from an especially critical detail: blood in the urine as a *primary complaint* is a key indication that a patient should be referred to a urologist. Instead, blood is seen as evidence of a UTI and is thus normalized. I repeat that diagnosis of a UTI is the "single strongest independent predictor of delay in diagnosis of bladder cancer" (Cohn et al. 2014, 560) because it underlines how identification works. When doctors move from a symptom to a diagnosis, the process of discovery is over. Once blood in the urine is seen as evidence of a UTI, referral to a urologist is unlikely. UTIs in men, however, are uncommon; there is nothing "normal" about blood in the urine for men and, consequently, male patients are 65 percent more likely to be referred to a urologist with a finding of blood in the urine (Katz and Steinberg 2009, 12).

According to Ratcliffe (2005), identification is driven by metaphor (62–64). Medical diagnosis is based on algorithms and prototypes, and the cultural emphasis on women as reproductive beings is made possible and very powerful through the trope of metaphor. Many rhetoricians of health and medicine have interrogated the power of metaphor. For instance, Judy Segal (2005) argues that metaphors used in the medical field create contexts that determine health policy (115) and even that diagnosis itself is a metaphor (116). In her discussion of pandemic flu, Elizabeth Angeli (2012) concludes that the language used to report on swine flu sharply influenced the way the public made medical decisions (219). I want to build on these uses of metaphor, demonstrating how the everyday discourse of women's health constructs the rhetorical space within which misdiagnosis becomes common.

From a clinical perspective, women are conflated with being potential mothers. Blood in the toilet—an alarming finding for a man—is identified with menstrual blood for women through the powerful metaphor of motherhood. The coercive function of this particular metaphor invites women to interpret blood in the urine—a symptom of bladder cancer that is the same in men and women and is always abnormal—as normal. Women, who are (erroneously) understood to be categorically capable of reproduction, fertile, and heterosexual are associated with the regular presence of blood in their lives, and blood becomes a sign of health. When we are compelled to find commonality, we seek metaphors to help us name how we are alike, which also requires us to ignore what doesn't comfortably fit. Metaphor normalizes this omission because of its power to create community, categories, and diagnoses. In the case of bladder cancer, seeing women through the context of a mother metaphor uses blood to create identity, and as a consequence, to ignore it as a symptom. Blood helps construct the metaphor, but the power of the metaphor diminishes the significance of blood as a symptom; worse, it is seen as positive evidence of women as reproductive beings. Seeing women's health through a metaphorical lens of motherhood invites both women and practitioners into misdiagnosis. This metaphor exerts powerful diagnostic influence on doctors, and this particular identification affects women themselves. Seeing blood in the toilet just doesn't set off alarm bells for women in the way it does for men, so women delay their own access to diagnosis. Clearly, practitioners and women understand the difference between menstrual blood and blood in the urine, but metaphors are powerful. We learn from an early age that blood is a sign of "becoming a woman" and consequently conflate maturity and gender identity with the ability to bear a child. Its regular presence in our lives is seen as healthy, underwritten even further by the powerful sway of social legitimacy motherhood bestows on women.

NONIDENTIFICATION, METONYMY, AND RHETORICAL LISTENING

In light of troubled identifications, Diana Fuss argues for the power of nonidentification, which compels us to turn our attention to differences and away from commonalities because of identification's power to replace and erase. In her words, "To be 'like' the other is to be different from the other, to be precisely *not* the same" (quoted in Ratcliffe 2005, 64). Where Burke (1950) finds hope in identification, bridging untenable divisions through consubstantiation, commonalities, patterns, and categories of overlap, Fuss finds erasure and alienation. Identification is always driven through with division: as it includes, it also excludes because we have taken our eyes away from the critical places where we don't have identification, diminishing and masking them. As an antidote, nonidentification turns attention to the margins, to the spaces where we don't share commonalities (cited in Ratcliffe 2005, 72–73).

Fuss's concept of nonidentification can be seen in some instances of medical and health research, which sees the importance of the margins and differences. For instance, in the case of diagnosing heart attack, it became evident that women's symptoms were different from men's and that rates of heart attack were increasing in women. Algorithms needed to account for these differences. While the disease itself is not gendered, education campaigns such as the public service announcement (PSA) found on WomensHealth.gov emphasize nonidentity, setting aside women's symptoms as unique and also making sure symptoms are not dismissed because they are linked to other diagnoses. Hot flashes are not only a symptom of menopause, and shortness of breath doesn't always indicate a woman is out of shape, the PSA reminds us. They can both be an indication of heart attack. However, Caitlin Leach, in this volume, observes how the Go Red for Women campaign, which brings attention to women's heart attack symptoms, performs its own kind of troubled identification by using normative classifications that erase people of color and transgender people (US Department of Health and Human Services 2017). She reminds us that women as a subgroup are not heterogenous.

Ratcliffe (2005) wants to avoid these problems by developing Fuss's concept of nonidentification—switching tropes, moving away from metaphor, and offering metonymy instead. In doing so, she enables differences and commonalities to be noticed: "The differences between these two figures are important. Metaphor foregrounds resemblances based on commonalities, thus backgrounding differences; metonym foregrounds resemblances based on juxtaposed associations, thus foregrounding both commonalities and differences" (68). Consider, for instance, the metaphor of an idea as a light bulb. As I imagine it, the idea lights up the way the bulb in my closet does when I pull the chain. There is darkness and then, suddenly, there is light. This is certainly a productive way of thinking about some kinds of ideas. This metaphor does, however, mask the kinds of ideas pieced together from fragments of others, like puzzle pieces, and over a long period of time; in those instances, there is not a single "lightbulb" moment.

Metonymy lends itself to a more complicated interpretation, and, Ratcliffe (2005) argues, invites us more openly into listening to differences. A classic example of metonymy is the phrase *the pen is mightier than the sword*. The pen stands in for the concept of words as the sword stands in for the concept of violent force. However, their close association to the concepts they represent invites juxtaposition and foregrounds both similarity and difference. The pen supplements the concept of words rather than replaces it, as the sword supplements force, and we must return to *words* and *force* themselves in order to understand how the pen and sword are functioning as tropes. This trope invites us into an active cognitive state. If we merge the conceptualizations of Groopman and Ratcliffe, we can by means of metonymy complicate diagnoses and encourage curiosity rather than shutting down the cognitive process by means of anchoring with metaphor.

I would like to return to my personal experience to illustrate how identification, nonidentification, and metonymy can work in a simple way. When my doctor directed my attention to an image of the urinary bladder on a chart of male anatomy, I think he was more distressed than I was. I was in the early stage of diagnosis and too overwhelmed to pay close attention. However, since he had called attention to the problem, months later I searched for a chart of the urinary bladder depicted in female anatomy as a gift for him. While searching I found charts that illustrated the urinary tract out of its gendered anatomical context—a bladder, ureters and kidneys in an empty cavity, absent the sexual organs. This chart creates identification, seeing the bladder as a commonality and masking differences. I also found a beautifully drawn chart of the bladder set in female anatomy, which I gave to him. The strategy of having two separate charts puts nonidentification to use. Looking at these charts in isolation—for instance, if he were to show men the male chart and women the female chart—emphasizes the uniqueness of the urinary system according to gender. I noticed some months later, however, that my doctor replaced the chart I originally saw of male anatomy with a chart using two images side by side, one male and one female. This strategy invites comparison and contrast, which is the beginning of metonymy.

Charts and illustrations matter for helping patients understand their disease. A genderless chart, for instance, obscures important differences between men's and women's experiences. The most common procedure bladder cancer patients encounter is the cystoscopy, in which a tube with a camera is inserted through the urethra to allow visualization of the bladder. While the general procedure is the same for both sexes, the male urethra is much longer than the female one, making cystoscopy a more difficult and more painful procedure for men. A nongendered image or a gender-specific chart of only one sex is insufficiently informative in other ways, particularly if an individual's treatment requires the removal of the bladder. Women lose more organs than men do during a radical cystectomy (bladder removal surgery).

Creating better charts does very little, however, to untangle the many strands of troubled identifications, disidentification, and nonidentification involved in diagnosis of bladder cancer in women. The critical concern is how to respond rhetorically to these rhetorical problems, how to disrupt the powerful metaphor of the mother that gives rise to problems. Following Ratcliffe (2005), I argue we need to empower doctors, patients, caregivers, and our larger communities to listen rhetorically. Ratcliffe's concept emphasizes neither division nor identification. Instead, it requires us to be attentive to both differences and shared spaces, seeing them side by side, illustrating the need for curiosity and dialogue. Rhetorical listening is a *techne* to map nonidentity, laying images and stories side by side, a sort of listening that should happen before identification, which results in persuasion, or in the case of health, in diagnosis. For Groopman (2007), it translates into doctors allowing patients time to tell their stories, uninterrupted, before the heuristics and algorithms are applied. It means stepping back from the lens provided in a patient's chart and looking for the ways a previous diagnosis doesn't explain current findings, of cataloguing what remains outside the prototype and keeping it in mind. It means surrendering the certainty identification and statistically based algorithms construct. Groopman writes, "When physicians shift from a theoretical discussion of medicine to its practical application, they do not acknowledge the uncertainty inherent in what they do," and he believes they should feel obligated to admit uncertainty (152). Groopman also urges patients to participate in this process by asking doctors questions that work against cognitive traps and that invite doctors to reflect on their ways of coming to conclusions (174).

Katz and Steinberg (2009) believe also that better training in medical schools will help, specifically with the diagnosis of bladder cancer. Medical students are not required to do a urology rotation, so primary care physicians may not be prepared to effectively diagnose urological issues (12). Further, the general public needs to be more aware of the disease. Both of these inadequacies conspire to eliminate the urgency for referral to urologists for blood in the urine. Steinberg also recommends a relatively simple change in the algorithm for general practitioners treating UTIs. After the course of antibiotics is given, patients should have follow-up blood tests. Presence of blood in that follow-up should immediately prompt a referral to a urologist. (G. Steinberg, pers. comm., April 14, 2015)

It is a matter of listening in the gaps and acknowledging that women's and men's diagnoses diverge in ways that harm women. It is a way of listening rhetorically for nonidentification. This brings me, in conclusion, back again to the personal and individual. I was diagnosed in January 2012 with a UTI. Some of the symptoms persisted, and in March I called to discuss this with my GP's nurse. Instead of making an appointment, my GP called in another round of antibiotics for me. At the same time, I was going through perimenopause, for me a time of unpredictable menstrual cycles. From day to day, I never knew what to expect, but I took comfort in the fact that this unpredictability was normal, based on what I'd read. Between March and August there may have been noticeable blood in my urine, but if so, I misidentified it as part of an irregular menstrual cycle. By the end of August, it occurred to me that the amount and circumstance of the blood was abnormal, and I went to my GP again. This time they took a urine sample, but never analyzed it or examined me, instead sending me directly to the ER.

My case is a sort of prototype in itself for how diagnosis goes astray, following the pattern reported in research very closely, though the delay did not result in a life-threatening prognosis. If, in March, my primary care doctor had examined me, and if I had discussed both the "UTI" symptoms and perimenopause with her, she may have noticed important differences between "UTI" symptoms and my symptoms. These conversations take time, more than the twenty seconds Groopman describes to plug symptoms into an algorithm. In order to create opportunities for such conversations, we need both patient education and education for

GPs. We need to create discourse that breaks away from the dominating metaphors of women as mothers or reproductive beings in order to listen to them rhetorically.

Finally, it is critical that I mention another aspect of the disparities in healthcare around bladder cancer. African American men are more likely than white men to die of bladder cancer. African American women are more likely than white women to die of bladder cancer. Further, both African American men and women opt less often for bladder removal, which is clearly linked to higher mortality rates. If I am to listen metonymically, as Ratcliffe (2005) recommends (78–100), I am compelled to investigate these disparities, to resist seeing all women with bladder cancer as a subgroup. Leach's piece in this volume reminds me that Black women and transgender people (a group not even mentioned in the bladder-cancer literature) are erased in these discussions. There is much work to do.

REFERENCES

Angeli, Elizabeth L. 2012. "Metaphors in the Rhetoric of Pandemic Flu: Electronic Media Coverage of H1N1 and Swine Flu." *Journal of Technical Writing and Communication* 42 (3): 203–222. http://dx.doi.org/10.2190/TW.42.3.b.

Burke, Kenneth. 1950. *A Rhetoric of Motives.* Upper Saddle River, NJ: Prentice-Hall.

Cohn, Joshua A., Benjamin Vekhter, Christopher Lyttle, Gary D. Steinberg, and Michael C. Large. 2014. "Sex Disparities in Diagnosis of Bladder Cancer after Initial Presentation with Hematuria." *Cancer* 120 (4): 555–561. http://dx.doi.org/10.1002/cncr.28416.

Groopman, James. 2007. *How Doctors Think.* New York: Houghton Mifflin.

Katz, Mark H., and Gary D. Steinberg. 2009. "Sex and Race in Bladder Cancer: What We Have Learned and Future Directions." *Cancer* 115 (1): 10–12. http://dx.doi.org/10.1002/cncr.23997.

Meloncon, Lisa, and Erin A. Frost. 2015. "Charting an Emerging Field: The Rhetorics of Health and Medicine and Its Importance in Communication Design." *Communication Design Quarterly* 3 (4): 7–14.

Mungan, N. Aydin, Katja K.H. Aben, Mark P. Schoenberg, Otto Visser, Jan-Willem W. Coebergh, J. Alfred Witjes, and Lambertus A.L.M. Kiemeney. 2000. "Gender Differences in Stage-Adjusted Bladder Cancer Survival." *Urology* 55 (6): 876–880. http://dx.doi.org/10.1016/S0090-4295(00)00523-9.

National Cancer Institute, Surveillance, Epidemiology, and End Results Program. 2016. Cancer Stat. Facts: Bladder Cancer. http://seer.cancer.gov/statfacts/html/urinb.html.

Ratcliffe, Krista. 2005. *Rhetorical Listening: Identification, Gender, Whiteness.* Carbondale: Southern Illinois University Press.

Scott, J. Blake, Judy Z. Segal, and Lisa Keranen. 2013. "The Rhetorics of Health and Medicine: Inventional Possibilities for Scholarship and Engaged Practice." *Poroi* 9 (1): 1–6. http://dx.doi.org/10.13008/2151-2957.1157.

Segal, Judy Z. 2005. *Health and the Rhetoric of Medicine.* Carbondale: Southern Illinois University Press.

US Department of Health and Human Services. 2017. *Make the Call. Don't Miss a Beat.* https://www.womenshealth.gov/heartattack/index.html.

SECTION IV

Digital Medical Rhetorics

9

BRAS, BROS, AND COLONS
How Even the Mayo Clinic Gets It Wrong Gendering Cancer

Miriam Mara

Feminist responses to inadequate healthcare for women in the 1970s articulated questions about access and led to the subsequent opening of women's health centers. Jennifer Nelson (2015) documents the history of early efforts to create equitable healthcare in her book *More Than Medicine*. Calls to conduct clinical trials with women as well as men and worries about dosing based on an average male body later followed (Liu and Dipietro Mager 2016, 708). Other work from Laura Purdy (2001) analyzes moves to medicalize and sometimes pathologize natural female processes like menstruation and childbirth. Recent scholarship by Karla Holloway (2011) and Tasha Dubriwny (2013) notes how medicalization and other biomedical tactics can lead to loss of autonomy for women in healthcare settings. In Mary Assad's chapter in this collection on the American Medical Association's Go Red campaign, she details how the effort to bring attention to heart disease in women both tries to associate gender with a health malady and reifies troubling assumptions about women's social identity within a health campaign. Her analysis fits with my understanding of how biases about women and their bodies creep into healthcare contexts. Despite this critical attention, problems with gender persist in healthcare, and biases about women's inherent weakness or (in)ability to handle pain affect encounters with medicine.

Cancer care, specifically, reflects such biases in the metaphors used to describe cancer, like cell *reproduction*, which links cancer with processes only female bodies carry out. Tammy Duerden Comeau (2007) traces nineteenth-century efforts to classify cancer, showing that scientists and clinicians used first tumor structures then growth patterns to define cancer, always defining it as female disease. She claims, "The portrayal of cancer as reproductive implied that it implicitly belonged in female bodies and reaffirmed cancer as primarily a 'woman's disease'" (175). Popular attention to breast cancer, in part brought by the Susan Komen

DOI: 10.7330/9781607329855.c009

pinkification campaigns, also contributes to current beliefs that women are more prone to cancer and notions that female reproductive organs automatically *turn on them* as they age.

To identify and question those biases about women's bodies and their probability of developing cancer, this chapter analyzes the rhetorical approach to cancer care on the Mayo Clinic website. The tab Patient Care & Health Info resides on the Mayo Clinic main page to the far left (Mayo, Home). To understand the Mayo Clinic website, first I examine alternate ways attention paid to breast cancer versus prostate cancer has been interpreted in contemporary feminist and men's-rights communities. I analyze the Mayo Clinic site—especially in terms of breast, prostate, and colon cancer—and show how new research about colon cancer's gendered age of incidence can help understanding. The Mayo Clinic website information reinforces false beliefs that women's bodies are more prone to cancer and in need of discipline—like screening—than men's bodies. That same underlying belief about the weakness of women's bodies can also translate into differing levels of autonomy granted to male patients versus female ones. Writing aimed at specific gendered groups reveals assumptions about each group's ability to choose appropriate care, undercutting autonomy for women.

Readers might note the possibility of tension between autonomy and standard of care. As Vivian M. Woodward (1998) explains, "Overemphasis [on autonomy] may confuse and suppress beneficent intervention" (1046). Patient refusal of treatments or procedures (noncompliance) becomes an easy way to identify how bioethical ideals like autonomy can come into conflict with providing the perceived best care or the bioethical principle of beneficence. Beneficence involves medical practitioners' duty to provide care that increases wellness or well-being, and sometimes clinicians desire to foster wellness or augment length of life for patients, even when such treatment and procedures are painful or harmful in other ways. Although the principle of autonomy maintains that patients can always refuse screenings or treatments against medical advice, healthcare professionals can struggle with accepting absolute patient autonomy.

Unfortunately, the willingness to recognize patient autonomy can be affected by demographic factors, including gender. As Holloway (2011) finds, all four bioethical tenets (autonomy, beneficence, nonmaleficence, and justice) are sometimes undercut by race and gender. In this collection, Caitlin Leach's chapter examining intersectionality in patienthood also maintains a focus on this conflict between patient decision-making and biomedical language of compliance, medical jargon for expectations that patients assent to all recommended procedures, take all recommended medicines in the prescribed manner, and alter their lifestyles in response to medical recommendations. She highlights the power structure and hierarchy between health professionals and patients and questions the perceived rightness of all health instructions and therapies. For my examination of Mayo's patient rhetoric, better understanding of the biases about groups can help professionals find balance among bioethical principles.

PINK IS EVERYWHERE: UNEQUAL ATTENTION TO BREAST CANCER VERSUS PROSTATE CANCER

To understand how gender affects medical contexts, reproductive cancers have become a popular site of analysis because sex, if not gender, connects directly to disease risk and outcomes for those diseases. Indeed, comparisons are made about attitudes toward—and spending on—breast cancer in relation to prostate cancer. The level of research funding for breast cancer far exceeds that of prostate cancer. Some feminist health rhetoricians attribute such differences in attention to prostate cancer and breast cancer to a willingness in biomedicine, as in the larger society, to surveil, screen, discipline, and constrain women's bodies. As Dubriwny (2013) explains, "Women are represented as part of an inherently at-risk group that must engage in a constant monitoring and management of risk" (13). Such monitoring includes cancer screening, as "some feminists have noted the increasing surveillance of women's bodies by biomedicine through prevention and early detection" (Pitts 2001, 22). This willingness to *protect* and thus surveil women's bodies creates dual effects, as women are expected to attend screening visits and men are able to avoid them and choose when to participate, maintaining autonomy over their bodies. When prevention gets equated with surveillance, women are expected to regularly get their unruly bodies observed, palpated, and regulated.

The gendering of cancer in service to regulation of women becomes clear in the campaign to fight breast cancer. As one of the largest cancer incidences among women, breast cancer is in fact a legitimate health concern. Yet the preponderance of cancer marketing in the world is for breast cancer. Cancer marketing includes consumer products connected through charitable organizations to breast cancer research, public health campaigns to encourage mammograms, and literature themed on breast cancer tragedies and victories. Laurie Gilmore Selleck (2010) explains that "breast cancer is the health threat about which women are most aware" (121–122). While some examples of male cancer narratives exist—Walter White's ungendered lung cancer diagnosis, for example—there is no subgenre of prostate cancer narratives. This cultural, as well as medical, attention to breast cancer seems to support feminist claims about regulation and discipline of women's bodies.

Despite swimming in cancer marketing and narratives skewed only to breast cancer, gender-specific, reproductive cancers create fear in men, not just women, and "males and females reported less perceived risk and less frequent worry for colon cancer than for gender-specific cancers" (McQueen et al. 2008, 69). Furthermore, opinions differ about the reasons for unbalanced attention to breast cancer. Feminists read all the attention to breast cancer as attempts to regulate female bodies, but men's-health advocates such as the Prostate Cancer Foundation notice differences in medical and cultural attention to breast cancer versus attention to prostate cancer and attribute them to discrimination against men (Brower 2005, 1014). Their argument suggests society does not mind if men die from prostate cancer. On the National Coalition for Men website, Ray Blumhorst (2011) claims, "The disparity in annual, government research funding between the two cancers is striking and discriminatory, illustrating yet again the institutionalized misandry existing in Western societies." Such contentions have led to increased public attention to both prostate cancer and testicular cancer with popular movements like Movember, when men grow mustaches during the month of November to raise money for research. Yet the differences in funding persist, and men's-rights groups believe those differences are the result of anti-male sentiment. These alternate readings of the differences in attention paid to breast cancer versus prostate cancer—as either attempts to discipline women or apathy about men's heath—present a very real variance in explanatory frames and provide an area of inquiry for health rhetoricians. Incorporating nonreproductive colorectal cancers into an analysis of rhetorics of cancer on the Mayo Clinic website provides a useful way to nuance the rhetorical choices about breast and prostate cancer and better understand gendered differences in cancer recommendations and screening.

INCIDENCE AND MORTALITY

In order to evaluate the rhetoric about breast, colorectal, and prostate cancer, it is helpful to see incidence and mortality rates. The Centers

Table 9.1. Incidence and mortality rates from CDC

Cancer Site	Breast cancer	Prostate cancer	Colon cancer	Total of all three sites
Incidence women	230,815		65,020	295,835
Incidence men	2,109	176,450	71,099	249,658
Total incidence	232,924	176,450	136,119	409,374
Mortality women	40,860		24,583	65,443
Mortality men	464	27,681	27,230	55,375
Total mortality	41,324	27,681	51,813	120,818

for Disease Control and Prevention (CDC) provides these statistics, and recent complete numbers from 2013 are found in table 9.1. While breast cancer incidence is highest at 230,815 female and 2,109 male new diagnoses, colorectal cancer has the highest mortality, with 51,813 deaths, including 27,230 men and 24,583 women (Centers, "Breast," n.d., "Colorectal," n.d.). Breast cancer mortality totals 40,860 women and 464 men, killing more women than colorectal cancer does (Centers, "Breast," n.d.). Prostate cancer has the lowest total mortality rate but kills more men than colorectal cancer does, with 27,681 deaths in 2013 (Centers, "Prostate," n.d.).

METHODS

With these numbers in mind, and by collecting screenshots of the patient-information pages on the Mayo Clinic website for breast, prostate, and colorectal cancer and comparing the language and appearance of those pages, I evaluate how the rhetorical treatment of the three types of cancer constructs notions of agency and autonomy. I pay attention to the language use, sentence structure, and emphasis created by visual cues, looking for fear appeals and passive sentence construction as tactics. For each cancer, the Mayo Clinic patient pages include several tabs, like Symptoms and Causes (which includes a list of risk factors) and Diagnosis and Treatment, which have multiple subheadings, like "Overview," "Definition," "Diagnosis," and "Treatment." I compare rhetorical choices in the pages for breast, prostate, and colon cancers to show subtle and obvious differences in similarly organized information. Finally, for risk factors, I create four categories or codes including *behavioral, genetic, demographic,* and *other.* The *other* category mostly includes comorbid conditions that indicate risk, as well as anything else that did not fit in the remaining three categories.

DISCIPLINING UNRULY BODIES: MAYO
TESTS AND PROCEDURES PAGES

The Mayo Clinic website provides useful health and medical information, and the patient pages remain a reliable source for lay people. Like all medical writing, the site reflects the culture from which it springs, including attitudes about gender. Earlier in this collection, in her chapter on gendered inequalities in medical attention to sexual pleasure, Colleen A. Reilly also interrogates "inadequacies" of the Mayo Clinic website, especially in their choice to treat female pleasure only in the context of illness (FDS). She highlights how the Mayo site reinforces outdated and harmful ideas about women's bodies by downplaying "insufficient stimulation" as a reason for lack of orgasm. This additional analysis of the Mayo-site information dovetails well with my critique of its rhetorical choices about cancer.

In keeping with those harmful ideas about female bodies, the Mayo site uses more dramatic language about breast cancer than about colon or prostate cancer. "Tests and procedures," for example, introduces mammograms, explaining their "key role in early breast cancer detection and help[ing] decrease breast cancer *deaths*," a description loaded with fear (Mayo, "Mammogram," n.d., para. 1; emphasis added). While writers later admit that "how often you should have a mammogram depends on your age and your risk" (para. 3), they do not mention any possible harms from mammogram, harms from radiation, pain, or mental harms of fear and false positives. Nor do they acknowledge any possibility that one might never have a mammogram. Thus, they create fear about breast cancer and elide possible negative effects of screening and treatment.

Conversely, the available screenings for prostate cancer foreground questions of overdiagnosis and iatrogenic (ill effects caused by examination or treatments) possibilities. The page about the prostate-specific antigen (PSA) test specifically names overdiagnosis as a "limitation" of PSA (Mayo, "PSA Test," n.d.). It begins by claiming, "Whether to test healthy men with no symptoms for prostate cancer is controversial" (Mayo, "Prostate," Diagnosis, n.d., para. 1). Important, it leads with a question word "whether," ends with the term "controversial," and describes men as *healthy*, neglecting to create fear of prostate cancer and foregrounding possible problems with screening. The colon cancer screening page still applies fear tactics, claiming that "choosing a colon cancer screening test may not be an easy decision, but it's a potentially lifesaving one" (Mayo, "Colon Cancer Screening," n.d., para. 26). Yet the language in this section about colorectal cancer screening remains less strident and more open to bodily autonomy than the mammography section, yet less willing to grant bodily autonomy than the prostate cancer screening section.

FOSTERING OR DOWNPLAYING FEAR: MAYO "DEFINITIONS" SECTIONS

While the Tests and Procedures pages reflect gender differences in screening recommendations, the Diseases and Conditions pages for breast, prostate, and colon cancer follow similar rhetorical patterns, especially in their handling of emotion and the degree to which they respect patient autonomy. Here, each cancer has a "Definition" or "Overview" section that explains basics of the cancer. The prostate definition includes that prostate cancer is "one of the most common" but quickly reassures men by explaining "prostate cancer usually grows slowly." By foregrounding slow growth and suggesting prostate cancer "may need minimal or no treatment," the Mayo writers provide men with comfort and highlight the ability for men to eschew medical treatment, preserving their bodily autonomy (Mayo, "Prostate," Diagnosis, n.d., para. 2).

The breast cancer "Overview" section offers no such option. Writers communicate fear in the second sentence, reminding readers "breast cancer is the most common cancer diagnosed in women." There is no mention of overdiagnosis or the possibility for slow growth in some breast tumors. Indeed, the writers focus on "improve[ment in] the screening and diagnosis," attributing "the number of deaths steadily . . . declining" to "earlier detection." Of the three introductory pages for breast cancer, colon cancer, and prostate cancer, the breast cancer "Overview" is the section to use the term "death," in addition to the term "survival rates," using very clear fear appeals (Mayo, "Breast," Symptoms, n.d., para. 2). In this way, the breast cancer definition hides real issues with overdiagnosis and highlights fear, which encourages women to submit to screening.

The "Overview" section for colon cancer foregrounds the origins of most colorectal cancers as "small, noncancerous (benign) clumps of cells called adenomatous polyps" (Mayo, "Colon Cancer," Symptoms, n.d., para. 2). The page also reminds readers that polyps "produce few, if any, symptoms," leading to a recommendation for "regular screening tests" (Mayo, "Colon Cancer," n.d., para. 3). This introductory section, like the one on the breast cancer page, uses mild fear language—about lack of symptoms—to encourage "regular screening" and suggests treatment of "removing polyps before they can become colon cancer" (Mayo, "Colon Cancer," Symptoms, n.d., para. 3). This section, like the prostate cancer "Definition" section, eschews the terms *death* and *survival*. The colon and breast cancer pages use "screening" overtly, while the prostate definition section does not include the word, referring vaguely to "a better chance of successful treatment" when "detected early" (Mayo, "Prostate," n.d., para. 3). As in the screening pages for the three types of cancer, the introductory pages create more fear and expectation of screening for breast cancer, middling fear and some expectation of screening for colon cancer, which affects people of both genders, and little fear and no mention of screening for prostate cancer, which affects only men. Women's bodies are more rigidly disciplined in these rhetorical arrangements.

This pattern suggests gender might have some effect on the language about cancers, and that female cancers evoke the strongest language of surveillance and discipline. If one were comparing the breast cancer and prostate cancer language, the stronger fear rhetoric on the breast cancer page might be explained by mortality statistics. However, adding the colon cancer pages, which do not advocate screening or use fear at the same level as the breast cancer pages, despite higher incidence and mortality, provides a way to understand the language choices as responding to gender rather than merely responding to medical realities.

EMOTIONS HELP MEN MAKE DECISIONS: MAYO SYMPTOMS SECTIONS

The "Symptoms" sections for each cancer are similar, but they differ in suggested responses to symptoms, and the differences are gendered. Each contains a paragraph titled "When to see a doctor" where those differences appear. The breast cancer section for symptoms suggests, "If you find a lump or other change in your breast—even if a recent mammogram was normal—make an appointment with your doctor for prompt evaluation," providing little ground for autonomous decision-making (Mayo, "Breast," Symptoms, n.d.,). Any change in the breast must result in an appointment with a medical doctor. The prostate cancer symptom section conversely provides men with complete autonomy, suggesting, "Make an appointment with your doctor if you have any signs or symptoms *that worry you*" (Mayo, "Prostate," Symptoms, n.d. para. 3).

Allowing men to decide which symptoms worry them and when they will consult with medical professionals reinforces gendered assumptions that men make decisions about their bodies, whereas women are instructed very particularly. Interestingly, men's emotions, such as worry, are validated and even given authority to be used as arbiter of treatment decisions. The colon cancer symptoms section moves back toward lack of autonomy, directing, "If you notice any symptoms of colon cancer, such as blood in your stool or a persistent change in bowel habits, make an appointment with your doctor" (Mayo, "Colon Cancer," Symptoms, para. 3). The directive still includes more options for avoiding a doctor visit by limiting the need to contact an MD to when there are actual symptoms rather than vague language of "change in your breast." As on the other pages on the Mayo clinic site, the "Symptoms" sections provide the most autonomy to men on the prostate cancer page, a medium amount of autonomy in the gender-neutral colon cancer page, and the least amount of autonomy on the breast cancer page.

WHO DECIDES? MAYO TREATMENT SECTIONS

The treatment sections in the Mayo clinic patient portal for all three cancers foreground how gender affects the expectation of retaining control over decisions about one's own body. They each begin with a paragraph about differing treatment and the ways staging affects treatment options, although breast cancer introductory material is more detailed. The first sentence of the breast cancer "Treatment" section foregrounds the paternalistic attitude of biomedicine toward women, claiming, "Your doctor determines your breast cancer treatment." This sentence places the doctor as subject of the sentence and the actor, using a very strong verb, "determines." The next sentence reads, "Your doctor also considers your overall health and your own preferences" (Mayo, "Breast," Diagnosis, n.d. para. 1). As in the first sentence, the doctor retains all decision-making and merely "considers" what the patient might want as part of larger considerations.

Both the prostate cancer and colon cancer "Treatment" sections' first sentences use passive voice and make the treatment or options the subject of the sentence, meaning the actor is not necessarily named. For example, in the colon cancer "Treatment" section, the first sentence reads "The type of treatment your doctor recommends will depend largely on the stage of your cancer." This future tense verb "will depend" allows action from outside the sentence, perhaps from the patient, and places the doctor into the sentence as part of a modifying prepositional phrase with a weaker verb of "recommend." The word *doctor* does not appear in the first sentence of the prostate cancer "Treatment" section. It begins, "Your prostate cancer treatment options depend on several factors"; putting "your prostate" first provides a clearer message that the actor could be the patient, and using "options" as the subject of the sentence seems to place decision-making in "your," or the patient's, control (Mayo, "Prostate," Diagnosis, n.d., para.1). Like the colon cancer page, the main verb is "depend," much softer than the "determines" verb on the breast cancer page. The opening paragraphs place doctors in complete control of breast cancer treatment decisions, and mostly in control of colon cancer decisions, but places male patients more in control of prostate cancer decisions.

After the introductory paragraphs in the "Treatment" sections, the writers provide descriptions of the types of treatment and why/how they are done. The breast cancer page begins with surgery options in a bulleted list, first describing "Removing the breast cancer (lumpectomy)," which is the least invasive surgery. The last sentence of the lumpectomy bullet suggests the procedure "is typically reserved for smaller tumors," providing a hopeful beginning (Mayo, "Breast," Diagnosis, n.d., para. 4). Each of the treatment sections provides the least intrusive or least frightening option first. In the prostate cancer "Treatment" section, the least intrusive option listed is surveillance, a wonderful treatment option of doing nothing other than monitoring the tumor with follow-up tests. This option, with a subhead "Immediate treatment may not be necessary," helps male readers with a new diagnosis to remain in control of their bodies in culturally sanctioned ways (Mayo, "Prostate," Diagnosis, n.d. para. 2). Even though some research suggests certain breast cancers also grow slowly or regress (Zahl, Maehlen, and Welch 2008), there is no active surveillance option for breast cancer, not even for ductal carcinoma in situ (DCIS). The colon cancer "Treatment" section follows the short paragraph with a bulleted list of procedures under the subhead "Surgery for early-stage colon cancer." The pronouncement about surgery up front gets softened by language like "minimally invasive approach," and the list of options includes one that can be performed during a routine colonoscopy (Mayo, "Colon Cancer," Diagnosis, n.d. para.1).

Once the less intrusive options are covered, the writers explain more aggressive treatment options for each of the three cancers. The prostate cancer writers create a separate statement about surgery side effects, warning that "radical prostatectomy carries a risk of urinary incontinence and erectile dysfunction" (Mayo, "Prostate," Diagnosis, n.d. para. 14). This kind of cautioning serves to create fear in men of such "radical" options, rather than fear of disease. Conversely, the breast cancer surgery side-effects list is much less frightening and less comprehensive. The writers explain that "breast cancer surgery carries a risk of pain, bleeding, infection and arm swelling," but they leave out common longer-term side effects of mastectomy, lumpectomy, and even biopsy surgeries, such as infection and loss of motion in arms and shoulders (Mayo, "Breast," Diagnosis, n.d. para. 5). Such omission suggests the creators of the page do not want women to even consider the option of avoiding surgery, again limiting information and thus autonomy. The colon cancer "Treatment" sections do not have specific warnings about surgery side effects.

The "Treatment" sections, and especially the language of the introductory paragraphs, show how gender can affect the rhetoric of treatment choices, in this case to foreground choice for prostate cancer patients, who are men, to provide some autonomy for colon cancer patients, who are men and women, and to discipline breast cancer patients, who are primarily women. The rhetoric of the "Treatment" sections matches the messages from the larger pages for each cancer, which is to assume breast cancer is nearly inevitable for women and that they must aggressively treat it according to instructions from healthcare professionals with little information about the iatrogenic possibilities of such treatment. In opposition, the assumption is that prostate cancer affects men very little, that it can be treated without penetration of male bodies, and that men remain autonomous even when they develop illness. The colon cancer site finds middle ground between these versions of gendered reality, falling more toward encouraging treatment.

POSTDIAGNOSIS AUTONOMY CHECKS: MAYO COPING AND SUPPORT SECTIONS

The sections of the Mayo pages that include information about postdiagnosis psychological health for breast, prostate, and colon cancer patients subtly reinforce ideas about women's inability to manage emotions while simultaneously undermining women's bodily autonomy. The breast cancer "Coping and support" section begins with a simple sentence: "A breast cancer diagnosis can be overwhelming" (Mayo, "Breast," Diagnosis, n.d.). There is no human in the subject of the sentence, and the diagnosis is the actor, which overwhelms the disappearing human. The colon cancer section begins similarly, stating, "A cancer diagnosis can be emotionally challenging" (Mayo, "Colon Cancer," Diagnosis, n.d.). In this case, the nonpresent human is merely challenged rather than overwhelmed. The prostate cancer section states, "When you receive a diagnosis of prostate cancer, you may experience a range of feelings—including disbelief, fear, anger, anxiety, and depression" (Mayo, "Prostate," Diagnosis, n.d.). This sentence includes a human actor, "you," in both clauses, giving agency to men. Additionally, men with prostate cancer experience emotion, but they are not challenged and certainly not overwhelmed. The inconsistent diction and sentence structure for differently gendered cancers reflect attitudes about men's and women's ability to make medical decisions under emotional strain.

The first advice in the list for coping for each of the three cancers is learning about the disease. The prostate "Coping and support" section advocates "learn[ing] enough about prostate cancer to feel comfortable making treatment decisions" (Mayo, "Prostate," Diagnosis, n.d.). The colon cancer page uses exactly the same language following a bolded bullet that reads "Know what to expect" (Mayo, "Colon Cancer," Diagnosis, n.d.). The breast cancer version states, "Learn enough about your breast cancer to make decisions about your care," using softer words but also evading the idea that *treatment* decisions would be up to the patient (Mayo, "Breast," Diagnosis, n.d.).

In the breast cancer bullet about learning in the "Coping and support" section, the only source listed is "your doctor," (Mayo, "Breast," Diagnosis, n.d.), while on the prostate cancer page, "Your doctor, nurse, or health care professional" can "recommend reliable sources of information." For the colon cancer page, "Ask your doctor" is followed by a sentence suggesting you "look for information in your local library and on reliable websites" (Mayo, "Colon Cancer," Diagnosis, n.d.). One type of advice, found only on the breast cancer site, is shockingly paternalistic, and it oddly works against pinkification efforts to *educate*. The final two sentences in the "learn enough" bullet on the breast cancer page read, "Still, some *women* may not want to know the details of their cancer. If this is how you feel, let your doctor know this too [emphasis added]" (Mayo, "Breast," Diagnosis, n.d.). Neither the colon cancer pages nor the prostate cancer pages include this advice about not wanting to know, suggesting the advice is not necessary for patients with other cancers and rather is pointedly aimed at women, whom the writers consider too feeble to handle difficult medical information. The creators of the page may wish to intimidate women away from learning about breast cancer, asking difficult questions, and/or making decisions with which medical practitioners may not agree. Rather than acknowledging emotions as helpful in treatment decision-making—like the prostate cancer example of using men's "worry" as the arbiter of care—women's emotions are used to remove them from treatment information and decisions. Singling out breast cancer and naming women specifically (since

2 percent of breast cancer incidence is in men) reinforces the Mayo site's willingness to make gendered assumptions about women's ability to handle emotion and to bypass autonomy for women.

SINS OF OMISSION: MAYO RISK FACTORS SECTIONS

Some of the most salient rhetorical choices reflecting gendered assumptions occur in the "Risk factors" sections. Each section includes information about the characteristics that statistically increase risk for the three types of cancer. These risk sections for colorectal and breast cancer are extensive, with thirteen risk factors listed for each. Each of them has risks in all four categories: behavioral, genetic, demographic, and other (Mayo, "Colon Cancer," Symptoms., n.d.). Prostate cancer, by comparison, has only four risk factors listed, and they are contained to demographics and genetics, with no behavioral risk factors to limit men's conduct (Mayo, "Prostate," Symptoms, n.d., para. 1). The higher incidence and mortality for colorectal cancer in males might make sex a demographic risk factor, but the site makes no mention of it. In other words, research showing incidence of colon cancer at a later age in women provides a way to talk about risk in more complicated ways the Mayo site fails to engage in.

In the section titled "Risk factors" for colorectal cancer, the Mayo clinic lists thirteen possible risk enhancers. They include behavioral, demographic, and genetic/personal factors. The "Risk factors" section includes a bulleted list with a word or phrase of bolded language followed by an extended description. Two of the risk factors involve other diagnoses comorbid with colorectal cancer, inflammatory intestinal conditions like Crohn's disease and genetic illness like familial adenomatous polyposis, which are logical inclusions. Only one of the risks in the colon cancer list is behavioral: a low-fiber, high-fat diet. Interestingly, writers elucidate risk from "diets high in red meat and processed meats," which is more specific than low fiber, high fat (Mayo, "Colon Cancer," Symptoms, n.d.). This shift from a larger category of fiber to the details about type of meat shows the rhetorical possibilities for specificity in recommendations.

Colon cancer risks differ by sex with higher incidence and mortality rates in men and an average higher age of incidence in women, yet Mayo does not differentiate risk or screening recommendation by sex or sex/ age ratio. Research suggests that "age-specific CRC [colorectal cancers] incidence and mortality are lower in women than in men, which implies that women reach comparable levels of CRC incidence and mortality at higher ages than men" (Brenner et al. 2007, 828). H. Brenner et al. (2007) clarify the age differences:

> Our analyses of age- and sex-specific incidence and mortality of CRC in the US and 10 other large countries from different parts of the world indicate that the lower incidence and mortality among women quite consistently translates to an age difference of approximately 4–8 years at which comparable levels of risk are reached. Colorectal cancer incidence and mortality at various ages are closely related to potential benefits of screening, which have to be weighed against costs and potential adverse side effects in choosing the age of screening initiation. Our analysis suggests that the balance in favour of screening is likely to be reached several years later among women than among men. (829–830)

Their findings are reinforced by Tzu-An Chen et al. (2012), who explain that "the age-standardized incidence rates of CRC are lower among women than men" (345). Jarslaw Regula, Anna Chaber, and Michael Kaminski (2012) mention the Brenner study, a study from Austria (Ferlitsch et al. 2011), and their own study, which all confirm a gender age difference of five to ten years in prevalence of advanced neoplasia and add that a "meta-analysis of 17 screening colonoscopy studies confirms findings from studies described above. The risk was significantly higher for men for advanced neoplasia (OR, 1.83) and colorectal cancer (OR, 2.02) across all age groups" (33). The odds ratio (OR) is a ratio of the odds an event, or illness in this case, will occur in one group to the odds it will occur in another group. It implies a comparison rather than simple risk analysis. A number above one suggests the event is more likely in the first group, in this case men. These studies and analyses agree that female risk remains lower than male risk in the same age group. Thus, women might not need screening for colorectal cancers as early as men do.

Other reasons for changing screening recommendations include the differences in the ways women experience colon cancer and colonoscopy. Some evidence suggests women's colorectal cancers more often present on the right of the colon and may be more difficult to treat. Yet these findings do not undercut the age difference and the overall higher incidence and mortality in men. All the evidence suggests that the later age at which women present might indicate a later age at which screening might begin. Regula, Chaber, and Kaminski (2012) also note that women are more likely to experience discomfort and complications from colonoscopy. Changing screening recommendations to reflect a later starting age for women would spare them uncomfortable screenings until they become necessary based on actual risk and would match public health recommendations to statistics. The hesitation to make changes in the screening recommendations implies reticence to surveil and discipline male bodies at an earlier age than female bodies, even when the science reflects need for such earlier screening.

In Mayo's risk list for colorectal cancers, neither sex nor a sex-to-age ratio factor is included. One explanation for excluding sex or a sex-to-age ratio as part of the risk factors could be discomfort with using demographic descriptors as risk factors, but the page creators include other demographic descriptors. Two risk factors on the list are demographic—older age and African American race—which shows the Mayo Clinic willingly includes demographic factors in risk assessment when it deems them appropriate (Mayo, "Colon Cancer," Symptoms, n.d. para. 13). While it might be uncomfortable to include racial markers as risk factors, the Mayo weighs the discomfort with the expedience of getting this information to people who might benefit from it. The other category of age also could be a health truth readers find difficult to acknowledge. The verbiage provides a number, suggesting that "older than 50" is the age when colon cancer occurs (Mayo, "Colon Cancer," Symptoms, n.d. para. 13). Yet gender, which is increasingly understood to alter the risk for colorectal cancer, is not included. In other words, there is no easy explanation for omitting male sex as a risk factor for colon cancer.

Still, the Mayo clinic suggests that "guidelines generally recommend that colon cancer screenings begin at age 50," with no suggestion that this recommendation could vary by sex (Mayo, "Colon Cancer," Symptoms, n.d. para. 13). The Mayo site also does not include gender or sex as a risk factor for colorectal cancers despite recognizing race as a factor. Shifting the screening age for women to fifty-five years and adding being male as a risk factor would reduce constraint on women's bodies by allowing them to avoid uncomfortable tests until an older age while simultaneously maintaining vigilant attempts to detect colorectal cancers in men. Unwillingness to make these slight shifts in screening recommendations and risk factors reinforces feminist arguments about biomedicine's enthusiasm for control over female bodies and undercuts suggestions that men are being unfairly targeted to assume health risks when more attention goes to fighting female reproductive cancers.

CONCLUSION

The Mayo Clinic pages for breast, prostate, and colon cancer provide evidence of gender bias about who is likely to contract cancer, as well as who has the ability or right to manage emotions and decisions. They evince such bias when granting or denying agency and autonomy in recommendations for screenings and treatment. The analysis reflects both a willingness to discipline and screen women's bodies even when evidence-based science does not support the screening recommendations and insistence upon autonomy for men. The inclusion of colon cancer with the gendered breast and prostate cancers helps show that feminist health critics better understand the emphasis on breast cancer in popular culture and advertising as a way to create fear and control women's bodies rather than as a willingness to put men at risk of death. The colon cancer screening recommendations give an appropriate age range to begin colonoscopy for men. However, they recommend screening women at an earlier age range than incidence and mortality support, showing lack of respect for women's bodily autonomy. Pretending men and women are equally at risk beginning at fifty years old allows men to get appropriately screened but pushes women into uncomfortable—for them—tests before they are clinically indicated. This willingness to screen women earlier than incidence rates project matches the rhetorical choices in the breast cancer information, which subtly undercut women's autonomy. Thus, the Mayo Clinic website reflects ideas about weakness in women's bodies and a complementary willingness to discipline those bodies and their attendant emotions through screening and treatment.

REFERENCES

Blumhorst, Ray. 2011. "Prostate Cancer Strikes One in Six Men but Gets Very Little Funding for Research." National Coalition for Men. https://ncfm.org/2011/08/news/mens-health/prostate-cancer-strikes-one-in-six-men-but-gets-very-little-funding-for-research/.

Brenner, H., Michael Hoffmeister, Volker Arndt, and Ulrike Haug. 2007. "Gender Differences in Colorectal Cancer: Implications for Age at Initiation of Screening." *British Journal of Cancer* 96 (5): 828–831.

Brower, Vicki. 2005. "The Squeaky Wheel Gets the Grease: Research Funding Is Not Necessarily Allocated to Those Who Need It Most." *EMBO Reports* 6 (11): 1014–1017.

Centers for Disease Control. n.d. "Breast Cancer." Last reviewed May 28, 2019. https://www.cdc.gov/cancer/breast/statistics/index.htm.

Centers for Disease Control. n.d. "Colorectal (Colon) Cancer Statistics." Last reviewed May 28, 2019. https://www.cdc.gov/cancer/colorectal/statistics/index.htm.

Centers for Disease Control. n.d. "Prostate Cancer." Last reviewed May 28, 2019. https://www.cdc.gov/cancer/prostate/statistics/index.htm.

Chen, Tzu-An, Hsiao-Yen Kang, Huan-Cheng Chang, Wen-Chu Lin, Tsung-Ming Chao, and Jorng-Tzong Horng. 2012. "Gender Differences in Colorectal Cancer during the Past 20 Years in Taiwan." *International Journal of Colorectal Disease* 27 (3): 345–353.

Comeau, Tammy Duerden. 2007. "Gender Ideology and Disease Theory: Classifying Cancer in Nineteenth Century Britain." *Journal of Historical Sociology* 20 (1–2): 158–181.

Dubriwny, Tasha N. 2013. *The Vulnerable Empowered Woman: Feminism, Postfeminism, and Women's Health.* New Brunswick, NJ: Rutgers University Press.

Ferlitsch, Monica, Karoline Reinhart, Sibylle Pramhas, Caspar Wiener, Orsolya Gal, Christina Bannert, Michaela Hassler, Karin Kozbial, Daniela Dunkler, Michael Trauner, and Werner Weiss. 2011. "Sex-Specific Prevalence of Adenomas, Advanced Adenomas, and Colorectal Cancer in Individuals Undergoing Screening Colonoscopy." *JAMA* 306 (12): 1352–1358.

Holloway, Karla F. C. 2011. *Private Bodies, Public Texts: Race, Gender, and a Cultural Bioethics.* Durham, NC: Duke University Press.

Liu, Katherine A., and Natalie A. Dipietro Mager. 2016. "Women's Involvement in Clinical Trials: Historical Perspective and Future Implications." *Pharmacy Practice* 14 (1): 708–717.

Mayo Clinic. n.d. Home. http://www.mayoclinic.org/.

Mayo Clinic Staff. n.d. "Breast Cancer." Diagnosis and treatment. http://www.mayoclinic.org/diseases-conditions/breast cancer/diagnosis-treatment/treatment/txc-20207949.

Mayo Clinic Staff. n.d. "Breast Cancer." Symptoms and causes. http://www.mayoclinic.org/diseases-conditions/breast cancer/home/ovc-20207913.

Mayo Clinic Staff. n.d. "Colon Cancer." Diagnosis and treatment. http://www.mayoclinic.org/diseases-conditions/colon-cancer/diagnosis-treatment/treatment/txc-20188274.

Mayo Clinic Staff. n.d. "Colon Cancer Screening: Weighing the Options." http://www.mayoclinic.org/diseases-conditions/colon-cancer/in-depth/colon-cancer-screening/art-20046825.

Mayo Clinic Staff. n.d. "Colon Cancer." Symptoms and Causes. http://www.mayoclinic.org/diseases-conditions/colon-cancer/home/ovc-20188216.

Mayo Clinic Staff. n.d. "Mammogram." http://www.mayoclinic.org/tests-procedures/mammogram/home/ovc-20230954.

Mayo Clinic Staff. n.d. "Prostate Cancer." Diagnosis and treatment. http://www.mayoclinic.org/diseases-conditions/prostate-cancer/basics/tests-diagnosis/con-20029597.

Mayo Clinic Staff. n.d. "Prostate Cancer." Symptoms and Causes. http://www.mayoclinic.org/diseases-conditions/prostate-cancer/basics/complications/con-20029597.

Mayo Clinic Staff. n.d. "PSA Test." http://www.mayoclinic.org/tests-procedures/psa-test/details/risks/cmc-20200313.

McQueen, Amy, Sally W. Vernon, Helen L. Meissner, and William Rakowski. 2008. "Risk Perceptions and Worry about Cancer: Does Gender Make a Difference?" *Journal of Health Communication* 13 (1): 56–79.

Nelson, Jennifer. 2015. *More Than Medicine: A History of the Feminist Women's Health Movement.* New York: NYU Press.

Pitts, Victoria. 2001. "Popular Pedagogies, Illness, and the Gendered Body: Reading Breast Cancer Discourse in Cyberspace." *Popular Culture Review* 12 (2): 21–36.

Purdy, Laura. 2001. "Medicalization, Medical Necessity, and Feminist Medicine." *Bioethics* 15 (3): 248–261.

Regula, Jaroslaw, Anna Chaber, and Michael F. Kaminski. 2012. "Should There Be Gender Differences in the Guidelines for Colorectal Cancer Screening?" *Current Colorectal Cancer Reports* 8 (1): 32–35.

Selleck, Laurie G. 2010. "Pretty in Pink: The Susan G. Komen Network and the Branding of the Breast Cancer Cause." *Nordic Journal of English Studies* 9 (3): 119–138.

Woodward, Vivian M. "Caring, Patient Autonomy and the Stigma of Paternalism." *Journal of Advanced Nursing* 28 (5): 1046–1052.

Zahl, Per-Henrik, Jan Maehlen, and Gilbert Welch. 2008. "The Natural History of Invasive Breast Cancers by Screening Mammography." *Archives of Internal Medicine* 168 (21): 2311–2316.

10

INTERROGATING RACE-BASED HEALTH DISPARITIES IN THE ONLINE COMMUNITY BLACK WOMEN DO BREASTFEED

Lori Beth De Hertogh

INTRODUCTION

Although rhetoricians of health and medicine are paying increased attention to intersections between health texts and online communities (Hinson 2016; Koteyko, Hunt, and Gunter 2015; Owens 2009, 2015; Persky, Sanderson, and Koehly 2013; Segal 2008, 2009; Willerton 2008), we have had few conversations in our published forums about how racial minorities use social media to interrogate health disparities, particularly regarding breastfeeding. How, for example, do African American women challenge and rewrite race-based health disparities that position them as inadequate when it comes to breastfeeding? In what ways do African American women use social media to create and circulate *their own* breastfeeding texts? And how might these texts create space for Black women to both resist and augment dominant medical narratives (such as those produced by the Centers for Disease Control and Prevention [CDC]) about breastfeeding?

This chapter draws on these questions and others to explore how the online breastfeeding community, Black Women Do Breastfeed, employs rhetorical strategies to respond to medical, discursive, and historical frameworks that position African American women as deficient at breastfeeding their children. In doing so, I argue that Black Women Do Breastfeed uses social media platforms to create activist health texts that challenge and rewrite race-based health disparities rooted in sociocultural and medical epistemologies that pathologize breastfeeding among Black women. As other chapters in this collection aptly illustrate, such pathologizing is often gendered and reflects biomedical and cultural assumptions about intersections among health, gender, and race.

DOI: 10.7330/9781607329855.c010

This chapter begins with an introduction to the Black Women Do Breastfeed community and the methods and methodologies that guided my research. I next offer an overview of the impact race-based health disparities have on breastfeeding practices among African American women, and in doing so, emphasize the ways health disparities are embedded in cultural and rhetorical practices that pathologize breast-feeding. I then briefly trace historical trends that have shaped African American women's breastfeeding experiences in order to provide socio-historical context for my analysis of how Black Women Do Breastfeed uses social media to interrogate race-based health disparities by producing what I call *counteractivist* and *parallel activist health texts*. I conclude by arguing that while social media and activist health texts can empower minority communities like Black Women Do Breastfeed, these platforms and strategies reflect medical, gendered, and racial biases that privilege some groups over others.

BACKGROUND, METHODS, AND METHODOLOGY

Black Women Do Breastfeed (BWDBF) is an online community (consisting of a blog, Facebook page, and Twitter feed) founded in 2010 by Nicole Sandiford, a Black woman who immigrated to the United States from Barbados. On the BWDBF blog homepage, Sandiford argues that "our breastfeeding stories and images are not easy to find online. In fact, it would seem as if the story of modern Black American women breastfeeding is limited. This blog seeks to highlight the many Black mothers in the United States (and beyond) who do indeed breastfeed their children. Despite the statistics that show a despairing picture of breastfeeding among Black mothers in the United States, there are many of us who have breastfed, are breastfeeding, and will breastfeed our children" (n.d.). From March 2015 to July 2016, I collected digital artifacts (e.g., blog posts, videos, tweets) primarily from the Black Women Do Breastfeed Facebook page in order to better understand how the community responds to the "despairing picture of breastfeeding among black mothers in the United States." I focused my data collection on the BWDBF Facebook page because it is the community's most active platform. Using purposive sampling, I selected data that best illustrate how BWDBF uses social media to produce *counter*activist and *parallel* activist health texts to rewrite race-based health disparities that pathologize breastfeeding.

I invited community members to participate in an IRB-approved online survey about social media, race, and breastfeeding in February

2016, but because the survey received insufficient responses, I did not include survey data here. While all content discussed in this chapter is publicly available online, I chose to not use personal images from the community (e.g., mothers breastfeeding their children) or individuals' names in an effort to protect group members' privacy. When discussing community members' posts, I use pseudonyms and/or general appellations like *mother, child,* or *infant.*

My data-collection process and analysis of the community's health texts is rooted in rhetorical analysis and guided by the Association of Internet Researchers' (AoIR) 2012 recommendations for conducting ethical online research. This chapter's methodology is also informed by Caroline Dadas's (2016) notion of "messy methods" for social media research, a methodological orientation that acknowledges the inherent "messiness of using social media as a method of participant recruitment and data collection" (63). Dadas's work, along with the AoIR's recommendations, guided me as I introduced myself to the Black Women Do Breastfeed community on Facebook and Twitter, gathered and analyzed digital artifacts, and invited members to participate in an online survey.

My analysis of how Black Women Do Breastfeed uses social media to rewrite "the story of modern black American women breastfeeding" ("Welcome page," n.d.) reflects my positionality and epistemologies as a heterosexual, white, middle-class woman. Thus, I do not claim to personally understand minority women's experiences with healthcare organizations or breastfeeding. But as a feminist rhetorician of health and medicine who studies childbirth and infant feeding, I am greatly concerned with the reproductive and perinatal health disparities experienced by women of color. I hope this chapter encourages rhetoricians of health and medicine specifically, and the field of technical communication more broadly, to pay closer attention to the health disparities minority women face. I also hope this chapter contributes to this edited collection's goal to encourage a deeper interrogation of the ways pathology operates as a form of meaning making that shapes women's health experiences.

RACIAL HEALTH DISPARITIES IN BREASTFEEDING

Unequal access to quality healthcare is a national epidemic. The Center for American Progress (Russell 2010) reports that 68 percent of Hispanics[1] had health coverage in 2009 compared to 88 percent of white Americans. The numbers for African Americans are slightly better, yet nevertheless worrisome: about 79 percent of African Americans had health coverage in 2009 compared to 88 percent of whites (1). National programs such as the Affordable Care Act, Healthy People 2020, and the National Institute on Minority Health and Health Disparities have increased minorities' access to healthcare. However, there remains an alarming gap—or what has come to be called a *health disparity*—across the United States. Healthy People 2020 defines a health disparity as "a particular type of health difference that is closely linked with social, economic, and/or environmental disadvantage. Health disparities adversely affect groups of people who have systematically experienced greater obstacles to health based on their racial or ethnic group; religion; socioeconomic status; gender; age; mental health; cognitive, sensory, or physical disability; sexual orientation or gender identity; geographic location; or other characteristics historically linked to discrimination or exclusion" (n.d.).

Healthy People 2020's definition emphasizes that health disparities are not simply about access to healthcare but are closely linked to systemic social, racial, and economic discrimination and inequalities. As rhetoricians of health and medicine have shown (Arduser 2013; Bellwoar 2012; Liz, this collection; Owens 2009, 2015; Segal 2009; Seigel 2013), discursive practices reinforce power structures and policies that diminish groups' and individuals' health agency, or their ability to meaningfully influence their own health experiences and outcomes. In short, health inequalities are not just the byproduct of biological, environmental, or technological circumstances but are also tied to rhetorical practices that reinforce racist, classist, and sexist social structures and epistemologies.

One important, yet understudied, aspect of race-based health disparities is breastfeeding among African American women. Research by the Centers for Disease Control and Prevention (2013) indicates that about 59 percent of Black women breastfeed, compared to 75 percent of whites and 80 percent of Hispanic women. The CDC's findings are supported by research from the US Department of Health and Human Services, which reports that African American breastfeeding rates are significantly lower than white and Hispanic rates. For example, the Surgeon General's 2011 "Call to Action to Support Breastfeeding" illustrates racial demographics in breastfeeding rates for infants born in 2007, indicating that only 12.5 percent of African American women still breastfeed at twelve months, compared to 24.7 percent of Hispanic women and 23.3 percent of non-Hispanic white women. While breastfeeding rates among Black women have increased over the last decade, there remains a significant gap between racial groups. The reasons for these gaps are myriad and include factors such as income, work environment, access to healthcare, and education (Jones et al. 2015).

Disparities in breastfeeding rates are an important health concern for African American women and their families. According to a 2014 study published in the *Journal of the National Cancer Institute*, parous women (i.e., women of childbearing age) who have not breastfed have an increased risk of developing breast cancer later in life (Palmer et al. 2014). Because breastfeeding rates are lower among African American women than among their nonwhite Hispanic counterparts, African American women are potentially at greater risk of developing breast cancer. Despite efforts by organizations like the African American Breast Cancer Epidemiology and Risk (AMBER) Consortium to increase breastfeeding among Black women, breastfeeding rates remain low. What, then, is a workable solution to this complex problem?

One possible solution is online breastfeeding communities like Black Women Do Breastfeed, which promote and support breastfeeding among African American women. A key way they accomplish this is by using social media to produce activist health texts that move beyond medical orientations toward breastfeeding and toward community-based ways of knowing. While official health organizations like the AMBER Consortium successfully use digital technologies to connect African American women with breastfeeding resources, these types of organizations navigate challenges informal advocacy groups like BWDBF do not. For example, according to a 2014 study by C. Lee Ventola, social media use by healthcare organizations can "present potential risks to patients and HCPs [healthcare providers] regarding the distribution of poor quality information, damage to professional image, breaches of patient privacy, violation of personal-professional boundaries, and licensing or legal issues" (491). Unlike organizations such as the AMBER Consortium, informal online health communities rarely negotiate such complex legal, ethical, and professional terrain, a feature that makes communities like Black Women Do Breastfeed important rhetorical sites for addressing race-based health disparities in nontraditional ways.

DEFINING ACTIVIST HEALTH TEXTS

I define the term *activist health texts* as communications produced by groups and individuals that resist and redefine rhetorical boundaries between official health communications produced by organizations like the Department of Health and Human Services (HHS), Centers for Disease Control and Prevention (CDC), and World Health Organization

(WHO), and "unofficial" health texts created by individuals, groups, and communities. As Miriam Mara's chapter in this collection suggests, these types of health organizations often produce health texts that rhetorically reinforce negative gendered assumptions about women's bodies, particularly in regard to their reproductive capabilities. My use of the term *activist health text* is informed by a growing body of scholarship in rhetorics of health and medicine (Arduser 2013; Bellwoar 2012; Dubriwny 2013; Koerber 2013; Lay 2000; Owens 2009; Seigel 2014) that examines how nonmedical individuals produce and circulate "unofficial" health texts such as social media posts, photos, or digital narratives.

In her work on everyday health texts, Hannah Bellwoar (2012) suggests that "in studies of medical discourse, the traditional cultural frame considers agency to be in the production of texts and the interpretation of information, tasks typically associated with medical professionals. Patients in this frame are not seen as participants or makers of knowledge in the production of health care texts" (325). Like Bellwoar, I argue that unofficial health texts produced by BWDBF are important communications that allow individuals to act as "makers of knowledge in the production of health care texts" (325). However, I expand Bellwoar's work to suggest that activist health texts are particularly important for disadvantaged groups, who often rely on alternative rhetorical strategies and tools to address race-based health disparities.

INTERROGATING RACIAL DISPARITIES IN BREASTFEEDING: A BRIEF LOOK AT PAST AND PRESENT

Over the last decade, healthcare providers and researchers have striven to better understand why Hispanic women—despite the fact that many share socioeconomic backgrounds similar to African American women—continue to have significantly higher breastfeeding rates than their Black counterparts. As I illustrate in the previous section, research by the CDC (2013) indicates that about 59 percent of African American women breastfeed compared to 80 percent of Hispanic women. The reasons for such a large gap between these groups are unclear. However, research by Chelsea McKinney et al. (2016) describes three possible factors that might drive such a disparity: first, Black women are more likely to be given formula by healthcare providers than are other racial groups. Second, Hispanic mothers typically have more family members who breastfeed. Third, Hispanic families have higher marital rates, which may give Hispanic women more familial support and time away from work to breastfeed.

These factors may help explain disparities between Hispanic and African American breastfeeding rates. However, they do not account for the medical and sociohistorical forces that have negatively shaped Black women's experiences with breastfeeding and perinatal care over the last two centuries. Consider, for example, the story of Anarcha, Lucy, and Betsey, three enslaved African American women treated by Dr. James Marion Sims, a nineteenth-century gynecologist. Sims performed surgeries on these women for labor-related injuries, often conducting procedures with neither consent nor anesthesia. In an interview on National Public Radio, Dr. Vanessa Northington Gamble describes Anarcha, Lucy, and Betsey's perinatal experiences this way: "These women were property. These women could not consent [to surgery]. They were performed without anesthesia. There was a belief at the time that Black people did not feel pain in the same way. They were not vulnerable to pain, especially black women" (Vedantam 2016). Although the perception that Black people are more tolerant to pain than whites seems anachronistic, recent studies indicate otherwise (Goyal et al. 2015; Hoffman et al. 2016; Young et al. 2013). Research by Kelly Hoffman et al. (2016), for example, demonstrates that both laypeople and individuals with medical training often assume Blacks have a higher pain tolerance than whites.

The history of racist gynecological- and perinatal-care practices by healthcare professionals and institutions remains embedded in the cultural consciousness of Black women today. A video entitled *A Black Woman Speaks . . . of White Womanhood, of White Supremacy, of Peace* recently circulated in several online breastfeeding communities such as Hey Facebook, Breastfeeding Is Not Obscene and Chocolate Milk Matters. The video, a reenactment of a poem written by Beah Richards (1975) for the 1951 American People's Peace Congress' in Chicago, shows a young Black woman speaking to white women about enslaved women's experiences as wet-nurses. In an unwavering voice, the narrator tells the audience that enslaved Black women often "gave suckle" to white children with the knowledge that they "nursed [their] own child's enemy" (min 1:40). Research by PhD candidate and certified nurse-midwife Stephanie Devane-Johnson suggests the practice of forcing enslaved women to nurse white children resonates with African American women today. For example, she underscores that some Black women continue to associate breastfeeding with the "image of a 'mammy'" who is forced to breastfeed a slave owner's children (quoted in Hoban 2016).

Devane-Johnson's research also indicates that social media facilitate the circulation of negative breastfeeding images and associations in ways potentially broader and more impactful than print-based media (Hoban 2016). On January 30, 2016, an online breastfeeding advocacy group called "I hate it when people act like breastfeeding is obscene, GET OVER IT!" shared the following Facebook post, which accompanied an image (not included in this chapter due to copyright issues) of an enslaved woman breastfeeding a white child:

> Slavery, privilege, and racism persist today and although many steps mov-
> ing forward there is still a long way to go in terms of helping black or
> African Americans get the recognition and rights for equal rights, Black
> women's rights, peer support without people crying that it's "reverse rac-
> ism" (it's not and it doesn't exist). . . . When communities do better we all
> prosper. It's because of slavery that breastfeeding in the black community
> is looked down upon, but we know that looking at looking at [*sic*] vulner-
> able communities we need to support this to decrease the highest section
> of infant morbidity and mortality rates.

This post illustrates several important rhetorical maneuvers. One, it shows how online breastfeeding communities use social media to circulate historical (and in some cases, negative) breastfeeding images. Second, the circulation of troubling images like the one that accompanied this post may, as Devane-Johnson (2016) suggests, discourage African American women from breastfeeding because it rhetorically reinforces negative associations between racial oppression and infant feeding. The post's author points out this connotation, telling readers that "it's because of slavery that breastfeeding in the black community is looked down upon." Third, the written commentary accompanying the photo reveals Black women are well aware that attitudes toward breastfeeding are rooted in broader sociohistorical contexts that privilege white power. The author is careful to remind readers that "slavery, privilege, and racism persist today and although many steps moving forward there is still a long way to go in terms of helping black or African Americans get the recognition and rights for equal rights." This author's comment suggests an African American woman's decision to breastfeed is not simply a medical choice, but a decision inextricably linked to cultural and rhetorical power structures that reflect centuries of oppression.

While the dissemination of negative breastfeeding images via social media might discourage some women from breastfeeding, the rhetorical activities of the BWDBF community indicate that the circulation of *positive* historical images might, by contrast, encourage it. For example, a 2014 post to the BWDBF Facebook page called "There is nothing new except what has been forgotten" shows what appears to be a twentieth-century image of a black woman breastfeeding her infant. The post received 2,500 likes, was shared over two hundred times, and received dozens of positive comments. Community members' supportive reactions to this and similar posts suggest positive historical texts about breastfeeding shared via social media may help destigmatize breastfeeding in African American communities.

In their work "Racial and Ethnic Disparities in Breastfeeding," Katherine Jones et al. (2015) argue that recognizing "the historical challenges that African American women have faced" is critical to understanding and reducing social barriers that negatively impact breastfeeding among Black women (189). In the introduction to this collection, Erin Frost and Michelle Eble likewise underscore the historical and contemporary ways women's health is both gendered and racially mediated, noting that public health institutions and their associated policies "have historical patterns" that respond to "particular kinds of bodies in unjust and inequitable ways" (8). By acknowledging the sociohistorical contexts that have shaped and continue to shape intersections between race and breastfeeding, as well as the larger biomedical and public health practices that enact health disparities, rhetoricians of health and medicine are better positioned to understand why communities like Black Women Do Breastfeed create and circulate activist health texts.

COUNTERACTIVIST HEALTH TEXTS

For many members of the Black Women Do Breastfeed community, breastfeeding is an act that either implicitly or explicitly counters medical rhetorics that position African American mothers as inadequate or deficient at breastfeeding. These individuals' discursive activities suggest that an alternative narrative exists—one in which Black women proudly and successfully breastfeed their children. For example, in a July 9, 2016, post to the BWDBF Facebook timeline, one mother shares an image of herself breastfeeding, followed by the tagline: ". . . no shame proud to be a beautiful black women and breastfeeding [my baby] loves her chocolate milk." In a similar post on July 7, 2016, a young mother proudly tells the community that her son "only takes breast no formula." And in July 5, 2016, post, a mother shares a picture of herself breastfeeding her child, followed by the celebratory remark: "I breastfed my oldest baby girl and now she gets to see me nurse her baby sister just like I watched my mom. I am building a legacy of black women who breastfeed."

The above narratives embody *counter*activist health texts—that is, texts and narratives that explicitly resist, subvert, and rewrite official health texts (such as those produced by the CDC and WHO) that pathologize breastfeeding and situate Black women as lacking. The first woman's statement that she is "proud to be a beautiful black women and breast-feeding" followed by the second mother's comment that her son "only takes breast no formula" suggest these mothers *reject* the idea that Black women rely too heavily on formula or dismiss breastfeeding altogether. The last mother's statement that she and her daughter are "building a legacy of black women who breastfeed" further reinforces the idea that African American mothers—despite discouraging reports by the CDC, AAP, and other organizations—are in fact actively breastfeeding their children as well as "building a legacy" of breastfeeding among Black women. These counteractivist health texts resist medical narratives that suggest breastfeeding is a pathology that must be corrected by medical intervention and instead argue breastfeeding is best supported by famil-ial and community-based ways of knowing.

My use of the term *counteractivist health text* to describe these mothers' breastfeeding narratives builds on Lora Arduser's (2013) use of the term "counternarratives," or narratives that help groups and individuals chal-lenge the ways healthcare institutions frame conversations about health and bodies. I draw from Arduser's concept of counternarratives to argue that Black Women Do Breastfeed uses social media to produce and cir-culate counteractivist health texts that rewrite racial health disparities about breastfeeding. While *parallel* activist health texts (as I illustrate in the next section) occur alongside and augment sanctioned health communications, counteractivist health texts run counter to dominant health narratives.

My notion of counteractivist health texts builds on, yet departs from, other rhetorical frameworks for understanding intersections between health communication and rhetorical agency. One influential concept is Mary Lay's (2000) notion of "boundary spanning," which she defines as a process that "involves rhetors' attempts to establish authority within their own or another's community and often to challenge dominant jurisdictional borders. Resisting the labels of deviant or amateur, bound-ary spanners often attempt to prove their authority by demonstrating their ability to use the techniques and vocabulary of the dominant pro-fession or community" (78).

The concept of counteractivist health texts offers a somewhat dif-ferent view of this rhetorical process; rather than adopt the language and epistemologies of official health communications, counteractivist health texts enact rhetorical agency by openly resisting and rewriting dominant medical narratives, a process that becomes particularly fluid in digital environments. The ability to produce counteractivist health texts is especially important for minority communities like Black Women Do Breastfeed because it allows community members to assert rhetorical authority over their own health experiences and ways of knowing.

Breastfeeding stories and their attendant hashtags provide useful examples for examining how this process works. In the following May 26, 2016, post to the BWDBF Facebook page, a mother describes her experience with breastfeeding her son, followed by the hashtags #bwdbf and #wedothis: "I love seeing all these amazing sisters creating a bond with their babies and helping to normalize breastfeeding! #bwdbf #wedothis." In a similar post on May 30, 2016, another woman shares her breastfeeding story, telling readers that "I absolutely love your page. I have relatives that shame breastfeeding, but too bad! It makes me so proud to see other strong black women feeding babies the way they were meant to be fed! #bwdbf #wedothis."

These posts rhetorically interrogate the idea that Black women are physically and culturally disengaged from breastfeeding. The first woman's comment, "I love seeing all these amazing sisters . . . helping to normalize breastfeeding!," and the second mother's statement, "It makes me so proud to see other strong black women feeding babies," underscore that many African American women *do* in fact breastfeed their children and are empowered by it. Moreover, community members' use of the hashtag #wedothis rhetorically counters the idea that Black women do not actively breastfeed their children, despite data produced by WHO and the CDC that indicate low breastfeeding rates.

Counteractivist health texts like those shared above can circulate via any medium or mode. Social media platforms, however, support this type of rhetorical activity in unique ways. For example, by clicking on the #wedothis hashtag, users can easily connect with other BWDBF community members, access images of Black women breastfeeding, and comment on others' tweets and posts. Clicking on this hashtag also connects users to related online communities such as NormalizeBreastfeeding .org and Hey Facebook, Breastfeeding Is Not Obscene. Unlike print-based modes of communication, social media allow BWDBF community members to quickly connect with others and join cross-community conversations about breastfeeding.

For poor women and women of color, social media are particularly important tools for countering dominant medical narratives that pathologize breastfeeding, largely because these platforms are free and can be accessed from a range of devices and applications. Although some argue social media activism (or what has been derisively labeled as *slacktivism*) is ineffective or a poor substitute for meaningful engagement, virtual activism is critical for marginalized communities because it is often a critical medium for challenging social, political, and economic infrastructures and policies that mediate their health experiences. As civil rights activist and political organizer DeRay Mckesson points out, social media enable Black communities to tell their own stories, transform "'a history of erasure,'" build community, and demand accountability (quoted in Berlatsky 2015). Similarly, social media platforms help communities like Black Women Do Breastfeed create counteractivist heath texts that challenge healthcare organizations' positioning of African American women as disengaged from breastfeeding.

While counteractivist health texts are important tools for rhetorical activism, so too is the physical act of breastfeeding. In her book *Breast or Bottle?*, Amy Koerber (2013) stresses that breastfeeding can be an important form of rhetorical resistance or, as she puts it, a way of "bucking the system" (116). Drawing from interviews with members of the international breastfeeding organization La Leche League, Koerber argues that community members used breastfeeding to assert "their own authority in the context of disciplinary rhetorics that interfere with breastfeeding. Such actions often involved resisting faulty medical advice or continuing to breastfeed even when friends and relatives discouraged it" (117). In a similar manner, BWDBF community members use personal narratives, comments, and hashtags like #wedothis and #bwdbf to circulate counteractivist health texts that "buck" official reports and medical narratives that pathologize breastfeeding and that situate Black women as lacking or deficient.

PARALLEL ACTIVIST HEALTH TEXTS

Social media sites like Instagram, Twitter, and Facebook provide rich rhetorical and technological platforms for online breastfeeding communities to create and distribute *parallel* activist health texts, or texts that occur alongside (and in some cases augment) official health communications about breastfeeding produced by organizations such as the CDC, WHO, and La Leche League. Consider, for example, the following post shared on March 15, 2016, on the BWDBF's community's Facebook page:

> My daughter just turned 6 months and I am going through a lot of pain from her biting and pulling!! I am tempted to wean. I don't know what to do!!! HELP PLEASE!!!

This post prompts an extended conversation among community members about ways this mother can minimize her breastfeeding discomfort. One commenter advises the mother to momentarily push the baby's head into her breast when she starts biting; this advice is echoed by several other individuals, one of whom states this method "works like a charm!"

These posts and comments function as parallel activist health texts that augment official health communications about breastfeeding. For example, the first commenter's suggestion that the mother might briefly restrict her baby's breathing to prevent biting supplements advice produced by established health organizations like La Leche League. On the organization's "What Should I Do If My Baby Bites Me?" web page, La Leche League offers numerous strategies to discourage biting (such as briefly pulling a baby's head in close to the breast), but they do not overtly suggest a mother might momentarily restrict her baby's breathing, a rhetorical maneuver likely designed to safeguard against legal action. Because organizations like La Leche League are bound to legal and professional guidelines that "unofficial" breastfeeding communities like BWDBF are not, these online communities are vital to the creation and circulation of parallel activist health texts that augment official breastfeeding literature.

IMPLICATIONS AND RHETORICAL LIMITATIONS

As this chapter illustrates, African American women strategically use social media to create "unofficial" narratives that both challenge and expand official health communications about breastfeeding. While such discursive maneuvers demonstrate African American women's enactment of rhetorical agency through the creation of "everyday" online health texts (Bellwoar 2012), it is important to remember such texts are mediated by digital platforms that are by no means free of racial or gendered biases. Indeed, as Kristin Arola (2010, 2012), Sherry Turkle (1997), Adam Banks (2006), and others have aptly illustrated, digital media are embedded with social, racial, and gendered biases that often invisibly privilege some groups over others. What this means for communities like Black Women Do Breastfeed is that while social media sites are powerful venues for the creation of activist health texts, these spaces can also invisibly marginalize the very communities who employ them.

What, then, does this mean for communities like BWDBF who use social media to interrogate race-based health disparities? Might such texts simply reinforce the very health disparities and gendered pathologies these communities seek to subvert? Can BWDBF and other online communities—despite Audre Lorde's (2007) warning that "the master's tools will never dismantle the master's house"—succeed in their efforts? Certainly, there are no clear-cut answers to these questions, but they remind us social media (and the rhetorical movements that emerge within them) are rooted in rhetorical, racial, and gendered frameworks that extend beyond the tools themselves.

Another rhetorical limitation to consider is the assumption by communities like Black Women Do Breastfeed that "the breast is best." Koerber (2013) argues that the widespread adoption of this mantra has grown out of national breastfeeding campaigns that describe formula as less healthy and "natural" than breastmilk. Rhetorically positioning formula as the lesser of two options can be problematic for African American women who might need to rely on formula more than their white or Hispanic counterparts do (often due to limited or no maternity leave, as well as a lack of cultural, workplace, and/or familial support) to nourish their children.

It is important, therefore, to remember that while "unofficial" activist health texts can be empowering, such texts still reflect the rhetorical values of influential healthcare organizations. These rhetorical overlaps are not inherently harmful; nevertheless, they enforce cultural biases that shape, guide, and sometimes limit the rhetorical strategies of advocacy groups. Because women in general—and women of color especially—are already disadvantaged by systemic sexism and racism, rhetoricians of health and medicine must be diligent about recognizing the ways health texts, even when they are produced by communities focused on social justice, can reify health disparities and practices that pathologize breastfeeding.

NOTE

1. The term Hispanic is used to maintain consistency with reporting data from government and national healthcare agencies and organizations. However, it should be noted that this is a contested term and carries with it personal, sociocultural, gendered, and political ramifications.

REFERENCES

Arduser, Lora. 2013. "The Care and Feeding of the D-Beast: Metaphors of the Lived Experience of Diabetes." In *Rhetorical AccessAbility: At the Intersection of Technical Communication and Disability Studies*, edited by Lisa Meloncon, 95–113. Amityville, NY: Baywood.

Arola, Kristin L. 2010. "The Design of Web 2.0: The Rise of the Template, the Fall of Design." *Computers and Composition* 27 (1): 4–14.

Arola, Kristin L. 2012. "It's My Revolution: Learning to See the Mixedblood." In *Composing (Media) = Composing (Embodiment)*, edited by Kristin L. Arola and Anne Frances Wysocki, 115–142. Logan: Utah State University Press.

Banks, Adam. 2006. *Race, Rhetoric, and Technology: Searching for Higher Ground.* Urbana, IL: NCTE.

Bellwoar, Hannah. 2012. "Everyday Matters: Reception and Use as Productive Design of Health-Related Texts." *Technical Communication Quarterly* 21 (4): 325–345.

Berlatsky, Noah. 2015. "Hashtag Activism Isn't a Cop-Out." *Atlantic,* January 7. http://www.theatlantic.com/politics/archive/2015/01/not-just-hashtag-activism-why-social-media-matters-to-protestors/384215.

Black Women Do Breastfeed. 2014. "There is nothing new except what has been forgotten." Facebook, October 21.

Black Women Do Breastfeed. 2016. "Hello! Would love for you to share this on your page! I love breastfeeding and I love this page!" Facebook, May 26.

Black Women Do Breastfeed. 2016. "I breastfed my oldest baby girl and now she gets to see me nurse her baby sister just like I watched my mom. I am building a legacy of black women who breastfeed." Facebook, July 5.

Black Women Do Breastfeed. 2016. "My daughter just turned 6 months and I am going through a lot of pain from her biting and pulling!! see me nurse her baby sister just like I watched my mom. I am building a legacy of black women who breastfeed." Facebook, March 15.

Black Women Do Breastfeed. 2016. "No Shame. I'd rather feed him than make him cry." Facebook, July 7.

Black Women Do Breastfeed. 2016. "Us at carowinds amusement park celebrating the 4th of July no shame proud to be a beautiful black women and breastfeeding she loves her chocolate milk." Facebook, July 9.

Breastfeeding a Nation: The History of My Chocolate Milk. 2015. *"A Black Woman Speaks . . .* of White Womanhood, of White Supremacy, of Peace." Facebook, August 2015. https://www.facebook.com/groups/BreastfeedingIsNotObscene/permalink/10152921648511533/?comment_tracking=%7B%22tn%22%3A%22O%22%7D.

Centers for Disease Control and Prevention. 2013. "Progress in Increasing Breastfeeding and Reducing Racial/Ethnic differences." *Morbidity and Mortality Weekly Report* 62 (5): 77–80.

Dadas, Caroline. 2016. "Messy Methods: Queer Methodological Approaches to Researching Social Media." *Computers and Composition* 40: 60–72.

Dubrivny, Tasha. 2013. *The Vulnerable Empowered Woman: Feminism, Postfeminism, and Women's Health.* Piscataway, NJ: Rutgers University Press.

Goyal, Monika K., Nathan Kuppermann, Sean D. Cleary, Stephen J. Teach, and James M. Chamberlain. 2015. "Racial Disparities in Pain Management of Children with Appendicitis in Emergency Departments." *JAMA Pediatrics* 169 (11): 996–1002.

Healthy People 2020. n.d. "Disparities." Healthypeople.gov. Updated April 20, 2020. https://www.healthypeople.gov/2020/about/foundation-health-measures/Disparities.

Hinson, Katrina. 2016. "Framing Illness through Facebook Enabled Online Support Groups." *Communication Design Quarterly* 4 (2): 22–31.

Hoban, Rose. 2016. "Distant Echoes of Slavery Affect Breast-Feeding Attitudes of Black Women." North Carolina Health News, March 3. http://www.northcarolinahealthnews.org/2016/03/03/distant-echoes-of-slavery-affect-breastfeeding-attitudes-in-black-women/.

Hoffman, Kelly M., Sophie Trawalter, Jordan R. Axt, and Norman M. Oliver. (2016). "Racial Bias in Pain Assessment and Treatment Recommendations, and False Beliefs about Biological Differences between Blacks and Whites." *Proceedings of the National Academy of Sciences* 113 (16): 4296–4301.

"I hate it when people act like breastfeeding is obscene, GET OVER IT!" 2016. "As an acknowledgement of Black History Month we are posing this, but also know that we support that black history is American History and that the education of it should not be segregated to one month alone." Facebook, January 6. https://www.facebook.com/Breastfeeding123/photos/a.315124538393.151638.308245108393/10154040536818394/?type=3&theater.

Jones, Katherine M., Michael L. Power, John T. Queenan, and Jay Schulkin. 2015. "Racial and Ethnic Disparities in Breastfeeding." *Breastfeeding Medicine* 10 (4): 186–196.

Koerber, Amy. 2013. *Breast or Bottle: Contemporary Controversies in Infant-Feeding Policy and Practice.* Columbia: University of South Carolina Press.

Koteyko, Nelya, Daniel Hunt, and Barrie Gunter. 2015. "Expectations in the Field of the Internet and Health: An Analysis of Claims about Social Networking Sites in Clinical Literature." *Sociology of Health and Illness* 37 (3): 468–484.

La Leche League International. 2012. "What Should I Do If My Baby Bites Me?" http://www.llli.org/faq/bite.html.

Lay, Mary. 2000. *The Rhetoric of Midwifery: Gender, Knowledge, and Power.* New Brunswick, NJ: Rutgers University Press.

Lorde, Audre. 2007. *Sister Outsider: Essays and Speeches.* Berkeley, CA: Crossing Press.

McKinney, Chelsea O., Jennifer P. Hahn-Holbrook, P. Lindsay Chase-Lansdale, Sharon L. Ramey, Julie Krohn, Maxine Reed-Vance, Tonse N.K. Raju, and Madeleine U. Shalowitz, and on behalf of the Community Child Health Research Network. 2016. "Racial and Ethnic Differences in Breastfeeding." *Pediatrics* 138 (2): 1–11.

Owens, Kim H. 2009. "Confronting Rhetorical Disability: A Critical Analysis of Women's Birth Plans." *Written Communication* 26 (3): 247–272.

Owens, Kim H. 2015. *Writing Childbirth: Women's Rhetorical Agency in Labor and Online.* Carbondale: Southern Illinois University Press.

Palmer, Julie R., Emma Viscidi, Melissa A. Troester, Chi-Chen Hong, Pepper Schedin, Traci N. Bethea, Elisa V. Bandera, Virginia Borges, Craig McKinnon, Christopher A. Haiman, Kathryn Lunetta, Laurence N. Kolonel, Lynn Rosenberg, Andrew F. Olshan, and Christine B. Ambrosone. 2014. "Parity, Lactation, and Breast Cancer Subtypes in African American Women: Results from the AMBER Consortium." *Journal of the National Cancer Institute* 106 (10): 1–8.

Persky, Susan, Saskia C. Sanderson, and Laura M. Koehly. 2013. "Online Communication about Genetics and Body Weight: Implications for Health Behavior and Internet-Based Education." *Journal of Health Communication* 18 (2): 241–249.

Richards, Beah. 1975. *Black Woman Speaks and Other Poems.* Bronx, NY: Inner City Press.

Russell, Lesley. 2010. *Fact Sheet: Health Disparities by Race and Ethnicity.* Center for American Progress. https://cdn.americanprogress.org/wp-content/uploads/issues/2010/12/pdf/disparities_factsheet.pdf.

Sandiford, Nicole. n.d. Home. *Black Women Do Breastfeed* (blog). blackwomendobreastfeed.org.

Segal, Judy Z. 2008. *Health and the Rhetoric of Medicine.* Carbondale: Southern Illinois University Press.

Segal, Judy Z. 2009. "Internet Health and the 21st-Century Patient: A Rhetorical View." *Written Communication* 26 (4): 351–369.

Seigel, Marika. 2014. *The Rhetoric of Pregnancy.* Chicago: University of Chicago Press.

Turkle, Sherry. 1997. *Life on the Screen: Identity in the Age of the Internet.* New York: Simon and Schuster.

US Department of Health and Human Services. 2011. "The Surgeon General's Call to Action to Support Breastfeeding." Washington, DC: US Department of Health and Human Services, Office of the Surgeon General.

Vedantam, Shankar. 2016. "Remembering Anarcha, Lucy, and Betsey: The Mothers of Modern Gynecology." *Hidden Brain.* NPR, February 16. http://www.npr.org/templates/transcript/transcript.php?storyId=466942135.

Ventola, C. Lee. 2014. "Social Media and Health Care Professionals: Benefits, Risks, and Best Practices." *Pharmacy and Therapeutics* 39 (7): 491–520.

"Welcome Page." n.d. *Black Women Do Breastfeed* (blog). https://blackwomendobreastfeed .org/.

Willerton, Russell. 2008. "Writing Toward Readers' Better Health: A Case Study Examining the Development of Online Health Information." *Technical Communication Quarterly* 17 (3): 311–334.

Young, Megann F., H. Gene Hern, Harrison J. Alter, Joseph Barger, and Farnaz Vahidnia. 2013. "Racial Differences in Receiving Morphine among Prehospital Patients with Blunt Trauma." *Journal of Emergency Medicine* 45 (1): 46–52.

11

GENDERED RISK AND RESPONSIBILITY IN THE AMERICAN HEART ASSOCIATION'S GO RED FOR WOMEN CAMPAIGN

Mary K. Assad

I found out that heart disease is the number one killer of women. How did I not know that? I found out that one in three women die from heart disease. How did I not know that? I couldn't just sit there and let this killer do to other women what it had done to me. I couldn't stand there and watch as this occurred to other women and not do anything. I had to empower myself to do something. I Go Red for every woman because it's time for us to make a change.

—Gloria, Go Red Woman

A slim, attractive woman sits before a camera and speaks directly into it, as if her closest friends and family are on the other side. She speaks with urgency and intense emotion, her eyes pleading with her audience to listen to her words. She wears a red dress with a deep V-neck that frames a fading, but still visible, scar in the middle of her chest. Although viewers may not know Gloria at the start of the clip, the health campaign that sponsors her message clearly hopes that by the end, viewers will identify not only with the woman in the red dress but also with the campaign and its larger cause.

Established in 2004 by the American Heart Association (AHA), the Go Red for Women (Go Red) campaign seeks to dispel the myth among the American general public that heart disease is a man's disease. Go Red has attempted to frame heart disease rhetorically as a women's health concern by articulating unique physiological risk factors and symptoms and also highlighting aspects of a woman's social identity that threaten her health. In other words, since its inception, Go Red has sought to gender heart disease. This goal has resulted

DOI: 10.7330/9781607329855.c011

in campaign messages that urge women to pay attention and take action. However, these messages reflect and perpetuate existing gender norms and stereotypes despite a larger rhetorical framework of female empowerment.

This chapter acknowledges the important work Go Red has accomplished in raising awareness of heart disease as a women's health issue but problematizes the notions of gender upon which the campaign relies. Through methods of rhetorical analysis, I examine the campaign's web-based messages to determine how the campaign frames heart disease as a women's health concern and what beliefs and actions the campaign seeks to induce in women. This analysis reveals that Go Red portrays a woman's tendency to care for others as a gender-specific risk factor that can be remedied through a reconceptualization of self-care but also harnessed and repurposed through engagement with practices of discursive care. This chapter first provides context to situate Go Red as a medical advocacy website that reflects the aims and ideologies of the new public health model. Then, the analysis focuses on the campaign's gendered articulations of risk and attributions of responsibility to demonstrate how Go Red seeks to persuade women heart disease is a relevant and urgent concern in their lives. The chapter concludes by considering the implications of Go Red's health media.

MEDICAL ADVOCACY WEBSITES AND THE NEW PUBLIC HEALTH

The increasing tendency for patients to consult the internet for health information underscores the need for close analysis of materials presented as trustworthy, authoritative, and objective. Marie Moeller (2014) observes that "the Internet has revolutionized the way users are able to interact with the medical establishment and to access medical information" (52). As a result, she emphasizes the need for rhetorical and technical communication scholars to continue analyzing "traditional sources" but also urges scholars to expand their notice to other, often overlooked sites of "medical technical rhetoric on the Internet" including medical advocacy sites (53). She notes that although such sites galvanize social recognition and monetary funds, "fundraising has never been the sole purpose of these sites"; rather, they also "support patients and patient-adjacent populations by providing access to general medical information . . . and a host of other technical medical information" (53). Moeller argues that the discourse produced by Susan G. Komen for the Cure exemplifies the dangerous tendency for the "medical charity model" (55) of health advocacy to produce and perpetuate problematic "harmful biopolitical logics" (54) the general public feels uncomfortable critiquing or resisting due to the organization's visible social presence as an altruistic and well-intentioned charity. While Moeller compellingly argues for the need to analyze and critique "the technical writing in medical advocacy websites" (60), I emphasize the need also to analyze the nontechnical writing found within those same spaces, particularly when such messages augment more technical discussions of health, illness, and the body. In other words, we must consider how medical advocacy websites often combine technical and colloquial language and genres within a single site to develop an ethos of humanized and approachable medical authority.

In fact, the desire to present such an ethos prompted the American Heart Association to establish Go Red. The campaign presents its history as a response to medical and rhetorical exigency, explaining, "In 2003, research revealed that heart disease was by far the No. 1 killer of women. . . . To save lives and raise awareness of this serious issue, the American Heart Association launched Go Red for Women" (Go Red, "About," n.d.). However, few users of the site may realize that Go Red was crafted by communication professionals as a marketing campaign. The Cone Communications website offers another perspective on the campaign's origins, explaining that Go Red was established to "infuse more passion and emotion into the AHA's brand, which was well-respected but largely recognized as clinical" (Cone, n.d.). Thus, Go Red was established with the dual goals of raising awareness of heart disease and rebranding the AHA, and both goals influence the content and presentation of the campaign's messages.

While Go Red's website can be considered a medical advocacy site of the type described and problematized by Moeller, the individual messages published on this site, as well as through print and on television, represent instances of "health media," or targeted messages that "reflect social values and norms" and are thus "important for understanding dominant meanings of health" (Davies and Burns 2014, 713). When viewed through Michel Foucault's analytics of governmentality, we might also "consider the ways in which health media *produces* and *governs* 'healthy' lifestyles and behaviors and establishes the norms and limits of 'healthy' subjectivities" (713). In other words, health media have the power to draw boundaries between health and disease as social concepts, to constrain bodies and identities according to particular social norms, and to determine the standards against which individuals evaluate and monitor their own behaviors.

Such social demarcations and subtle mechanisms of governance are key characteristics of the new public health, a model Alan Petersen and Deborah Lupton (1996) identify as an outgrowth of neoliberalism. They explain how the new public health model invites conformity to designated health regulations and norms, not by coercion but instead by suggesting individuals are autonomous, empowered agents who have control over their bodies and health and thereby encouraging individual processes of self-regulation (11–12). The desired norms are often established and articulated within a larger framework of risk assessment and management, wherein risks operate as "sociocultural constructs" that "inevitably include moral judgments of blame" (18). Thus, under the new public health model, populations are exhorted to monitor their behaviors even when free of apparent disease so as to navigate the various risks that threaten to overtake their bodies. Because "our understanding of these dangers and hazards, including their origin and outcomes, are constituted through social, cultural and political processes" (18), analysis of such processes—and in particular, the textual objects that animate these processes—becomes crucial for understanding how risks are articulated and addressed by various stakeholders. Medical advocacy websites, as increasingly prolific sponsors of health media, situate individuals in relation to risk and designate certain beliefs, practices, and bodies as particularly at risk. As a result, analyzing such sites can reveal how individuals are called upon to assess and manage risk at both the personal and social levels.

Informed by rhetorical theory, this analysis of Go Red's health media builds from the assumption that medical advocacy websites are inherently motivated by a desire to persuade. They not only provide descriptions of health and disease but also attempt to convince users to reorient themselves in relation to a particular risk or set of risk factors. In other words, these sites hope to change not only a user's perspective on a disease more broadly as a social and biomedical concern but also a user's personal, individual perception of and response to the risk(s) articulated by the website's messages. In this way, medical advocacy websites are rhetorical. Kenneth Burke (1969) defines the "basic function of rhetoric" as "the use of words by human agents to form attitudes or to induce actions in other human agents" (41). He explains that rhetoric "is not merely descriptive, it is *hortatory*. It is not just trying to tell how things are, in strictly 'scenic' terms; it is trying to *move* people" (41). The following analysis examines how Go Red seeks to move women in response to heart disease risk.

ARTICULATIONS OF RISK IN THE GO
RED FOR WOMEN CAMPAIGN

Although targeted heart disease research began on a large scale with the Framingham Heart Study in 1948, it was not until the late 1980s that researchers made a concerted effort to include women in heart disease studies; for decades, research had been performed exclusively on men, and findings were generalized to both men and women (Legato and Leghe 2010). This shift led to the development of "sex-specific cardiology" (151), or sustained research on heart disease in women.[1]

While sex-specific cardiology seeks to uncover physiological differences between men and women, Go Red articulates risk not only in these terms but also through language that shifts the focus away from a woman's physiological body and toward her social identity. In other words, Go Red articulates what I call *gender-specific risk*. In making this conceptual distinction, I use *sex* to refer to "a biological characterization based primarily on reproductive potential, whereas gender is the social elaboration of biological sex" (Eckert and McConnell-Ginet 2003, 10). While gender often "seems natural" and "beliefs about gender seem to be obvious truth," concepts associated with gender must be examined to explore what seems to many as common sense (9). Rather than being innate, gender is in fact "something we do" and "perform" (10). Therefore, I use the term *sex-specific risk factors* to refer to biological aspects of a woman's body that have been identified by medical professionals as putting her in danger of developing or dying from heart disease. I use the term *gender-specific risk factors* to refer to aspects of a woman's social identity, including her attitudes, beliefs, and behaviors, that have been identified by medical professionals, health campaigns, or the lay public as putting her in danger of developing or dying from heart disease.

Often, a woman's social identity involves adopting the role of a caregiver, and maintaining this role has been shown to compromise a woman's health. The Nurses' Health Study examined the effects of caregiving as a chronic stressor for cardiovascular disease in women and found that caregivers of children, grandchildren, or an ill spouse are at a higher risk of developing heart disease than noncaregivers (Bassuk and Manson 2010, 169). When caring for aging or ill loved ones, women must tend to specialized medical needs, manage medical equipment, and communicate with healthcare professionals (Abel and Nelson 1990). Penelope Eckert and Sally McConnell-Ginet (2003) observe that, despite the difficult tasks women must perform when caring for others, feelings of love and nurturing—or a woman's tendency to display emotional care—are often emphasized within society, while the "instrumental tasks" female caregivers perform are underappreciated in terms of social recognition as well as financial compensation (139).

Through many campaign messages, including its television feature and individual narratives, Go Red suggests a woman's tendency to care for others at the expense of herself puts her at risk for developing heart disease. However, Go Red's messages deemphasize caregiving as an *occupation* or practical duty and instead articulate caregiving as a *mental preoccupation*. By portraying caregiving less as an instrumental task and more as an emotion-driven tendency, the campaign depicts women as selfless and nurturing, an ideal of feminine identity that has long been a part of Western culture (Wood 1994). In the 2008 television feature *Choose to Live*, the narrator explains, "Sometimes women pump so much energy into their children or their careers that they forget themselves in the process, and that can have devastating consequences when it comes to their health and their risk for heart disease" (Choose to Live 2008). The phrase "forget themselves" could be interpreted in many ways. Does the campaign mean to suggest that women do not think about their own health at all? Or that they do think about it but do not take any related actions? In either case, by directly correlating a woman's tendency to "forget" herself with "risk for heart disease," Go Red distills a set of clinically established risk factors into an umbrella cause: self-neglect.

Highlighting this problem on an individual level, the campaign publishes short written narratives on a select group of women[2] each year. These texts are written by an unnamed campaign representative but often include direct quotations from the featured women. Through a process of qualitative analytic coding,[3] I identified emergent themes among forty-eight narratives published from 2008 to 2012 on the campaign website. Nearly half (twenty-three) include references to a woman's tendency to care for others at the expense of herself, and I offer some representative examples in this analysis.

These narratives often characterize a woman's tendency to care for others instead of herself as a lapse in mental focus or attention. Go Red Woman Kimberly states, "'Women, in particular, need to be reminded to take care of our bodies and pay attention when something is not right. . . . We tend to focus so much on how everyone around us is feeling that we forget about ourselves'" (Kimberly's Story, 2013). Echoing the language of *Choose to Live*, Kimberly suggests that women often "'forget'" themselves because they are preoccupied with thoughts about others. This line does not refer to instrumental caregiving tasks a woman might perform but rather to her vague concern for how others are "'feeling.'" Thus, Kimberly implies women are responsive not just to others' immediate needs but also to their general well-being and emotions. While Kimberly's narrative focuses on the identity of women more broadly, Liz's connects womanhood with motherhood in ways typical of many other campaign messages that construct women's identities in terms of their relationships. The narrator states, "Liz Tatham is a mom, and moms know how to fix things." However, Liz realized "that she was so busy fixing things for others, she ignored her symptoms" (Liz's Story 2011). Unlike the term *forget*, the word *ignored* suggests Liz may have noticed the existence of a health concern but purposefully chose not to take action in response because she felt her other obligations were more pressing.

The campaign emphasizes that this tendency to prioritize one's own health last is dangerous and can lead to a failure to perform necessary self-care. Theresa's heart attack made her realize she had been sacrificing too much. She explains, "As women we say, 'Oh, I have to make a doctor's appointment, but this week I have soccer games to attend, so I'll do it next week'" (Theresa's Story 2008). Her perspective suggests women defer their own needs for the benefit of their children. These sacrifices include failing to adhere to medical recommendations for diet, exercise, and doctor visits. Both Theresa and Kimberly use the term *women* to make generalizations about beliefs and behaviors they feel are typical of the female gender. Speaking more directly to her audience but making a similar generalization, Maricela states, "'You take care of your home, you take care of your children, you take care of your husband, you take care of everybody else but yourself. You come in last'" (Maricela's Story 2010). By including these women's quotations in the narratives, Go Red suggests their beliefs and tendencies are gender-specific and invites readers to identify with the women, their perspectives, and their struggles.

ATTRIBUTIONS OF RESPONSIBILITY IN THE GO RED FOR WOMEN CAMPAIGN

Although we might conclude the campaign is problematizing the tendency for a woman to care for herself last, and thereby critiquing the social pressures and assumptions that condition women to behave in these ways, other components of the campaign's messages invite women to continue to occupy these gendered social roles. Indeed, the campaign encourages women to reconceptualize self-care as an outwardly focused act. Whereas the new public health model highlights the need for individuals to monitor their "lifestyles . . . in such a way as to avoid illness" (Petersen and Lupton 1996, 15), Go Red urges a woman to view such monitoring as crucial for avoiding personal illness *so that* she can uphold her responsibilities to others. By focusing on a woman's role as mother and matriarch of her family, Go Red urges women to view self-care as a form of *other*-care, or a way to provide the emotional support that defines her role. Failure to perform self-care impacts not only her own health but also the physical health and emotional well-being of her loved ones.

The thirty-minute television feature *Choose to Live* offers anecdotes from several women's lives. Gail, a middle-aged mom of a teenage daughter, is overcome with emotion as she explains the moment she realized she needed to transform her unhealthy lifestyle: "[My daughter] came to me and said, the way you're going, you're not gonna be around for my children, and that really bothered me, 'cause my children mean everything to me." Gail then began monitoring her diet and training for a 5k, and the film follows her journey to the finish line. Cici, who experienced a heart attack at thirty-one, explains the thoughts and feelings her experience triggered: "My life flashed in front of me, and all I could think about were my two little girls and that I wanted to be around to raise them and take care of them. I just knew I needed to make some life changes." Whereas Gail's daughter's verbal comment served as her catalyst for change, for Cici, the simple thought of her daughters moved her to action.

The narratives of the Go Red women convey similar messages. For instance, "Loraine said it can be hard to find time to do things for herself. But she knows it's important to stay healthy for her family." A quotation from Loraine then explains her moment of change: "'When my father got sick, I decided to take the time because it will eventually help me take care of my children and my children's children'" (Loraine's Story 2008). Although the narrative does not clarify what Loraine will "'take the time'" to do, readers might assume she is referring to the time and effort related to exercise, dietary changes, and learning about heart disease. Loraine is a younger woman, yet she does not focus on immediate benefits of self-care. Instead, she presents lifestyle modifications as an investment in a healthier, more productive, and more caring self much further down the road. Similarly, "Maricela's goal in life is to improve her health so that she can live long and be there for her children and grandchildren" (Maricela's Story 2010). Michelle focuses more on immediate circumstances when she states, "'I *liked* to eat healthy foods and I *liked* to exercise, but I didn't make those things a priority. . . . I love my children with my whole heart, but I've found that the way to put them first is to take care of myself'" (Michelle's Story 2008). Just as other campaign texts emphasize a woman's lack of focus or attention as the root of her self-neglect, here, too, a woman's failure to prioritize properly is singled out as the problem. Here and elsewhere, though, the campaign messages do not explain how exactly a woman might be able to make such changes despite a demanding schedule. These messages assume a change in mental focus or an adjustment in priorities will be enough. Maria's narrative further brings this issue to light. She states, "'In the last three years, I've had no time for myself. I don't have the same energy I used to, but I know that if I don't take care of myself, I can't take care of my family'" (Maria's Story 2009). Despite feeling overwhelmed and exhausted, Maria believes she needs somehow to engage in self-care to maintain her caregiving role; however, she does not mention how she might find ways to do so, leaving the reader to wonder what options, if any, are available to her and other women in similar situations.

While some of the Go Red women's stories focus on the need to care for children or grandchildren, others emphasize the need to spare their children sorrow. Diagnosed with atrial fibrillation and a hole in her heart, and bearing a strong family history of heart disease, young Mary Leah describes the impact of her mother's illness: "'I cried when my mom was diagnosed because I couldn't imagine raising my daughter without her here'" (Mary Leah's Story 2013). In the 2011 short film, *Go Red Moms* (OfficialGoRed4Women 2011a), Jamie urges viewers to take the issue seriously because of the impact heart disease can have on their families. She lost her own mother to heart disease, and so she pleads, "Do this for your kids. If you're not gonna do it for yourself, then do it for your kids, so that they don't have to go through the pain of not having a mother, losing a mother." The conclusion of the 2013 *Go Red Moms* film includes a line of bold text across the screen that reads, "Putting your health first is the No. 1 way to care for your family" (OfficialGoRed4Women 2013). Viewers familiar with Go Red's messages will recognize "No. 1" is often used to refer to heart disease as the leading cause of death among women. Reusing this language in such a way, the campaign suggests women can claim power over this "silent killer" by engaging in self-care and, in so doing, protect not only their own bodies but also their families.

In addition to the responsibility of self-care, Go Red also suggests women need to perform acts of what I call *discursive care* by sharing medical facts and personal stories with others. Through an electronic media kit and other online resources, Go Red encourages women to engage in conversations about heart disease with their loved ones and others. These messages personify heart disease as a "killer" and emphasize the need to protect women from this deadly foe. The 2013 electronic media kit (Media Room) invites women to "Go Red by wearing red, living a healthy lifestyle and speaking red by spreading the message that heart disease is killing our mothers, daughters, sisters and friends." To "Go Red" thus involves visually identifying oneself with the cause, self-regulating one's behaviors, and engaging in awareness-raising communicative practices. This excerpt also defines a woman's identity in relation to her roles in others' lives.

The previous year's electronic media kit (Media Room) includes a similar message: "But the fight is not over. Because this No. 1 killer is still taking the lives of our mothers, sisters, daughters and friends. Because women we love are dying, and many more are impacted every day." Portions of this message are reproduced elsewhere on the website, including downloadable fact sheets. Some messages speak directly to the reader. For instance, the *Just a* Little *Heart Attack*[4] fact sheet (Just a *Little* Heart Attack 2011) warns, "Don't let the women you love become a statistic." By personalizing the numbers and risks, and by situating a global public health problem within the more immediate framework of "women we love," the campaign suggests heart disease is not just an issue for doctors and researchers to address; rather, it is a concern that can disrupt women's closest familial and social bonds. Therefore, the action of *speaking red* becomes one method for women to feel as if they have some power and control in response to a complex, often mysterious medical threat.

This emphasis on speaking to others about heart disease mirrors the viral marketing strategy typical of other health-promotion initiatives, including Merck's Tell Someone campaign (Davies and Burns 2014). Viral marketing encourages individuals to "pass on a marketing message to others creating the potential for exposure and growth of the message" (716). In order for such a strategy to succeed, individuals must have a personal stake and feel motivated to communicate the message. Cristyn Davies and Kelly Burns (2014) show how Merck's campaign "emphasizes individual women's personal responsibility to educate about HPV" and "positions girls and young women as powerful agents with the knowledge and desire to inform their networks about HPV and cervical cancer" (716). In attributing agency to individual women as communicators, however, the campaign inherently limits that agency by telling a woman exactly what she needs to say and do, placing the onus of responsibility on her shoulders, and inferring that if she does not act in accordance with this recommendation, others will suffer.

Go Red draws upon the viral marketing strategy by urging women to believe in the power and importance of their own voices for heart disease education. The campaign situates such communicative acts as a woman's personal responsibility but also as a behavior in line with her innate sense of nurturing and protectiveness. The sentiments expressed by Gloria in this chapter's epigraph (Gloria's Story 2009) represent the type of strong, urgent, and defensive emotional response Go Red hopes other women will feel and act upon. Indeed, Go Red does not simply encourage women to educate others, but to save them, by coining phrases such as "Speak Up to Save Lives"[5] that directly equate communication with prevention of death and imply silence is a failure of responsibility with heavy consequences.

IMPLICATIONS

As individuals continue to turn to the internet for medical knowledge and advice, medical rhetoricians must examine what kinds of resources are offered, by whom, and for what purposes in order to understand how these resources shape the beliefs and actions of particular populations. Gendered resources, specifically, can provide opportunities to uncover intersections between gender and illness both within and outside clinical contexts. This analysis of the Go Red for Women campaign points to the need for further research on such intersectionality with regard to four key topics: gender-specific risk, caregiving practices, the new public health model, and the pragmatics of self-care.

This chapter's definition of *gender-specific risk* can be expanded to include aspects of an individual's gender-based social identity, including attitudes, beliefs, and behaviors, that have been identified by medical professionals, health campaigns, or the lay public as raising the likelihood of disease. Such a definition allows us to read gender outside binary constructions and within a range of disease contexts. Analyzing medical advocacy sites and other health media with attention to such articulations of risk can help us understand how health campaigns reflect and reproduce dominant social norms related to gender. For instance, even though Go Red problematizes a woman's tendency to care for others before herself, it reinforces the caring role as a particularly female trait by encouraging women to engage in self-care for the benefit of others. Such discourse assumes many women could not be persuaded to care for themselves unless they believed the benefits of these actions would ultimately be unselfish. Further research might examine how aspects of gender, rather than sex assigned at birth, are identified as sources of disease risk and therefore causes for monitoring by the self and also by medical professionals.

Go Red's insistence that women view self-care as outwardly focused rests on the assumption that women are inherently caregivers, even though the campaign often defines caregiving as simply a vague and persistent concern about others rather than the performance of specific tasks. Analysis of this campaign's discourse reveals the need to examine the social constraints that shape women's caregiving work both instrumentally (such as caring for an ill family member or working in a nursing home) and emotionally (such as worrying about others' needs in ways articulated by Go Red). Since research has found associations between instrumental caregiving and heart disease risk in women (Bassuk and Manson 2010), we must not only find ways to reduce caregivers' risk but also interrogate the social conditions within which women are, by default, the carers. As Eckert and McConnell-Ginet (2003) observe, a societal emphasis on women's feelings of love and nurturing can lead to the perceptual and financial devaluation of their caregiving work. Thus, gender norms that persist over time can shape cultural views of gender roles and responsibilities while also relegating certain tasks to women simply because women are assumed to be naturally suited for them. By encouraging women to view self-care as a form of *other*-care, Go Red reinforces care as a typically female occupation and mental preoccupation and in turn misses an opportunity to empower a woman to view self-care as meaningful and worthwhile for herself. Without ignoring or minimizing the value of a women's love for her family, the campaign's messages about heart disease could be enriched by considering why women may feel they need to justify self-care or feel guilty for taking time for themselves. Further research might examine intersections between gender and caregiving in health campaigns and consider whether and how concepts of *care* emerge in messages aimed at men.

Gendered social norms should also be examined within the context of the new public health model. Within this model, contemporary health campaigns emphasize the individual's responsibility for maintaining health and preventing disease. While at times such messages are empowering, at other times they place blame on those who become sick and therefore must not have tried hard enough to be healthy. Such health media reflect the ideologies of the biomedical health system. As Caitlin Leach (this collection) emphasizes, this system articulates modifiable risk factors as problems an individual should be able to solve and in turn minimizes or ignores social context and structural factors that affect an individual's health-related beliefs and behaviors. These blame attributions may become amplified in the context of health messages that recast self-care as *other*-care and therefore suggest a personal health failure holds consequences beyond the self. This chapter acknowledges health campaigns can effectively motivate and inspire individuals to make changes that improve their health, self-efficacy, and outlook on life. However, it is important to consider how an overemphasis on individual responsibility might lead to guilt, blame, and a sense of defeat among individuals who cannot reach a desired health outcome. Furthermore, discourse that identifies women as prone to self-neglect implies women must be subjected to more rigorous disciplining, not only because their bodies are unruly, as Miriam Mara (this collection) discusses, but also because their judgment is unreliable. Further research could consider how personal responsibilities are assigned in health campaigns targeting a specific gender and what differences among campaigns suggest about gendered assumptions regarding responsibility and decision-making.

Finally, Go Red's framing of self-care as a necessary practice for women calls into question the pragmatics of such self-care and the limitations that a woman, or an individual of any gender, might face in the pursuit of it. Taking care of oneself is not as simple as remembering to go to the gym or understanding the basics of nutrition. Obstacles stemming from lack of financial resources, inadequate access to care, language barriers, preexisting medical conditions, lack of social support, and demanding work schedules, among other causes, impact one's ability to engage in self-care despite a desire to do so. Therefore, further research might investigate the extent to which gendered health-media messages acknowledge and unpack the pragmatics of self-care, either by inviting discussion of individuals' situations and challenges or by providing resources to address those challenges.

As a health campaign aiming to change the beliefs and behaviors of women at risk for heart disease, Go Red seeks to move women to action by persuading them they need to take care of themselves in order to care for others in their lives. By calling attention to the many demands placed upon women's time and energy, the campaign is poised to critique the social constraints and gender-based expectations women face. However, the campaign falls short of questioning these norms and instead reinforces them by urging a woman to perform self-care *so that* she can continue to occupy the caregiver role. Beth Boser (this collection) finds a similarly troubling celebration of traditional gender roles in postpartum-distress discourse. Her analysis of a self-help book on the topic reveals that even though the book suggests postpartum distress has social causes, it does not offer a satisfying critique of those causes or offer solutions for women to break out of socially imposed constraints, including the expectation to be an ideal mother. Instead, women are advised to manage those challenges effectively; thus, the solution is located at the individual level. In advising women to improve their level of self-care, Go Red similarly shifts the conversation away from problematic social constraints and toward individual self-management. Such self-management, the campaign suggests, will not only reduce a woman's risk for heart disease but also allow her to maintain her gendered identity. Further research should address the extent to which gendered health communication simultaneously problematizes and upholds traditional gender roles and stereotypes.

NOTES

1. Sex-specific cardiology has explored the effects of hormonal changes, menopause, and hormonal replacement therapies on women's heart disease risks; revealed differences between men's and women's artery size and cardiac-chamber size (Legato and Leghe 2010, 151–152); and uncovered that women's heart attack symptoms less often include the "crushing central chest pain" typical of heart attacks in men (Worrall-Carter et al. 2011, 529). Instead, women feel vague symptoms, a circumstance that often leads to delays in reporting and symptom recognition, misdiagnoses, and death (529–533). These symptoms include "back pain, indigestion, breathlessness, weakness, dizziness, and a general feeling of malaise or 'just not feeling well,' as well as pain in the chest, the arm, and the jaw" (American 2009, 4).

2. The campaign conducts a yearly "casting call" to choose women willing to share their heart disease stories. These women become the public faces and voices of the campaign, and their stories are presented in various forms throughout Go Red's web- and print-based materials. From 2008 to 2012, these women were identified as the Go Red Women. The campaign has since changed their designation to Real Women or Survivors.

3. I followed the procedures outlined by Emerson, et al. (2011) in *Writing Ethnographic Fieldnotes.*

4. The campaign released a brief film called *Just a* Little *Heart Attack* in 2011 as a promotional piece that uses exaggeration and humor to warn women of their risk for heart disease. Directed by and starring actress Jennifer Banks, the film depicts a busy working mom who fails to notice heart attack symptoms as she hurries to get herself, her husband, and her children ready in the morning (OfficialGoRed-4Women 2011b). This film is viewable through the campaign's YouTube channel.

5. In 2010, the campaign released a thirty-minute television special on NBC called *Speak Up to Save Lives* along with related promotional material, including a discussion guide for women to use when planning private fundraisers and discussion-centered events.

REFERENCES

Abel, Emily K., and Margaret K. Nelson. 2010. "Circles of Care: An Introductory Essay." In *Circles of Care: Work and Identity in Women's Lives*, edited by Emily K. Abel and Margaret K. Nelson, 4–34. Albany: SUNY Press.

American Heart Association. 2008. *Choose to Live*. www.goredforwomen.org. 1 June 2012.

American Heart Association. 2009. *Complete Guide to Women's Heart Health: The Go Red For Women Way to Well-Being and Vitality*. New York: Clarkson Potter.

American Heart Association. 2010. *Speak Up to Save Lives*. www.goredforwomen.org. 1 June 2012.

Cone. n.d. "Go Red for Women." http://www.conecomm.com/case-studies/aha-go-red-for-women/.

Bassuk, Shari S., and JoAnn E. Manson. (2010). "Gender-Specific Aspects of Selected Coronary Heart Disease Risk Factors: A Summary of the Epidemiologic Evidence." In *Principles of Gender-Specific Medicine*, 2nd ed., edited by Marianne J. Legato, 162–174. Burlington, MA: Academic Press.

Burke, Kenneth. 1969. *A Rhetoric of Motives*. Berkeley: University of California Press.

Davies, Cristyn, and Kellie Burns. 2014. "Mediating Healthy Female Citizenship in the HPV Vaccination Campaigns." *Feminist Media Studies* 14 (5): 711–726.

Eckert, Penelope, and Sally McConnell-Ginet. 2003. *Language and Gender*. Cambridge, MA: Cambridge University Press.

Emerson, Robert M., Rachel I. Fretz, and Linda L. Shaw. 2011. *Writing Ethnographic Fieldnotes*. Chicago: University of Chicago Press.

Gloria's Story. 2009. American Heart Association. www.goredforwomen.org. 8 June 2012.

Go Red for Women. 2013. American Heart Association. www.goredforwomen.org.

Go Red for Women. n.d. "About Go Red for Women." https://www.goredforwomen.org/en/about-go-red-for-women.

Just a *Little* Heart Attack Fact Sheet. 2011. American Heart Association. www.goredforwomen.org. PDF. 27 January 2014.

Kimberly's Story. 2013. American Heart Association. www.goredforwomen.org. 10 July 2013.

Legato, Marianne J., and Jaswinder K. Leghe. 2010. "Gender and the Heart. Sex-Specific Differences in the Normal Myocardial Anatomy and Physiology." In *Principles of Gender-Specific Medicine*, 2nd ed., edited by Marianne J. Legato, 151–161. Elsevier.

Liz's Story. 2011. American Heart Association. www.goredforwomen.org. 1 June 2012.

Loraine's Story. 2008. American Heart Association. www.goredforwomen.org. 8 June 2012.

Maria's Story. 2009. American Heart Association. www.goredforwomen.org. 8 June 2012.

Maricela's Story. 2010. American Heart Association. www.goredforwomen.org. 1 June 2012.

Mary Leah's Story. 2013. American Heart Association. www.goredforwomen.org. 10 July 2013.

"Media Room." American Heart Association. 27 January 2014. www.goredforwomen.org.

Michelle's Story. 2008. American Heart Association. www.goredforwomen.org. 8 June 2012.

Moeller, Marie. 2014. "Pushing Boundaries of Normalcy: Employing Critical Disability Studies in Analyzing Medical Advocacy Websites." *Communication Design Quarterly* 2 (4): 52–80.

OfficialGoRed4Women. 2011a. "Go Red Moms." *YouTube*. Web. September 19, 2011.

OfficialGoRed4Women. 2011b. "Just a *Little* Heart Attack." *YouTube*. Web. August 31, 2011.

OfficialGoRed4Women. 2013. "Go Red Moms 2013." *YouTube*. Web. September 13, 2013.

Official Yearly Narratives. American Heart Association. www.goredforwomen.org. See individual names.

Petersen, Alan, and Deborah Lupton. 1996. *The New Public Health: Health and Self in the Age of Risk*. London: SAGE.

Theresa's Story. 2008. American Heart Association. www.goredforwomen.org. 8 June 2012.

Wood, Julia T. 1994. *Who Cares? Women, Care, and Culture*. Carbondale: Southern Illinois University Press.

Worrall-Carter, Linda, Chantal Ski, Elizabeth Scruth, Michelle Campbell, and Karen Page. 2011. "Systematic Review of Cardiovascular Disease in Women: Assessing the Risk." *Nursing and Health Sciences* 13 (4): 529–535.

SECTION V

Textual Examinations

12

PATHOLOGIZING BLACK FEMALE BODIES
The Construction of Difference in Contemporary Breast Cancer Research

Jordan Liz

According to the Human Genome Project, all humans are 99.9 percent similar in our genetic makeup (2000). At the time this statement was issued, it provided further support to similar remarks made by UNESCO's 1950 "The Race Question," Richard Lewontin's 1972 observation that there is more genetic variation within than between groups, and the 1998 "Statement on Race" by the American Anthropological Association, to name a few (UNESCO 1950; Lewontin 1972, American Anthropological Association 1998). Indeed, it seemed to suggest that perhaps, finally, the myth of biological races was debunked (Roberts 2012; Sussman 2014; Yudell 2014). As Peter Chow-White writes, "With this evidence, many constituencies within and beyond the academy trumpeted the end of biological notions of race and the scientific validation of race as a social construction" (292). Nevertheless, some contemporary population geneticists posit that not only do the five racial groups—European, African, Native American, Asian, and Pacific Islander—correspond to discrete genetic clusters but additionally that some races are genetically more susceptible to certain diseases: African American women to breast cancer, African American men to prostate cancer, and Mexicans to type-2 diabetes (Palmer et al. 2013; SIGMA 2014; Han et al. 2015).

To elaborate further, a 2013 study found a statistically significant positive relationship between one's degree of African ancestry and a triple-negative breast cancer risk variant in the TERT gene (Palmer et al. 2013).[1] In their account, this correlation partially explains the differences in breast cancer prevalence between African American and white women. As the authors note, "In an African American population, that percent African ancestry is strongly associated with triple-negative breast

DOI: 10.7330/9781607329855.c012

cancer. This finding provides further evidence that genetic factors play a role in the disproportionately high prevalence of this breast cancer subtype among African American women and highlights the need for further discovery of variants that contribute to this disparity" (133). To be clear, this claim entails that, independent of socioeconomic factors, merely being a woman of African ancestry predisposes one to breast cancer at a higher rate than white women.

In this chapter, I aim to provide a critical philosophical examination of two recent case studies (Palmer et al. 2012; Palmer et al. 2013) concerning the genetic susceptibility of African American women to breast cancer. The purpose of this analysis is to unearth a series of assumptions regarding race, gender, and disease susceptibility operative in these studies. The goal, then, is to determine what assumptions are required in order to make the conclusions reached by these studies epistemically possible. Of particular interest is attempting to determine how African American and white femininity are constructed in relation to one another within this scientific discourse.

Now, it may be objected from the outset that an analysis of two studies is too limited to draw any major conclusions about the use of race within genetic studies broadly speaking. It is important, however, to recognize that the conception of race, sex, and disease deployed in these studies is part of the paradigm of contemporary population genetics. That conception is not isolated from the rest of the biomedicine sciences but rather is made possible by them. As a result, whatever conclusions may be drawn from an analysis of these two articles has implications for understanding how African American females are pathologized by geneticists and biomedical researchers beyond the women involved in the two studies directly examined in this chapter.

The sections of this chapter are organized as follows: (1) an overview of recent claims made by biomedical researchers concerning the genetic susceptibility of certain nonwhites to certain diseases, (2) a summary of the two case studies in detail followed by (3) an analysis of what those studies entail about how African American femininity is being implicitly conceived of within the biomedical discourse and, finally, (4) a concluding section that briefly summarizes the main points of this analysis.

SECTION 1: RACE, ETHNICITY AND GENETIC CLUSTERS

Before turning to the two specific case studies, it is helpful to begin by discussing how geneticists and biomedical researchers generate unique genetic clusters that correspond to the five racial groups. One prominent example is offered by a study conducted by Noah Rosenberg et al. (2002). As they note, while most studies of human variation begin with populations defined by culture or geography, such populations may not correspond to an underlying genetic relationship. Consequently, in their study they analyze the genetic similarities between a set of predefined populations and various genetic populations using samples from the HGDP-CEPH Human Genome Diversity Cell Line Panel. According to their account, determining whether these populations are genetically significant may contribute to studies in human evolution and epidemiology.

To perform this analysis, Rosenberg et al. (2002) performed a model-based clustering algorithm using the population analysis software called STRUCTURE. The software places individuals into K clusters, where K is equal to a preselected number of groups. Each increase in K produces a division of one of the clusters produced at the previous level. At each K, the algorithm was performed ten times; for the most part, each run produced results with nearly identical individual membership coefficients. The exceptions were four runs at $K=3$ that separated East Asia into a third category, instead of in Eurasia, and one run at $K=6$ that separated Karitiana instead of Kalash. At $K=2$, the clusters were anchored by Africa and the Americas, regions with large genetic distance. As Rosenberg et al. further note, "At $K=5$, clusters corresponded largely to major geographic regions. However, the next cluster at $K=6$ did not match a major region but consisted largely of individuals of the isolated Kalash group, who speak an Indo-European language and live in northwest Pakistan" (2382). Based on their analysis, Rosenberg et al. conclude that "predefined labels were highly informative about membership in genetic clusters, even for intermediate populations, in which most individuals had similar membership coefficients across clusters" (2384). Moreover, they further conclude that "for many applications in epidemiology, as well as for assessing individual disease risks, self-reported population ancestry likely provides a suitable proxy for genetic ancestry" (2384). They do note, however, that for studies using more recently admixed populations, the use of genetic clusters is more appropriate than self-reported ancestry.

SECTION 2: AFRICAN AMERICAN WOMEN IN BREAST CANCER DISCOURSE

Lisa Carey at al. (2006) performed a study to determine any genetic correlation between a female patient's race and her susceptibility to different breast cancer subtypes. Of particular interest was basal-like breast cancer, or triple-negative breast cancer. According to Carey et al., basal-like breast cancer is more prevalent in premenopausal African American women (39 percent) than in postmenopausal African American women (14 percent) or non-African American women (16 percent). Race was self-reported by the study's 496 participants (196 African American, 300 non-African American). While a mutation in the *BRCA1* gene is considered in part responsible for the appearance of basal-like tumors, none of the African American women in the study were identified as carriers of that mutation. As such, Carey et al. conclude that the absence of *BRCA1* carriers suggests "that genes other than *BRCA1* could predispose women to basal-like breast cancer; however, environmental and socioeconomic factors could also play a role in the observed distribution of breast cancer subtypes" (2501).

This study by Carey et al. (2006) presents one of the earliest since the Human Genome Project to posit a relationship between self-reported race and likelihood of developing breast cancer.[2] Still, already in this study is an important point about the nature of race and genetics—namely, that racial disparities in disease prevalence may be explainable by appeals to distinct genetic factors. As such, if breast cancer is more prevalent among African American women, despite the absence of the *BRCA1* gene, then some other genes may be responsible. While socioeconomic and environmental factors are not eliminated from consideration, the notion that one's self-reported race correlates to a specific genetic cluster makes it plausible to consider whether race-specific biological factors are affecting differences in disease susceptibility.

To explore this further, I now turn to two recent case studies, one by Julie Palmer, Deborah Boggs, Lauren Wise, Lucile Adams-Campbell, and Lynn Rosenberg, which was published in 2012, and another by Palmer, Edward Ruiz-Narvaez, Charles Rotimi, L. Adrienne Cupples, Yvette Cozier, Lucile Adams-Campbell, and Lynn Rosenberg, which was published in 2013, that examine this relationship between African American women and breast cancer susceptibility. While both cases examine breast cancer susceptibility among African American women, each has a distinct focus: the first focuses on the impact of socioeconomic status on racial disparities in breast cancer, while the second focuses more specifically on genetic factors. Given these differences, examining both sheds further light on how race, sex, and disease are formulated in the current paradigm of biomedical research.

Case 1: Breast Cancer, Socioeconomic Status, and Race

According to Palmer et al. (2012), several studies indicate breast cancer incidence is greater in areas of higher socioeconomic status. These studies note that women with higher socioeconomic status tend to have their first birth at a later age, low parity, and menopausal female-hormone use. However, such women also tend to have high levels of educational attainment. This raises the question, is it living in a wealthy neighborhood or is it a person's personal level of education (independent of their neighborhood) that raises the likelihood of developing breast cancer? To disentangle this effect, Palmer et al. distinguish between two measures of socioeconomic status: "individual SES," defined as self-reported level of education, and "neighborhood SES," defined as an index derived from six indicators of income and education (measures taken from the US Census). These indicators are meant to measure the environmental effects of socioeconomic status, on the one hand, and individual/personal effects on the other hand.

At the time of this Palmer et al. publication in 2012, only two studies had considered individual-level SES and neighborhood SES simultaneously; however, both of those focused exclusively on white women. One study found that, controlling for individual-level SES and breast cancer risk factors, white women living in the top quintile of neighborhood SES had 20 percent greater odds of developing breast cancer than women at the lowest quintile. The second study similarly found that the odds of developing breast cancer were 30 percent higher for those living in the highest socioeconomic neighborhood relative to the lowest, and 20 percent higher for those with the highest educational attainment relative to the lowest. Now, unlike their white counterparts, African American women with the same level of education and income as the white women studied tend to live in poorer neighborhoods—they have similar individual SES but differ in neighborhood SES. "Thus, it may be more feasible to disentangle the individual effects of personal and neighborhood SES on breast cancer incidence by studying African American women" (Palmer et al. 2012, 1141). In addition to overall breast cancer incidence, Palmer et al. (2012) examined the incidence of estrogen receptor-positive (ER+) and estrogen receptor-negative (ER-) breast cancer, given that each is associated with a unique set of risk factors.

For the 2012 Palmer et al. study, data on African American women were acquired from the Black Women's Health Study. The study was initiated in 1995 and included 59,000 African American women ages twenty-one to sixty-nine from seventeen states throughout the United States. Data from 55,896 women between 1995 and 2009 were included in the analysis. At the time, these women completed health question-naires that provided information on several factors including "medical history, height and current weight, weight at age 18 years, age at men-arche, parity, age at first birth, lactation, breast cancer in a first-degree relative, hours per week of vigorous physical activity, alcohol consump-tion, cigarette smoking, menopausal status, age at menopause, oral contraceptive use, supplemental female hormone use, mammography use, and years of education" (Palmer et al. 2012, 1142). In 2003, the questionnaire was updated to include questions concerning fam-ily income. Follow-up questionnaires were sent to participants on a biennial basis. Information on disease incidence and risk factors was updated through these follow-ups. Reports of cancer diagnosis were validated through hospital pathology data and/or state cancer regis-tries. Records were acquired for 85 percent of these cases, of which 99 percent were confirmed.

Through geocoding, participants' addresses were linked to the 2000 US Census block data that included twenty-nine variables representing wealth and education. From these twenty-nine variables, the six most representative variables were selected to measure neighborhood SES. The variables selected were (1) median household income, (2) median housing value, (3) percentage of households receiving interest, divi-dend, or net rental income, (4) percentage of adults twenty-five years or older that have completed college, (5) percentage of employed persons aged sixteen years or older that are in occupations classified as manage-rial, executive, or professional specialty, and (6) percentage of families with children not headed by a single female (Palmer et al. 2012, 1142). These variables were used to construct an overall neighborhood SES score, with higher scores corresponding to wealthier neighborhoods. Of the 1,406 confirmed cases of breast cancer, 1,343 were success-fully geocoded and linked to the 2000 Census block data. Information about estrogen status (whether positive or negative) was available for 1,006 cases. The neighborhood SES score was updated every two years, depending on whether the person moved or, if she did not, if the score of the neighborhood had increased or decreased.

According to their statistical analysis, both neighborhood SES and individual SES were positively correlated with incidence of estrogen-receptor-positive breast cancer, after adjusting for age. However, two variables—parity (i.e., the number of greater-than-twenty-weeks births) and age at first birth—highly correlated with both measures of socioeconomic status. After controlling for these variables, the associa-tion between the SES variables and ER+ breast cancer was no longer statistically significant. Controlling for additional risk factors brought the association even closer to the null. Given that ER+ breast cancer is less common among African American women, this finding may explain why previous studies focusing predominately on white women found strong positive correlations between socioeconomic status and breast cancer incidence. That said, with regard to ER– breast cancer, "there was little evidence in the present study of a positive association of ER– cancer incidence with individual or neighborhood SES" (Palmer et al. 2012, 1145). More specifically, the analysis indicated a weak positive correlation between ER– cancer incidence and personal level of education, and a weak inverse correlation with neighborhood SES. Both of these associations, however, were statistically insignificant. In summary, then, while individual and neighborhood SES were positively correlated with the incidence of ER+ breast cancer, both were uncorrelated with the incidence of ER– breast cancer (1146).

Case 2: Racial Genetic Susceptibility to Breast Cancer

Genome-wide association studies (GWAS) performed on European and Asian-ancestry populations have found more than thirty single nucleotide polymorphisms (SNPs) related to breast cancer.[3] Most of these, however, are more strongly associated with ER+ breast cancer, which is the breast cancer subtype most prevalent in these populations. At the time of the 2013 Palmer et al.'s study's publication, no new genetic loci for ER+ breast cancer had been discovered from an African-ancestry population. However, GWAS performed on African-ancestry and European-ancestry populations identified a variant in the TERT gene associated with ER– breast cancer (Palmer et al. 2013). Moreover, studies of European-ancestry populations have identified a few more SNPs related to this particular breast cancer subtype. In the United States, ER– breast cancer is twice as common in women of African ancestry compared to other ancestral groups and is the most prevalent kind of cancer in Africa (Palmer et al. 2013). For this reason, it is vital to determine whether genetic loci from European- and Asian-ancestry populations contribute to the onset of ER– and triple-negative breast cancer among African American women.

Palmer et al. (2013) analyzed twenty-four SNPs that had reached genome-wide significance in either European- or Asian-ancestry populations to examine their association with overall breast cancer incidence and with specific subtypes. Moreover, to determine whether these genetic factors contribute to the higher incidence of these breast cancer subtypes in African American women, they "examined the relation of global ancestry (African versus European) to subtype of breast cancer" (128). In addition, thirty ancestry-informative markers (AIMs) were used to estimate and control for "population stratification due to European admixture" (128).

Data for this study were derived from the Black Women's Health Study. DNA samples were acquired from 26,800 of the participants. This subset of participants tended to be older but was still representative with respect to geographic location, education, body mass index, and family history of breast cancer. For this study, the case group consisted of participants who had provided a sample and been diagnosed with breast cancer since 2010. Controls consisted of participants who had provided a sample and had not been diagnosed with breast cancer as of 2010. The analysis also controlled for age and geographic region (Northeast, South, Midwest and West) (Palmer et al. 2013, 128). In total, the analysis included 1,199 breast cancer cases (336 classified as ER+; 229 as ER−; 81 as triple-negative), and 1,948 controls.

Of the twenty-four SNPs identified in European- and Asian-ancestry populations, five were present in the African American sample. Of particular note, the risk allele rs10069690 in the TERT gene had previously been associated with ER− breast cancer. Palmer et al. (2013) found this variant in higher frequency (0.57) in women of African ancestry than in those of European ancestry (0.27) and concluded that "the observed association likely explains part of the excess incidence of ER− breast cancer in African American women" (131). They further noted that, assuming the effect size is similar, this genetic locus may account for 15 percent of the greater incidence of triple-negative breast cancer in African American women, compared to those of European ancestry. That said, it seems possible that the effect size is actually larger in African American women, which would entail that this locus would account for upwards of 26 percent of the higher incidence of triple-negative breast cancer (131).

In addition to rs10069690 and rs8170, an SNP in the *BABAM1* gene—which prevents the expression of estrogen receptors traditionally associated with European ancestry—was found to be present in populations with African ancestry. The risk allele appears in a frequency of 0.25 in cases of triple-negative breast cancer and is associated with a 48 percent risk increase. Important, however, this variant was found in similar frequencies in African American and European samples and thus is unlikely to explain differences in incidence between the populations. Three additional SNPs were replicated in the African American sample: an SNP at the 10q26 locus associated only with ER+ breast cancer and two SNPs at 19p13 associated only with ER– breast cancer. While these results differed from other studies, Palmer et al. (2013) note that such "results may be due to chance" (132).

The study also found that African American women with a greater degree of African ancestry were much more likely to develop both ER– and triple-negative breast cancer. More specifically, "relative to women with ER+/PR+ breast cancer, women with ER-/PR- cancer were twice as likely to be in the highest quintile of African ancestry and women with triple-negative breast cancer were 3 times as likely to be in that quintile" (Palmer 2013, 132). These numbers suggest there may be risk variants unique to those of African ancestry that increase their genetic susceptibility to these breast cancer subtypes. Thus, the study concludes that "in an African American population, that percent African ancestry is strongly associated with triple-negative breast cancer. This finding provides further evidence that genetic factors play a role in the disproportionately high prevalence of this breast cancer subtype among African American women and highlights the need for further discovery of variants that contribute to this disparity" (133). As such, in addition to attempting to replicate risk variants found in European and Asian populations in African-ancestry populations, further research is needed to discover those unique risk variants. Such studies will help shed new light on the pathogenesis of these breast cancer subtypes in African-ancestry populations.

SECTION 3: THE PATHOLOGIZATION OF AFRICAN AMERICAN WOMEN

In the previous section, I summarized the methodology, analysis, and conclusions of two recent case studies. While brief, these overviews provide much insight into how claims concerning race, sex, and genetic susceptibility are constructed. In this section, I articulate three problematic assumptions operative in their accounts.

First Assumption: The Classed Racial Body

In the first article examined above, Palmer et al. (2012) sought to disentangle the differing effects of what they termed "individual SES" and "neighborhood SES" on breast cancer incidence. Specifically, however, their analysis is focused on breast cancer rates among white women. Because white women tend to live in neighborhoods that mirror their personal educational and income level, the individual effects of these SES variables become intertwined. In other words, focusing on white women, it is difficult to determine the extent of the effect of each specific variable on the onset of breast cancer. There is a problem of endogeneity. However, unlike white women, a noticeable discrepancy between these two variables is observed among African American women. As Palmer et al. note, given educational and income levels similar to white women, African American women tend to live in poorer socioeconomic neighborhoods. Because of this, they constitute the ideal group for measuring the differing effects of these two variables.

The framing of this problem is significant as it reveals that despite not being part of the study population, understanding cancer rates among white women is the true objective of this analysis, and a concern over the cancer rates of white women motivates this project. African American women are, then, only a means by which this can occur; they are a convenient object that allows us to disentangle the effects of these two distinct ways of understanding socioeconomic status. Now, this objectification may not seem entirely problematic. After all, it is the nature of scientific analysis to objectify individuals or populations for the sake of acquiring knowledge about some topic. That said, it may be argued that this instance of scientific objectification is particularly problematic for a few reasons. Most important, perhaps, it glosses over the fact that the reason women of color with equal educational and income status nevertheless live in poorer neighborhoods than white women is due to a legacy of institutional racism and sexism in the United States (Collins 1993; Crenshaw 1991; Guillaumin 2004). As a result, it fails to understand the limitations of any socioeconomic status that does not attempt to account for the lived experience of marginalized minorities (Williams, Priest, and Anderson 2016).

Indeed, the 2012 Palmer et al. article presupposes that variables for socioeconomic status may be neutrally constructed absent racial considerations—perhaps this presupposition is why the article does not take into account the educational level or income of one's parents when attempting to determine individual SES. In doing so, they seem to construct a variable best suited for measuring this status among white women and, more specifically, those of the upper-to-middle class. After all, if the goal is to disentangle the effect of neighborhood SES and individual SES, then race did not need to be introduced. While it is the case that African Americans tend to be poorer than white people, and that their poverty tends to be structurally different, there are nevertheless wealthy African Americans living in poor neighborhoods and impoverished white people living in affluent neighborhoods (Jargowsky 2013). Recognizing this is important because, within this medical discourse, one's self-reported race corresponds to a distinct racial genetic cluster. As a result, the use of race as a proxy for socioeconomic factor is made problematic insofar as race is also a biological category. Its usage here then seems to suggest an implicit commitment that white people are wealthy and African Americans are not, thereby erasing women of both races who do not fit this narrative.

Second Assumption: The Mechanical Racial Body

One of the conclusions of the first article (Palmer et al. 2012) is that both individual SES and neighborhood SES only weakly correlate with incidence of ER– breast cancer. However, both correlations are statistically insignificant, thereby revealing that these two measures have no effect on the incidence of this subtype of breast cancer in African American women. This finding is significant since, as the article emphasizes, ER– breast cancer is the most common subtype affecting this group of women. Here the problem of framing mentioned above is important: the researchers begin with a question concerning the cancer rates of white women and, more specifically, how those rates are determined by the women's socioeconomic status. Next, to analyze the differing effects of individual versus neighborhood SES, they examine how those variables affect the incidence of breast cancer in African American women. Ultimately, they determine neither variable contributes to that incidence. The initial assumption seems to be that the breast cancer of white women is determined, at least in part, by their socioeconomic status. However, important, their conclusion seems to suggest that those environmental factors play little role with regards to African American women.

To further elaborate, within these medical discourses, race is being used as a biological marker to describe certain biological phenomena and, more specifically, to address certain problems in the study of disease, such as the problem of "missing causality"—the underlying reason disease incidence differs between racial minority groups (Skim et al. 2015). As discussed in the previous sections, several studies point to certain genetic features found more commonly in a racial group's genetic make-up as a way of explaining differences between populations in the prevalence of a disease. The issue, however, is whether enough attention is being given to how these problems are being articulated. As Janet Skim et al. (2015) note, in discussing the problem of "missing causality," for example, geneticists and biomedical researchers already assume the answer has both environmental and genetic elements. Perhaps more important, geneticists and biomedical researchers seem to assume those

genetic elements are distinct from socioeconomic factors. The presump-
tion is that, if socioeconomic factors were the sole contributor to these
kinds of complex diseases, variables measuring such factors would yield
complete explanatory power. Their failure to do so indicates genetics
must be involved. Therefore, by incorporating a biological understanding of race (as opposed to a sociopolitical understanding of race) into
these discussions, the relationship between race and disease prevalence
seems to be geneticized from the outset.

According to this dichotomy of environment versus genetics, in
Palmer et al. (2012) the conclusion that neither measure of socioeconomic status is correlated with the incidence of ER– breast cancer entails
that African American women's greater disease burden is due solely to
genetic factors. As Palmer et al. (2013) note, certain risk variants, such as
rs10069690 in the TERT gene, are found in greater frequency in African
American women and thereby may help partially explain the disparity
in incidence. Indeed, this risk variant, by their estimates, potentially
accounts for a 15 percent higher incidence in triple-negative breast
cancer. Important, this estimate assumes this variant has the same effect
size in African American women as it does in white women. Palmer
et al. (2013), however, speculate the effect size is actually greater in
African American women and thereby may account for 26 percent of
the higher incidence. Now, to be clear, these genetic differences are
characterized in such a way that their presence is not a byproduct of
their environment but rather of some inherent particularity of their
racial genetic substructure. The source of this genetic uniqueness, then,
is not regarded as potentially deriving from the unique characteristics
of African American culture and/or an environment influencing the
expression of certain genes.

This characterization is significant because, as Sandra Soo-Jin Lee
(2008) argues, it shifts the responsibility from public health campaigns
directed at improving the conditions of poor communities to the
already disenfranchised and discriminated-against person of color.
However, aside from the ethical and political implications, this shift is
important for how we conceptualize difference and disease within the
biomedical sciences.

Third Assumption: The Abnormal Racial Body

How is genetic susceptibility understood? According to the World
Health Organization (WHO), any individual born with a greater risk of
acquiring a disease has a genetic predisposition or susceptibility to it,

as "the genetic susceptibility to a particular disease due to the presence of one or more gene mutations, and/or a combination of alleles need not necessarily be abnormal" (World 2016). The final phrase of that statement—"need not necessarily be abnormal"—is worth considering in more detail. It entails that having a genetic susceptibility to some disease is not itself abnormal. Given that members of all racial groups show some degree of susceptibility to a disease, this may not seem surprising. Moreover, the medical sciences routinely establish distinctions between the normal and the pathological, between the healthy body and its diseased (or in this case extrasusceptible) opposite. The medical sciences understand these concepts as being not only unproblematic but also necessary for their practice; after all, if health is the goal of these sciences, they must be able to identify illness.

However, that the genetic susceptibility of some can be regarded as abnormal is significant. As French philosopher of medicine Georges Canguilhem (1991) argues, the concepts of the normal and the pathological cannot be interpreted as simply a statistical mean; rather, they are concepts deeply intertwined with political, economic, and technological significance. What is "normal" from the perspective of the biological sciences is never discovered, nor is it discoverable because a living system does not operate according to a strict mathematical law. That is, unlike the objects of the physical sciences (e.g., physics or chemistry), the objects of the life sciences should not be reduced to mechanical and technical models—the organism is not a machine. The normal and the pathological are, then, designations made upon biological objects. Moreover, as Canguilhem further notes, to establish clear-cut distinctions between these concepts presupposes not only a mechanistic understanding of the body but in addition a homogeneity among bodies. Both of these assumptions are, for Canguilhem, unfounded. If that is the case, however, the normal and the pathological are contingent. Disease, then, is never a neutral concept. It is, as with every other scientific concept, influenced by a matrix of social, political, economic, and technological factors.

But, what exactly is the normal in discussions of racial genetic susceptibility? And, more important, why is it the norm? As others, such as historian Anne Pollock (2012) and anthropologist Michael Montoya (2011) have noted, the normal population appears to be European. In both studies discussed above, the abnormal prevalence of ER– breast cancer in African American women is established in direct comparison to white women. Moreover, both proceed to explain this by beginning with the data gathered from studies concentrated primarily on

Europeans and then determining what is present in African Americans in addition to the Eurasian risk variants. These additional risk variants, "novel" to the African American group, are then taken to explain the difference in disease prevalence. Even the determination of lower or higher risk is not neutral given that these terms are always relative to others. It is only in comparison to a white baseline that members of other racial groups are labeled more susceptible.

Now, it may be objected that the European is only the norm, or the baseline, because so much research has been performed on that group. The question then, however, is why was so much more research and study performed on that population, especially if the prevalence of diseases such as breast cancer in the European population is so low compared to other groups? Part of the issue here is that normal is self-reinforcing. Once a group is defined as normal, that norm perpetuates beyond that local medical discourse. In the case of race, this association must be given serious attention not only because of its potential impact on racial minorities but also because it serves to maintain non-whites as medically abnormal.

SECTION 4: CONCLUSION

In this chapter, I attempt to unearth three implicit assumptions operating within the contemporary discourse surrounding African American women and breast cancer by drawing on two recent case studies from the biomedical literature. In concluding, I want to emphasize a point made in this chapter's introduction, which is that some may object that this project presumes too much in drawing such serious implications from an analysis of two journal articles. While conclusions about the presuppositions of the authors that contributed to the projects may be drawn, no general conclusions concerning the conceptualization of racial thinking within the discourse of genetics may be established from such a limited sample. Now, in addition to perhaps more obvious replies concerning the number of authors of each study or that both reports are peer reviewed and thus represent work that has been critically engaged with by a number of experts in the field, this kind of objection ultimately fails to recognize the interconnectedness of scientific discourse. The assumptions apparent in these studies do not emerge in a vacuum, nor are they random. Indeed, these assumptions help clarify why biomedical researchers understand and interpret race in the way they do. Each study, then, represents a microcosm of the discipline and thus, while limited, provides us valuable resources for understanding how race currently operates in biomedical research.

NOTES

1. Triple-negative breast cancer is a particularly aggressive and difficult form to treat, as it does not express the genes for estrogen receptors, progesterone receptors, or the human epidermal growth factor receptor 2 (HER2). These receptors are the standard targets of most chemotherapies (BreastCancer.org 2015; National Breast Cancer Foundation Inc. 2012).

2. While beyond the scope of this chapter, it is important to note that medical accounts of race and cancer, including breast cancer, have existed in the United States since the early twentieth century. At the time, white women were thought extrasusceptible to cancer. However, over time, the discourse shifted and African American women became designated as biologically more susceptible (Wailoo 2011).

3. Single nucleotide polymorphisms (SNPs) are variations at a single nucleotide base (whether A, C, G, or T) within a sequence of DNA. Although any given SNP may not cause a disease, some SNPs are associated with the onset of various diseases. As such, they are commonly used by geneticists to determine whether an individual is genetically susceptible to a given disease (Keats and Sherman 2013).

REFERENCES

American Anthropological Association. 1998. "AAA Statement on Race." *Anthropology Newsletter* 39 (9): 3–3.

BreastCancer.org. n.d. "Triple-Negative Breast Cancer." BreastCancer.org. http://www.breast cancer.org/symptoms/diagnosis/trip_neg.

Canguilhem, Georges. 1991. *The Normal and the Pathological*. Translated by Carolyn R. Fawcett in collaboration with Robert S. Cohen. New York: Zone Books.

Carey, Lisa A., Charles M. Perou, Chad A. Livasy, Lynn G. Dressler, David Cowan, Kathleen Conway, Gamze Karaca, Melissa A. Troester, Chiu Kit Tse, Sharon Edmiston, Sandra L. Deming, Joseph Geradts, Maggie C.U. Cheang, Torsten O. Nielsen, Patricia G. Moorman, H. Shelton Earp, and Robert C. Millikan. 2006. "Race, Breast Cancer Subtypes, and Survival in the Carolina Breast Cancer Study." *JAMA* 295 (21): 2492–2502.

Chow-White, Peter. 2013. "Genomic Databases and an Emerging Digital Divide in Biotechnology." In *Race after the Internet*, edited by Lisa Nakamura and Peter Chow-White, 291–309. New York: Routledge.

Collins, Patricia Hill. 1993. "Toward a New Vision: Race, Class, and Gender as Categories of Analysis and Connection." *Race, Sex and Class* 1 (1): 25–45.

Crenshaw, Kimberlé. 1991. "Mapping the Margins: Intersectionality, Identity Politics, and Violence against Women of Color." *Stanford Law Review* 43 (6): 1241–1299.

Guillaumin, Colette. 2002. *Racism, Sexism and Power and Ideology*. New York: Routledge.

Han, Ying, Lisa B. Signorello, Sara S. Strom, Rick A. Kittles, Benjamin A. Rybicki, Janet L. Stanford, Phyllis J. Goodman, Sonja I. Berndt, John Carpten, Graham Casey, Lisa Chu, David V. Conti, Kristin A. Rand, W. Ryan Diver, Anselm J.M. Hennis, Esther M. John, Adam S. Kibel, Eric A. Klein, Suzanne Kolb, Loic Le Marchand, M. Cristina Leske, Adam B. Murphy, Christine Neslund-Dudas, Jong Y. Park, Curtis Pettaway, Timothy R. Rebbeck, Susan M. Gapstur, S. Lilly Zheng, Suh-Yuh Wu, John S. Witte, Jianfeng Xu, William Isaacs, Sue A. Ingles, Ann Hsing, PRACTICAL Consortium, ELLIPSE GAME-ON Consortium, Douglas F. Easton, Rosalind A. Eeles, Fredrick R. Schumacher, Stephen Chanock, Barbara Nemesure, William J. Blot, Daniel O. Stram, Brian E. Henderson, and Christopher A. Haiman. 2015. "Generalizability of Established Prostate Cancer Risk Variants in Men of African Ancestry." *International Journal of Cancer* 136 (5): 1210–1217.

Jargowsky, Paul A. 2013. *Concentrations of Poverty in the New Millennium: Changes in Prevalence, Composition and Location of High Poverty Neighborhoods*. Century Foundation and Rutgers Center for Urban Research and Education Report. https://tcf.org/assets/downloads/Concentration_of_Poverty_in_the_New_Millennium.pdf.

Keats, Bronyja J.B., and Stephanie Sherman. 2013. "Population Genetics." In *Emery and Rimoin's Principles and Practice of Medical Genetics*, 6th ed., edited by David Rimoin, Reed Pyeritz, and Bruce Korf, 1–12. London: Churchill Livingstone.

Lewontin, Richard. 1972. "The Apportionment of Human Diversity." *Evolutionary Biology* 6: 381–398.

Montoya, Michael J. 2012. *Making the Mexican Diabetic: Race, Science and the Genetics of Inequality*. Berkeley: University of California Press.

National Breast Cancer Foundation. n.d. "Triple Negative Breast Cancer." National Breast Cancer Foundation, Inc. http://www.nationalbreastcancer.org/triple-negative-breast-cancer.

National Human Genome Research Institute. 2000. "President's State of the Union Address Refers to Human Genome Project." https://www.genome.gov/10002102/2000-state-of-the-union-and-hgp.

Palmer, Julie R., Deborah A. Boggs, Lauren A. Wise, Lucile L. Adams-Campbell, and Lynn Rosenberg. 2012. "Individual and Neighborhood Socioeconomic Status in Relation to Breast Cancer Incidence in African-American Women." *American Journal of Epidemiology* 176 (12): 1141–1146.

Palmer, Julie R., Edward A. Ruiz-Narvaez, Charles N. Rotimi, L. Adrienne Cupples, Yvette C. Cozier, Lucile L. Adams-Campbell, and Lynn Rosenberg. 2013. "Genetic Susceptibility Loci for Subtypes of Breast Cancer in an African American Population." *Cancer Epidemiology, Biomarkers and Prevention: A Publication of the American Association for Cancer Research, Cosponsored by the American Society of Preventive Oncology* 22 (1): 127–134.

Pollock, Anne. 2012. *Medicating Race: Heart Disease and Durable Preoccupations with Difference (Experimental Futures)*. Durham, NC: Duke University Press.

Roberts, Dorothy. 2011. *Fatal Invention: How Science, Politics and Big Business Re-create Race in the Twenty-First Century*. New York: New Press.

Rosenberg, Noah, Jonathan K. Pritchard, James L. Weber, Howard M. Cann, Kenneth K. Kidd, Lev A. Zhivotovsky, and Marcus W. Feldman. 2002. "Genetic Structure of Human Populations." *Science* 298 (5602): 2381–2385.

SIGMA Type 2 Diabetes Consortium. 2014. "Sequence Variants in SLC16A11 Are a Common Risk Factor for Type 2 Diabetes in Mexico." *Nature* 506 (6): 97–101.

Skim, Janet K., Katherine Weatherford Darling, Sara L. Ackerman, Sandra Soo-Jin Lee, and Robert A. Hiatt. 2015. "Reimaging Race and Ancestry: Biomedicalizing Difference in Post-Genomic Subjects." In *Reimagining (Bio)Medicalization, Pharmaceuticals and Genetics: Old Critiques and New Engagements*, edited by Susan E. Bell and Anne Figert, 56–78. New York: Routledge.

Soo-Jin Lee, Sandra. 2008. "Racial Realism and the Discourse of Responsibility for Health Disparities in a Genomic Age." In *Revisiting Race in a Genomic Age (Studies in Medical Anthropology)*, edited by Sandra Lee, Barbara Koenig, and Sarah Richardson, 342–358. New Brunswick, NJ: Rutgers University Press.

Sussman, Robert W. 2014. *The Myth of Race: The Troubling Persistence of an Unscientific Idea*. Cambridge, MA: Harvard University Press.

UNESCO. 1950. "The Race Question." https://unesdoc.unesco.org/ark:/48223/pf0000128291.

Wailoo, Keith. 2011. *How Cancer Crossed the Color Line*. Oxford: Oxford University Press.

Williams, David R., Naomi Priest, and Norman Anderson. 2016. "Understanding Associations between Race, Socioeconomic Status and Health: Patterns and Prospects." Health Psychology 35 (4): 407–4011.

World Health Organization (WHO). 2016. "Genes and Human Disease." *Genomic Resource Centre*. http://www.who.int/genomics/public/geneticdiseases/en/index3.html.

Yudell, Michael. 2014. *Race Unmasked: Biology and Race in the Twentieth Century*. New York: Columbia University Press.

13

OVERCOMING POSTPARTUM DEPRESSION
Individual and Social Gendered Pathology in Self-Help Discourse

Beth L. Boser

Self-help is ubiquitous. A more than $11 billion industry in the United States offers improved relationships, social efficacy, professional performance, physical health, and psychological well-being, among others, marketed across a range of contexts (Lindner 2009). Self-help discourse comprises seminars, films, podcasts, websites, magazines, and books. Despite the rise of new forms of self-help, the self-help-book industry remains massive and exhibits strong and steady growth with unit sales increasing by 13 percent from 2015 to 2016 and another 18 percent from 2016 to 2017 (Milliot 2017, 2018). The diverse genre covers everything from instruction and information giving to self-transformation, consciousness raising, and political action (Kline 2009).

A prominent subgenre of self-help comprises texts on mental distress. Such texts provide sites wherein meanings relating to mental health are shaped and reinforced. The nature of self-help and the relationship of self-help audiences to texts make such discourse explicitly pedagogical and rhetorical, providing readers with symbolic frameworks through which to understand and interpret problems and to conceive of action. Like other types of discourse in health and medical contexts, expert voices in self-help encourage readers to "consider some conditions as pathological and others not" and hold the potential to "condition outcomes" (Derkatch and Segal 2005, 138–139). Furthermore, "the popularity of self-help books makes the authors' messages or guidance seem important, right, or truthful" (Zimmerman, Holm, and Starrels 2001, 165). The influence of self-help necessitates critical consideration of how such discourses shape understandings of pathology. Here, I am concerned with how gender and motherhood intersect with mental health and pathology; thus, I conduct a critical rhetorical analysis of

DOI: 10.7330/9781607329855.c013

the bestselling book *This Isn't What I Expected: Overcoming Postpartum Depression* by Karen Kleiman and Valarie Davis Raskin (2013). My analysis joins a handful of others in this volume that consider how women's reproductive health is pathologized and explore the tensions between experiential knowledge and medical discourse (see Anglesey; De Hertogh; and Novotny and Horn-Walker, this collection).

This bestselling book constructs postpartum distress as having both individual/biological and collective/social causes, which suggests solutions should be implemented on both individual and social levels. This depiction potentially enriches biomedical understandings of postpartum distress predominant in other discourses. Prior scholars argue that understandings of postpartum distress intersect sociocultural norms of gender and motherhood (Dubriwny 2013, 2010; Taylor 1996). Moreover, Marika Seigel (2014) demonstrates that texts providing instructions to women have symbolic and material consequences in that they have the power to make connections among ideas and images in ways that argue for proper action. I build on this work by exploring instructions provided to women suffering with postpartum distress and the ways in which those instructions encourage readers to understand and act upon their suffering. Prior to elaborating upon this argument, I provide an overview of scholarship on self-help, postpartum distress, and ideal motherhood.

SELF-HELP DISCOURSE

The diversity of self-help rhetoric necessitates that critics attend to specific instances as opposed to making general statements about the whole genre. Prior scholarship presents a complex and sometimes contradictory picture of self-help, as various studies yield both criticism and optimism regarding the emancipatory potential of self-help. Critics of self-help argue that it excessively focuses on the individual, exerts control, and pathologizes women. Heidi Rimke (2000) argues that self-help "exalts the individual over the social" and "teach[es] a subject to rely exclusively on oneself" (62). In self-help, the author claims, "all human conflicts are . . . psychological problems" that can "be set right at the level of psychical individual self-discipline" (73). Maureen Ebben (1995) offers the critical feminist perspective that self-help assigns responsibility to individual women and neglects economic and cultural factors. Individualized subjects become objects of control, as citizens are deemed psychologically healthy as long as they are carefully (self-)regulated in a range of ways (Rimke 2000). Furthermore, gendered pathologizing is rampant. Victoria DeFrancisco and Penny O'Connor (1995) lament the reduction of gendered problems to "a result of communication or cross-cultural difference" and claim that in self-help, "women and men . . . are not just from different cultural groups, but hierarchically, women exist in a less well-adjusted group" (222). Self-help tends to pathologize women's traditional and expected roles (Ebben 1995).

Disagreement comes from those who resist painting self-help with a broad brush. Some argue productive self-help scholarship resists reinforcing the binary conclusion that self-help is *either* oppressive *or* emancipating (Kline 2009; Neville 2012). Historically, self-help groups supported activism through sharing lived experience, particularly among marginalized groups—feminist consciousness raising is a quintessential example. Furthermore, self-help provided space in which oppressed groups resisted surveillance by the medical establishment (Kline 2009). Thus, analyses should attend to particular discursive characteristics of specific self-help discourses to determine their complex potentials and problems.

Accordingly, my purpose is not to forward a sweeping claim about a genre but rather to look at one particular example wherein self-help bridges the medical, the personal, and the social in contexts of postpartum distress in ways that may be empowering in some respects and limiting in others. In *This Isn't What I Expected: Overcoming Postpartum Depression* (Kleiman and Raskin 2013), the individualization observed in prior feminist analyses is complicated by emphasis on social context. However, constructions of gender in such discussions foreclose much of the text's resistive potential. Social expectations placed upon mothers are acknowledged along with biological causes; ultimately, such expectations are pathologized as individual women's failings, cutting off potential for collective acts of social healing. Prior work on postpartum distress and expectations of ideal motherhood provide a framework for this analysis.

POSTPARTUM DISTRESS AND PATHOLOGICAL MOTHERHOOD

In a groundbreaking study of postpartum self-help groups, Verta Taylor (1996) notes that postpartum distress is "the ultimate expression of maternal contradictions," wherein mothers experience extreme anguish during a supposed time of great joy (2). Biomedical frameworks dominate popular understandings of postpartum distress, as women are diagnosed with a particular form of postpartum disorder (e.g., postpartum depression, postpartum anxiety) and placed on a spectrum from mild (i.e., "baby blues") to severe (postpartum psychosis). From a medical perspective, symptoms of postpartum depression are similar to depression (e.g., feeling sad, hopeless, worthless, or helpless; experiencing loss of interest or energy; changes in sleep or appetite; having thoughts of suicide) but also include increased crying, social withdrawal, feeling disconnected from the baby, worrying about hurting the baby, or having guilt associated with feelings of not being a good mother (Centers, "Symptoms of Depression," n.d.; "Symptoms of Postpartum," n.d.). Although psychologists indicate that literature on prevalence is not conclusive, Michael O'Hara (2009) notes that the "most adequate" of prior studies found that as many as 7.1 percent of women experience a "major depressive episode" within three months of giving birth. The rate increases to 19.2 when minor depression is included.

Discourses of postpartum distress comprise a rhetorical blending of the biologically determined and the socially constructed, evidenced in descriptions of causes. No single agreed-upon cause exists; however, professional medicine indicates both "physical and emotional issues" are involved (Mayo "Postpartum Depression," n.d.). "Physical issues" include postchildbirth hormone level drops. "Emotional issues" include sleep deprivation, feeling "overwhelmed," "anxious about your ability to care for a newborn," "less attractive," and/or that "you've lost control," and struggling with "your sense of identity" (Mayo "Postpartum Depression," n.d.). Vacillation between biological and social in these features is striking, and complex constructions of postpartum distress spur competing perspectives about the best ways to understand the causes of—and potential solutions to—postpartum distress.

Most frequently, postpartum distress is understood as a mental illness best treated with medication. Feminist scholars critique this medicalized perspective. Rachel Liebert (2010) calls hormonal explanations for women's higher rates of depression "particularly insidious," as hormones are explicitly gendered and attributed to the very making of females; they pathologize women simply for being. An alternative perspective on causes of postpartum distress emphasizes sociocultural difficulties faced by mothers. These difficulties are driven by constructions of ideal motherhood (Dubriwny 2013).

The myth of ideal, Western, motherhood comprises practices, images, and identities that construct overall understandings of "good" motherhood (e.g., Hundley and Hayden 2016). Adrienne Rich (1986) first noted that motherhood is a patriarchal institution set to control women's reproductive power, and Sharon Hays (1996) elucidated characteristics composing "intensive mothering" (14), which are created and maintained through discourses about motherhood that construct specific expectations for women (Dubriwny 2013, 69). Ideal motherhood demands that mothers enact the role of primary constant caregiver, put the needs of children first, and fully give themselves to their children (Hays 1996). Furthermore, ideal mothers are overwhelmingly represented in media as white, middle- or upper-middle class, heterosexual, and mentally fit (Boser 2016; Dubriwny 2010, 2013). Hegemonic notions of this "good" motherhood depend on the opposing construct of the monstrous "bad" mother, who damages her child psychologically or physically (Dubriwny 2013; Ehrenreich and English 2005). Sarah Hayden and Heather Hundley (2016) summarize: "In the contemporary United States, we assess maternal practices as starkly good or bad and [these assessments] offer lessons for real-life moms about how they are expected to behave" (2).

Feminist perspectives suggest that sociocultural constraints placed upon mothers are largely responsible for postpartum distress. Prior work indicates such distress may be understood as a justified reaction to difficulties experienced by new mothers, or a response to unrealistic expectations of motherhood (e.g., Ussher 2010). Christine Everingham, Gaynor Heading, and Linda Connor (2006) found that women with postpartum depression had high expectations for living up to the cultural ideals of motherhood and experienced "some setback in these expectations" (1749); these mothers understood their experience through "perceptions of the 'good mother'" (1751). Rebecca Godderis (2010) notes that risk factors in psychiatric literature, such as "single marital status" and "ambivalent feelings about motherhood," reinforce the constructed standard of the good mother. Still, postpartum distress persists in being understood, overwhelmingly, as a mental illness. Moreover, the use of the psychiatric "postpartum triad"—wherein baby blues, depression, and psychosis are placed on a continuum—collapses distinctions among women who have "normal" experiences and those who are ill and places nearly all mothers within the purview of increased medical surveillance (Godderis 2010). Critics agree such medicalization negates potential for postpartum distress to challenge oppressive expectations of motherhood (Dubriwny 2010; Ussher 2010).

Yet, these critics acknowledge a bind. Liberating women from injustices associated with medicalization and ideal motherhood requires that sociocultural explanations for postpartum distress be emphasized; at the same time, suffering women require immediate assistance and care that may be most readily found within professional medicine. Women's health advocates helped medicalize postpartum distress as they demanded treatment, which depended on recognizing it as a "real" illness (Taylor 1996). However, acknowledging the problems of pathologizing women and critiquing motherhood expectations "is *not* synonymous with invalidating" women's pain (Liebert 2010, 5). Evidently, effective solutions for postpartum distress should involve engaging women as whole beings, in context. However, this is a challenging undertaking. Prior work suggests mental-health professionals readily understand the *problem* of postpartum distress as both biological and social. Simultaneously, they are "lacking in both language and schema" to articulate both biological and social *solutions* (Lloyd and Hawe 2003, 1783).

Frameworks for such social solutions—or at least for social resistance—may lie outside the realm of professional medical discourse. Tasha Dubriwny (2010) analyzed television news stories on postpartum distress to explore the potential therein of opening "discursive space in which mothers, activists, and social critics can critique the institution of motherhood and offer a new vision of mothering" (288–289). Unfortunately, the space offered by alternative discourses does not necessarily result in resistance, as decontextualization and individualization can occur just as readily in the news as in medical discourse (Dubriwny 2010). Yet, the resistive potential of postpartum discourses outside the strictly medical has only begun to be explored.

CONSTRUCTING POSTPARTUM DISTRESS

Self-help discourse potentially provides a nuanced understanding of postpartum disorder that blends medical information and women's lived experiences. This analysis of *This Isn't What I Expected: Overcoming Postpartum Depression* (Kleiman and Raskin 2013) contributes to scholarly conversations on self-help discourse within the larger context of rhetorics of health and medicine, and understandings of gendered postpartum pathology, by examining the extent to which self-help's positioning as intentionally therapeutic and potentially empowering offers a more well-rounded construction of postpartum distress. The book's subtitle, *Overcoming Postpartum Depression*, indicates a focus on solutions, and the content of the text suggests "overcoming" must occur on both individual *and* social levels. From the perspective of feminist critics, social healing is a productive step; however, *how* such individual and social "overcoming" is achieved, according to the book, matters. In mapping the contours of causes and symptoms of postpartum distress, the book problematizes both individual and social dimensions of distress and motherhood. However, promise implicit in this construction is unrealized, as "overcoming" is rhetorically reduced to individual women more effectively navigating social causes as opposed to collectively challenging them. Specifically, ideal motherhood is simultaneously critiqued *and* supported. In what follows, I consider the book's complication of professional medical understandings of postpartum distress through the blending of medical/individual and social pathology. Then, I illustrate how the resistive potential of such complications for "overcoming" postpartum distress on both individual and social levels is thwarted by the book's reliance on traditional gender roles that, paradoxically, are situated as both cause of *and* solution to postpartum distress.

This Isn't What I Expected: Overcoming Postpartum Depression provides comprehensive information on postpartum distress, leading readers through stages of defining, recognizing, understanding, treating, and recovering. Chapters center on, for example, types of postpartum distress, strategies to deal with negative thoughts, medication, therapy, social support, and motherhood expectations. Medical information abounds, including information on hormones and brain functioning, benefits and side effects of medications, and different approaches to psychotherapy. In this way, much of the "help" offered is inextricably connected to acceptance of medicalization. However, the totality of the text is not so one sided, as medical and social intermix throughout.

Medical and Social Pathology

The book emphasizes that postpartum disorders are *real* illnesses. In accordance with prior findings (e.g., Dubriwny 2013), the authors of the book advocate for combatting stigma by establishing that postpartum distress is no different than any other physical sickness. The authors use analogy to illustrate. They compare postpartum distress to other conditions including anemia (Kleiman and Raskin 2013, ix, 102), infected milk ducts (ix), bronchitis (52), and diabetes (49). Although comparisons place postpartum distress in the medical realm, the stated purpose is not submission to medical authority; rather, understanding that postpartum distress is the same as any other illness is framed as empowering. The discourse of the "real" illness suggests the importance of official institutional recognition for providing timely relief to severe distress. A degree of power to take control and act, on an individual level, accompanies the pronouncement that an illness is "real" (Graham 2009). Lack of understanding is presented as a "major source of frustration" (Kleiman and Raskin 2013, 4); therefore, the authors indicate that when a woman realizes she has a real illness, she experiences great relief. Joseph Gemin (1997) notes the act of identifying oneself as disordered "becomes in itself a remedy of sorts" (250), and Davi Johnson (2008) illustrates that claiming a diagnosis validates and affirms an individual's identity (33). Furthermore, such acknowledgment resists self-blame. Kleiman and Raskin state, "PPD [postpartum depression] is a real illness; it is not some sort of punishment for moral weakness, self-indulgence, a wish for a boy when you had a girl, a wish for a girl when you had a boy, nor is it anyone's fault" (10). Women would be ostensibly subject to allegations of personal fault were postpartum distress not a "real" illness, which suggests real-life consequences in relation to how distress is understood.

Once postpartum distress is established as "real," *This Isn't What I Expected: Overcoming Postpartum Depression* provides opportunities to self-diagnose, manage, control, and treat the illness in ways reminiscent of Michel Foucault's (1994, 1995) inspecting and medical gazes. The book is full of inventories and checklists, inviting readers to detail, and thus construct, the contours of their own pathology. Kleiman and Raskin state that the lists are for purposes of self-assessment "so you can then take the steps needed to recover" (5). By offering readers menus of symptoms to reflect upon, agency and responsibility to determine and assess the features of one's pathology are implied. Upon completing these inventories, readers may engage exercises through which they are encouraged to work on, for example, replacing negative and "self-defeating" thoughts with "realistic" ones (33). Shifting from medical diagnoses to mental exercises, these inventories and exercises suggest it may be within the individual woman's power to heal; in fact, the book indicates the first step in the "typical pattern of recovery" is to "try to use your internal resources to support yourself as much as possible" (27). Statements such as these that cast the management of postpartum distress as primarily an individual, albeit not entirely medical, endeavor are complicated by elements of the text that extend distress beyond the individual.

For example, the book's introduction sets up a well-rounded discussion of the postpartum context. The following passage illustrates rhetorical blending of the medical with the social in its discussion of the pressures of "perfect" motherhood, workplace support for families, and dissociation of mothers' love from willingness to sacrifice professional endeavors. The authors state their hopes:

> Mothers wouldn't feel so much pressure to be perfect, the link between hormones and postpartum depression would be well understood, new medications would work quickly and without side effects, and society

would support young families, as is done in some parts of the world, with generous parental leaves and flexible work schedules. Maternal love wouldn't be evaluated by whether a woman works in the home full time, not at all, or something in between. Women with postpartum depression and anxiety wouldn't be judged as either trying too hard or not trying hard enough. Every obstetrician would know that postpartum emotional disorders are the most frequent medical complication of childbirth, and therefore all new parents would be screened and educated about this disorder. (ix)

Such blending advocates a rich contextualization of postpartum distress and resists the tendency to reduce women to nothing more than medicalized objects for expert surveillance. Acknowledgement of social aspects of postpartum distress alongside medical explanations holds the potential to shift the discursive terrain of conversations about postpartum distress to include possibilities for causes and courses of action that could afford women agency. The theme of socially embedded postpartum distress persists throughout the book.

One of the primary ways this manifests is in *This Isn't What I Expected: Overcoming Postpartum Depression*'s new category of distress: "postpartum stress syndrome." According to Kleiman and Raskin, along with the one in five women who experience something from the full range of disorders encompassing postpartum depression, anxiety, panic, obsessive-compulsive disorder, or traumatic stress disorder (xi), they indicate that an additional 20–30 percent of mothers who do not "meet diagnostic criteria for PPD" will experience postpartum stress syndrome (xi). The newly coined syndrome provides a vast and flexible space for interpretation, as it "falls between the relatively minor baby blues and the relatively severe PPD" (14). This syndrome is "marked by feelings of anxiety and self-doubt coupled with a deep desire to be a perfect mother" (15), implicating both biology and ideology. The notion that postpartum stress syndrome is related to a "deep desire to be a perfect mother" (15) suggests social components of pathology related to normative understandings of ideal motherhood. Moreover, the syndrome's name distinguishes it from other forms of postpartum distress. For example, overwhelmingly, causes of "depression" and "psychosis" are attributed to physiological and neurological elements—that is, changes in the brain, brain chemistry, hormones, or genetically inherited traits (Mayo, "Depression," n.d.)—in other words, these conditions are rhetorically contained, by medical definitions, primarily within the individual body. Even discussions of baby blues do not extend beyond the body, as the associated "temporary moodiness," "sadness," and "irritability" (Kleiman and Raskin 2013, 13) seem to reside internally. In contrast, "stress" is

commonly understood to be a response to difficult or demanding circumstances. "Stress" implies some sort of relationship with a context.
Hence, much as Kenneth Burke (1969) suggests that a name carries with
it a whole world of meaning, the naming of this novel syndrome opens
up a range of social and ideological possibilities for consideration as part
of the problem of and solution to postpartum distress.

Along with possibilities come reasons to be skeptical. Despite the
fact that Kleiman and Raskin distinguish stress syndrome from severe
postpartum disorder, they also indicate throughout the text that postpartum stress syndrome falls under the heading of "PPD." However, they
also align it with baby blues in terms of recovery in that neither stress
syndrome nor baby blues should be treated with medication. Rather,
recovery should take nonmedical forms. Postpartum stress syndrome
thus becomes a rhetorical bridge spanning what otherwise might be
more clearly distinguishable illness and non-illness. Given the description of the syndrome, conceivably just about every new mother might
feel included. This expansive approach is further complicated by the
authors' assertion that 60–80 percent of mothers experience the brief
postpartum moodiness of baby blues. Even though baby blues "is not
actually an illness" (13), the authors note it is readily confused with postpartum disorder because the conditions all share common symptoms.
Such indications of overlap coupled with fuzzy and hugely encompassing statistics hearken to the hopes and fears of prior critics. As Dubriwny
(2013) notes, drawing parallels between symptoms of disorder and
normal experiences of motherhood both normalizes and problematizes
postpartum disorder. At the same time, Godderis (2010) argues that
such a fluid spectrum pathologizes normal experiences.

A broad community of parents is brought into the realm of postpartum distress through a range of textual features. Kleiman and Raskin
frequently point out experiences common across the full range of the
postpartum spectrum, and beyond. They state, "Most people agree that
a certain level of anxiety during the postpartum period is evolutionarily
adaptive. . . . Anxiety is an instinctive response to threatening triggers"
(21). Apparently, one major symptom of the illness is part of every single
parent's DNA. The notion that much of what is understood to be postpartum disorder is "normal" and that differing diagnoses are a matter
of degree, not kind, is emphasized. Moreover, the authors recommend
coping through "positive statements" that emphasize commonalities
among mothers with and without postpartum distress, such as, "All
mothers of new babies feel tired, irritable, or stressed at times" (37).
Indeed, the authors state that much of what they discuss is applicable to

"every mother, whether or not she has PPD" (231), as many experiences are "universal" (243). Thus, a significant part of the self-help prescribed by the book entails recognition of how social contexts of motherhood contribute to widely shared symptoms of what is commonly recognized as postpartum disorder but could, in many cases, simply be symptoms of motherhood.

By situating particular symptoms as both associated with postpartum distress *and* universal, *This Isn't What I Expected: Overcoming Postpartum Depression* discursively erases boundaries between those with "real" illness and all other mothers. From one perspective, this practice extends pathology; from another, it opens up space to critique the broad range of social causes for such negative experiences. Once such a space is created, strategies to resist and change those social causes are warranted. Therefore, the following section unpacks the extent to which the book delivers on its seeming promise to critique problems with the institution of motherhood and articulate social paths to overcoming those problems.

Motherhood as Problem and Solution

Gendered concerns relating to motherhood expectations are repeatedly linked to postpartum distress in various contexts throughout the book. Thus, on the surface, the content of the book suggests overcoming postpartum distress must occur in numerous ways at the social level. However, the authors do not conceive of ways to break out of the acknowledged, limiting, harmful system of ideal motherhood; instead, solutions are reduced to more effective navigation of the system as-is, by individual women. Even while the book continually acknowledges the challenging contexts of motherhood, it concurrently promotes and even celebrates intensely traditional constructions of motherhood that are exclusionary and restrictive.

Sections specifically devoted to motherhood provide evidence. *This Isn't What I Expected: Overcoming Postpartum Depression* critiques ideal motherhood and the binary of good/bad motherhood when it states,

> Our culture and media play a powerful role in shaping our expectations. And these expectations, in turn, create enormous pressure on mothers to strive for perfection . . . television shows that center on family life . . . overglamorize motherhood, placing it high on a pedestal . . . or reinforce the illusion that we can all strive for supermom status. (227)

Kleiman and Raskin indicate that such expectations "create a potential for PPD to develop if a woman is biochemically predisposed" (226). However, they then dismissively comment, "When producers of television programming or movies respond to the criticism that these 'Hollywood' depictions of mothers do not represent realistic portrayals, they typically justify their position by claiming that if it were realistic, it wouldn't be 100 percent entertaining. How true!" (227–28). Problems with the cultural demands of motherhood are reduced from diminishing agency and inducing illness to merely failing to accurately reflect reality.

Along with the dismissal of ideal motherhood constructions as mere entertainment—and hence, that such constructions have serious consequence—the problematic ways these constructions play out in real women's lives are recast as unrealized individual fantasies. "Fantasies" are what "set us up to believe that we have to behave and respond and feel a certain way" (Kleiman and Raskin 2013, 230). Despite earlier indications of ideological sources, the fantasies apparently originate from women's own mothers:

> By the age of two or three, little girls start to identify with their mothers and see themselves as potential mothers. The expectation of becoming mothers when we grew up permeated our childhood play—before we even knew where babies came from, most of us were dressing up as Mommy and playing "house." (228)

As the passage continues, the responsibility shifts away from mothers:

> Watch a young girl play now. As mothers of daughters, we can tell you that things haven't changed so much. Though we may try to expose our daughters to toys with little or no specific gender orientation, our daughters wear the fanciest pretty clothes, never forget lipstick or nail polish, and have perfectly coordinated and compliant baby dolls who gaze lovingly at their "Mommies" while peacefully resting in their "cribs." (228)

Seemingly, then, no one is responsible for the "fantasies;" they are simply the product of a deeply essential gendered identity. The blame for sociocultural conditions that underpin women's postpartum distress swiftly moves from a social system, to a familial relationship, to no one at all.

Failure to live up to ideal motherhood is blamed on "romanticized" ideas; hence, a woman's pain is caused by discrepancies between her own "memory" of the perfect mother she wanted to be as a child and her impression of herself as a "real" mother (231). Kleiman and Raskin state, "When you expect perfection, you are setting yourself up for failure" (238), recasting the social construction of motherhood as individual readers' perfectionism. Moreover, *This Isn't What I Expected: Overcoming Postpartum Depression* intimates that only giving up on "narcissistic desires" of ideal motherhood will allow a woman to "give [her]self completely to [her] child" (252). In other words, only if women accept that they cannot enact ideal motherhood will they be able to fulfill the key tenet of ideal motherhood. The underlying dynamic of this paradox is evidenced elsewhere in this collection and relies upon and supports gendered stereotypes; in a range of contexts, women are encouraged to take better care of themselves so they can better take care of others (see Assad, this collection).

Thus, effectively navigating the social gendered constraints surrounding postpartum distress does not include challenging them. Instead, the solution is understanding how to better navigate such constraints. The acceptance of ideal motherhood as an individualized pathology is paired with the quintessential feminine constraint—ideal beauty. Aligning with D. Lynn O'Brien Hallstein's (2011) observation that media add the "quickly slender postpartum" body to the barrage of expectations placed upon new mothers, *This Isn't What I Expected: Overcoming Postpartum Depression* maintains that attending to appearance is vital to recovery. According to the authors, one mother "shocked herself by gaining eleven pounds in the first three months [of pregnancy]. . . . In later months, she couldn't resist her cravings for ice cream and donuts. . . . By the time her daughter was born, [she] had gained forty-two pounds" (87). Because of this, the mother felt "unattractive," which was "related to having postpartum stress syndrome" (87). The solution, in this case, was the gym: "Her old gym didn't mind her bringing the baby to class with her," so she was able to "get back to her routine of working out four or five days a week" (88). Normalizing the presence of infants in a range of places is certainly a component of challenging ideal motherhood expectations; however, the primary purpose here is to discipline the postpartum body. Other "suggestions for making yourself feel more attractive during the postpartum period" (96) include, "Get dressed. . . . Wearing your nightgown all day is definitely the easiest route, but no one looks or feels fit or pretty in [that]" and "Put a little makeup on. . . . You deserve to look pretty, just for yourself" (96). Simultaneously, women must "beware the perfection trap" (97); appearing to have "stepped out of a *Vogue* advertisement" indicates they should "[ease] up a little" by "cutting back on the time [spent] on makeup, or wearing jeans more often" (97). Ostensibly, women must look pretty in just the right amount to appropriately navigate beauty expectations in postpartum contexts. Elsewhere in this collection, Maria Novotny and Elizabeth Horn-Walker argue that infertility is constructed as a failure of femininity; similarly, here, postpartum distress is associated with a failure to properly enact feminine norms.

These elements craft an image of appropriate motherhood that paradoxically evinces awareness of harms of such expectations while simultaneously resigning to—and even promoting—their inevitability. Readers are encouraged to recognize that motherhood expectations exacerbate postpartum distress and then to uphold and embody those expectations in the interest of healing. Motherhood is both the problem and the solution. In its persistent devotion to such contradiction, the book suggests attempts to resist motherhood expectations are futile. In this way, overcoming postpartum distress becomes a purely individual endeavor. Social potentialities are stopped short by the authors' refusal to challenge traditional gender norms in any meaningful way.

CONCLUSION

This analysis offers a glimpse of a self-help text that promises to treat postpartum distress as both individual and social. Descriptions of postpartum distress that include a range of biological and ideological contributors, along with a category of distress that posits a nonmedical framework for the postpartum period, create the potential to rework common understandings of pathology and critique social expectations of motherhood. However, as the book fleshes out postpartum contexts, strategies for "overcoming" emerge built upon a foundation of stereotypical representations. Thus, this analysis suggests maintaining a hopeful yet critical posture, recognizing self-help offers a context wherein medical *and* social explanations for postpartum distress hold the potential to be empowering for women, but such empowerment is not guaranteed. Opening space for resistance does not equal resistance, as is evidenced by prior analyses, as well as my own. So, critics must examine these openings and assess their merits. In doing so, critics should resist the urge to take a one-sided negative view and dismiss a whole range of texts as harmful or to reproduce an either/or binary (Kline 2009; Taylor 1996). Critique is necessary to deconstruct oppressive institutions and discourses and should be put to work by rhetoricians of health and medicine to find pragmatic ways to improve the lives of women.

In terms of *This Isn't What I Expected: Overcoming Postpartum Depression* and similar books, practical improvements are warranted. Outmoded gender constructions must be replaced with multifaceted perspectives on individual and social challenges of the postpartum period that resist individualizing the social in the interest of offering simple "solutions." For example, the book insists it is okay for women to decide to go back to work, or not, after having a baby. Of course, women's professional actions should not be judged or stigmatized. However, a social matter of such importance should not be reduced to a personal lifestyle preference. Instead, an in-depth discussion of the necessity of social and political support for mothers' career pursuits is needed. Work is not simply a choice for women who do not have the financial freedom to mother full time. A more thorough discussion of the complex challenges faced by a diverse range of women would be one way to more adequately work toward social recovery.

Furthermore, a more nuanced, intersectional approach is desperately needed in this text and others like it. A consideration of varying economic constraints should inform descriptions of women's postpartum realities, and examples should be drawn from a broad range of women beyond those who are middle class and white. Attention should be paid, for example, to the fact that low-income women receive substandard treatment for postpartum distress and that women of color receive particularly substandard care (Kozhimannil et al. 2011). Texts should explore differential care received, as well as the contextual reasons some women are more susceptible to postpartum distress than others. Authors should avoid implying all mothers have disposable income and make use of opportunities to advocate for more equitable family policies. Authors should encourage acceptance and normalization of diverse family structures. The self-help genre provides ample opportunities to do so; one of the benefits of self-help groups identified by Taylor (1996) is that participants "hear confirmation of their feelings in the voices of other women" (8). A more empowering self-help book would provide this experience to the broadest possible audience of readers.

Finally, authors of such texts should persist in reminding readers (and others in the professional health and medical community) that recognizing postpartum distress as a *real* problem does not mean it must be framed as an exclusively—or even primarily—individual biological problem. Alternatively, women need to be better supported in all aspects of life. Feminist frameworks that avoid placing the social into opposition with the biological may be useful in negotiating what sometimes seems to be a necessary clash between the two realms (Blencowe 2011). Ultimately, collective overcoming of postpartum distress necessitates continued work to come to grips with the complexities of the collective, with goals of improving women's lives holistically in both the short and long term.

REFERENCES

Blencowe, Claire Peta. 2011. "Biology, Contingency and the Problem of Racism in Feminist Discourse." *Theory, Culture and Society* 28 (2): 3–27.

Boser, Beth L. (2016). "'I Forgot How It Was To Be Normal': Decompensating the Binary of Good/Bad Motherhood." In *Mediated Moms: Contemporary Challenges to the Motherhood Myth*, edited by Heather L. Hundley and Sarah Hayden, 161–81, New York: Peter Lang.

Burke, Kenneth. 1969. *A Grammar of Motives.* Berkeley: University of California Press.

Centers for Disease Control and Prevention, Division of Reproductive Health. n.d. "Symptoms of Depression." Last reviewed December 5, 2019. https://www.cdc.gov /reproductivehealth/depression/.

DeFrancisco, Victoria Leto, and Penny O'Connor. 1995. "A Feminist Critique of Self-Help Books on Heterosexual Romance: Read 'Em and Weep." *Women's Studies in Communication* 18 (2): 217–227.

Derkatch, Colleen, and Judy Z. Segal. 2005. "Realms of Rhetoric in Health and Medicine." *University of Toronto Journal* 82 (2): 138–142.

Dubriwny, Tasha N. 2010. "Television News Coverage of Postpartum Disorders and the Politics of Medicalization." *Feminist Media Studies* 10 (3): 285–303.

Dubriwny, Tasha N. 2013. *The Vulnerable Empowered Woman: Feminism, Postfeminism, and Women's Health.* New Brunswick, NJ: Rutgers University Press.

Ebben, Maureen. 1995. "Off the Shelf Salvation: A Feminist Critique of Self-Help." *Women's Studies in Communication* 18 (2): 111–122.

Ehrenreich, Barbara, and Deidre English. 2005. *For Her Own Good: Two Centuries of the Experts' Advice to Women.* New York: Random House.

Everingham, Christine Rosemary, Gaynor Heading, and Linda Connor. 2006. "Couples' Experiences of Postnatal Depression: A Framing Analysis of Cultural Identity, Gender and Communication." *Social Science and Medicine* 62 (7): 1745–1756.

Foucault, Michel. 1994. *The Birth of the Clinic: An Archaeology of Medical Perception.* New York: Vintage Books.

Foucault, Michel. 1995. *Discipline and Punish: The Birth of the Prison.* New York: Vintage Books.

Gemin, Joseph. 1997. "Manufacturing Codependency: Self-help as Discursive Formation." *Critical Studies in Media Communication* 14 (3): 249–266.

Godderis, Rebecca. 2010. "Precarious Beginnings: Gendered Risk Discourses in Psychiatric Research Literature about Postpartum Depression." *Health* 14 (5): 451–466.

Graham, S. Scott. 2009. "Agency and the Rhetoric of Medicine: Biomedical Brain Scans and the Ontology of Fibromyalgia." *Technical Communication Quarterly* 18 (4): 376–404.

Hayden, Sarah, and Heather L. Hundley. 2016. "Introduction: Challenging the Motherhood Myth." In *Mediated Moms: Contemporary Challenges to the Motherhood Myth*, edited by Heather L. Hundley and Sarah Hayden, 1–13. New York: Peter Lang.

Hays, Sharon. 1996. *The Cultural Contradictions of Motherhood.* New Haven, CT: Yale University Press.

Hundley, Heather L., and Sarah Hayden, eds. 2016. *Mediated Moms: Contemporary Challenges to the Motherhood Myth.* New York: Peter Lang.

Johnson, Davi A. 2008. "Managing Mr. Monk: Control and the Politics of Madness." *Critical Studies in Media Communication* 25 (1): 28–47.

Kleiman, Karen R., and Valarie Davis Raskin. 2013. *This Isn't What I Expected: Overcoming Postpartum Depression.* Boston: De Capo.

Kline, Kimberly N. 2009. "The Discursive Characteristics of a Prosocial Self-Help: Revisioning the Potential of Self-Help for Empowerment." *Southern Communication Journal* 74 (2): 191–208.

Kozhimannil, Katy Backes, Connie Mah Trinacty, Alisa B. Busch, Haiden A. Huskamp, and Alyce S. Adams. 2011. "Racial and Ethnic Disparities in Postpartum Depression Care among Low-Income Women." *Psychiatric Services* 62 (6): 619–625.

Liebert, Rachel. 2010. "Feminist Psychology, Hormones and the Raging Politics of Medicalization." *Feminism and Psychology* 20 (2): 278–283.

Lindner, Melanie. 2009. "What People Are Still Willing to Pay For." *Forbes*, January 15. http://www.forbes.com/2009/01/15/self-help-industry-ent-sales-cx_ml_0115selfhelp.html.

Lloyd, Beverly, and Penelope Hawe. 2003. "Solutions Foregone? How Postnatal Professionals Frame the Problem of Postnatal Depression." *Social Science and Medicine* 57 (10): 1783–1795.

Mayo Clinic Staff. n.d. "Depression (Major Depressive Disorder)." http://www.mayoclinic.org/diseases-conditions/depression/basics/causes/con-20032977.

Mayo Clinic Staff. n.d. "Postpartum Depression." http://www.mayoclinic.org/diseases-conditions/postpartum-depression/basics/symptoms/con-20029130.

Milliot, Jim. 2017. "Adult Nonfiction Stayed Hot in 2016." *Publishers Weekly*, January 13. https://www.publishersweekly.com/pw/by-topic/industry-news/publisher-news/article/72501-adult-nonfiction-stayed-hot-in-2016.html.

Milliot, Jim. 2018. "Nonfiction Categories Continued to Grow in 2017." *Publishers Weekly*, January 19. https://www.publishersweekly.com/pw/by-topic/industry-news/bookselling/article/75877-nonfiction-categories-continued-to-grow-in-2017.html.

Neville, Patricia. 2012. "Helping Self-Help Books: Working Towards a New Research Agenda." *Interactions: Studies in Communication and Culture* 3 (3): 361–379.

O'Brien Hallstein, D. Lynn. 2011. "She Gives Birth, She's Wearing a Bikini: Mobilizing the Post-Pregnant Celebrity Mom Body to Manage the Post-Second Wave Crisis in Femininity." *Women's Studies in Communication*. 34 (2): 111–138.

O'Hara, Michael W. 2009. "Postpartum Depression: What We Know." *Journal of Clinical Psychology* 65 (12): 1258–1269.

Rich, Adrienne. 1986. *Of Woman Born: Motherhood as Experience and Institution*. 2nd ed. New York: W. W. Norton.

Rimke, Heidi Marie. 2000. "Governing Citizens through Self-Help Literature." *Cultural Studies* 14 (1): 61–78.

Seigel, Marika. 2014. *The Rhetoric of Pregnancy*. Chicago: University of Chicago Press.

Taylor, Verta. 1996. *Rock-a-by Baby: Feminism, Self-Help, and Postpartum Depression*. New York: Routledge.

Ussher, Jane M. 2010. "Are We Medicalizing Women's Misery? A Critical Review of Women's Higher Rates of Reported Depression." *Feminism and Psychology* 20 (1): 9–35.

Zimmerman, Toni Schindler, Kristen E. Holm, and Marjorie E. Starrels. 2001. "A Feminist Analysis of Self-Help Bestsellers for Improving Relationships: A Decade Review." *Journal of Marital and Family Therapy* 27 (2): 165–175.

14

MAKING BODIES
Medical Rhetoric of Gendered and Sexed Materiality

Sage Beaumont Perdue

INTRODUCTION

The fleshy site of the body oftentimes depends upon the sight of others, sanctioning the perceptual sight of the body as the signifier, wherein the flesh becomes the signified. In this sanctioning moment of making the body visible, bodies that do not quite fit the gendered and sexed expectations or "norms" of bodily appearance, then, present challenges with and against normative understandings of gender and sex, especially in a medical context. This chapter, "Making Bodies," concerns itself with the ways medical rhetoric and fixed notions of bodily appearance reduce materiality as both *site* and *sight*, evading particular phenomenological experiences of the clinical encounter and nonnormative ways of being-in-the-world. In this vein, the chapter centers transgender, nonbinary, and gender-nonconforming embodiment, momentarily suspending normative structures of gendered and sexed materiality and instead focuses on the ways nonnormative bodily appearance is often reduced to normative structures of gendered and sexed norms in a clinical encounter. What is lost in the clinical encounter when a physician misrecognizes the gender-nonconforming patient? What goes amiss when we inscribe gendered and sexed norms upon transgender bodies in the clinical encounter? That is, how are transgender, nonbinary, and gender-nonconforming bodies misperceived?

This chapter is divided into three sections to consider the problem of gendered and sexed conflation upon the body and, important, how this conflation plays out in the clinical encounter for some transgender, nonbinary, and gender-nonconforming individuals, particularly those individuals who might not "pass" as a "recognizable" male or female, man or woman. The conflation of gender/sex works to ensure both gender and sex are perceived as natural, interchangeable, and biologically real. Section 1, "The *Atmosphere* of (In)visibility," reviews a brief history

DOI: 10.7330/9781607329855.c014

of theoretical perspectives on the normative idealizations of gender and sex and questions the meaning of flesh through Gayle Salamon's reading of Maurice Merleau-Ponty's phenomenology of the body. Salamon and Merleau-Ponty, when read together, proffer a new way of thinking about our encounters in a world where we live amongst each other. Section 2, "Testosterone, Masculinity, Mattering," reimagines the notion of masculinity, questioning the medical rhetoric of standards of care for female-to-male transition. I analyze one transition-related medical document, which meets the standards placed on transition by the World Professional Association for Transgender Health (WPATH), wherein the description seems to reduce the process of female-to-male transition to standards and norms of masculinity. Here, I question whether or not administering testosterone is a question of masculinity.[1] The closing remarks, "Narrative Medicine Ruminations," coalesce in understanding how the materiality of the body is a contumacious substrate we must begin to grapple with, particularly in illness, disease, death, and, indeed, gender/sex embodiment.[2] "Making Bodies" makes the necessary call for the purview of narrative medicine to honor not only stories of illness and dying but also narratives of gender and sex in the clinical encounter. The final ruminations place somewhat utopic demands upon narrative medicine, and medicine more broadly, to come to recognize the boundless multitude of gendered and sexed lived realities. At best, this includes trans/gender women and trans/gender men but also those subject-bodies who identify as gender nonconforming, genderqueer, nonbinary, and/or agender.

THE *ATMOSPHERE* OF (IN)VISIBILITY

In this limited space, we certainly cannot trace all theories that have attempted to undo or rethink the gender/sex system; perhaps, though, we ought to name a few. Judith Butler's *Gender Trouble* (1990) destabilizes the category of sex insofar as the notion of "women" becomes interchangeable with biological sex, maintaining the heterosexual political discursive domain; in this domain, gender and sex work in an odd symbiotic relation to naturalize each other. Does sex presuppose gender? Or does gender presuppose sex? Who is "women" for? These are only a few questions *Gender Trouble* struggles both with and against. Butler seeks to set aside the coherent or fully formed subject, introducing her performative theory of gender. In a 1992 interview, Butler lays bare the stakes of gender performativity: "Performativity has to do with the repetition, very often with the repetition of oppressive and painful gender norms to force them to resignify. This is not freedom, but a question of how to work the trap that one is inevitably in" (Butler and Kotz 1992, 82–89). Rather acutely, Butler writes that the intense governing of normative gender treats the "body as a *site* of investment" (2011, 8; emphasis added). The governing of normative gender and the body as a site of investment, in turn, allows for some bodies to matter and for others to be *seen* as not worthy of livable investment at all. Teresa de Lauretis (1987), discusses how gender—"the technology of gender"—depends upon sexual difference. Simone de Beauvoir (1953) intimates in *The Second Sex* that the notion of woman is not a naturalized fact; woman is a historical idea (38). Anne Fausto-Sterling's (1997) essay "How to Build a Man" (247) asks what precisely it takes for one to become a man. Fausto-Sterling presents the ways biology and biomedicine reproduce constructions of masculinity through the materiality of intersex infants by surgically assigning normative sex and thus gender. Her influential work points to the violent medical and scientific phenomenon of assigning sex in order to ensure normative gender in the name of medicine, scientific truth, and epistemological absolutism—universal standards of the gendered and sexed body. That is, the *sight* of specific genitalia affords the clinical encounter space the ability to transmogrify the body into a *site* of naturalizing the body.

Paul Beatriz Preciado, in *Testo Junkie* (2013), continues in this vein, writing from within philosophy and critical theory, using the space of the text to trace affect, molecular becoming, and somatechnic experimentation throughout the undertaking of the text itself while self-administering testosterone. Preciado's "body-essay" reveals the complicated web of becoming, subjectivity, and human existence insofar as the text, similar to testosterone administration, summons bodily transmutation at the molecular level but also presses the philosophical, theoretical, and political implications of the gender/sex system. Preciado remarks, "As a body—and this is the only important thing about being a subject-body, a technoliving system—I'm the platform that makes possible the materialization of political imagination" (139).

Preciado (2013) exposes how hormone consumption enters one's biomolecular makeup, altering the *site* of how the trans body appears in the visual field of perception whereby medical rhetoric of gender/sex inscribes the materialization of the visible body. Instead of asserting transgender embodiment is akin to subversion, although subversive acts of gender or "performances" of the body, in fact, do continue to innovate the domain of gender, Preciado recognizes the intensity of gender's performativity in the material and endocrinological domains.

Materiality is turned inside out, outside in, and technologically remote. Along these lines of thinking of the subject-body as similar to a "technoliving system," Donna Haraway (1991), in her essay "A Cyborg Manifesto," pushes against totalized ontological claims of identity while renouncing antiscience discourse in order to make sense of human life and "all of our parts" (181). Haraway reminds us how the human body is implicated in the structures, categories, and rhetorics of the spatiotemporal horizon of materiality but also how materiality and the body are implicated in other living processes with other materialities, bodies, and technologies, belaboring the process of making and becoming bodies, as well as being seen and not being seen. By calling upon these and other philosophical, theoretical, and applied conceptualizations of gender/sex, we can begin to contextualize transgender, nonbinary, and gender-nonconforming materiality as not limited to biological, visible, and palpable matter.

In an effort to move away from the epistemological and ontological certainty of materiality of the body, this chapter situates phenomenology as a necessary vessel from which to think about what it means to *be* or *become* transgender, nonbinary, and gender nonconforming. Gayle Salamon (2010), in *Assuming a Body*, grapples with embodiment through Maurice Merleau-Ponty's phenomenology, psychoanalysis, and queer theory to bridge these philosophic modes of thought with transgender studies. This approach to thinking on the thinking of embodiment, then, without thinking of the body as an irreducible site in material resolution, negotiates betwixt and between materiality and, consequently, how materiality is "present to consciousness" (2). Salamon's reading of Merleau-Ponty points to the question at hand: How does contemporary medical rhetoric conflate the imposition of gender/sex inscribed upon transgender, nonbinary, and gender-nonconforming bodies? Primarily in chapter 2, "The Sexual Schema," Salamon takes Merleau-Ponty as her guide, focalizing the interstices of the body, materiality, and consciousness, pointing to how identitarian ontologies are always already an amalgamation of mind and matter but not only of the two insofar as the horizon of materiality is not limited to mind and matter of the self. Salamon attempts to relieve transgender, nonbinary, and gender-nonconforming ways of being from the limits of visibility and the body as pure material. Let me explain, following Salamon as my guide.

Salamon (2010) calls attention to, and this is critical here, Merleau-Ponty's (2012) phenomenology of the body to call into question the *flesh* and what I consider to be an ethic of human embodiment—*encounters with others, human and nonhuman, and the impact this may have on recognizing transgender, nonbinary, and gender-nonconforming subjects.* In other words, Salamon, through Merleau-Ponty, urges us to think about the flesh relationally. Transgender embodiment, indeed, takes place beneath the visible body, as well as beyond what can be seen. To be clear, to make the call that transgender embodiment goes beyond what can be seen does not mean to denote a purely transcendent subject in whom the gender/sex system has been magically unlocked. Rather, transgender embodiment enables us to continuously seek questions in which normative gender/sex discourse is at work without consistently reducing transgender people to the visible body (i.e., What does your genitalia look like? Why don't you pass? Do you want to pass?). In this way, transgender, nonbinary, and gender-nonconforming embodiment is not always locatable upon the physical site of the body, or inside it for that matter (what a challenge for the clinical encounter!). Salamon poignantly notes, "Merleau-Ponty is insisting that sexuality is not located in the genital nor even in one specific erotogenic zone, but rather in one's intentionality toward the other and toward the world" (53). At first glance, it appears problematic for Salamon to consider transgender embodiment on the beginning notes of sexuality insofar as transgender often pushes against queer theory, which has primarily focused on non-normative sexualities, erotics, and play (Edelman 2004; Freeman 2010; Love 2007). Nonetheless, Salamon, in an attempt to reconsider the transgender self first, thinks through sex and desire in order to understand gender and transgender materiality *not reduced to anatomical systems* and that which appears in the material form we nominally refer to as *the human body.* Deploying Merleau-Ponty's examination of intentionality toward the world shifts the focus from the confines of human anatomy and its biological codes and standards. Instead, "flesh" in this sense does not reduce flesh to a material thing; and in fact, this flesh we are speaking of here seems to be far more expansive.

When I say something like "Sage Perdue in the flesh!," I am simply speaking on the material body of "Sage," or claiming that "I" (Sage) have a material existence. *The Phenomenology of Perception* (Merleau-Ponty 2012) almost forces its reader to understand the flesh as this everyday human body but also something else entirely. The body is not space or time, nor is the body *in* space or time; rather, the body *inhabits* both space and time (2012, 140). The body with its world inhabits and enters another world, one "always surrounded by indeterminate horizons that contain other points of view" (2012, 141), such as psychic and phenomenological experiences meaningful for one's corporeality. Like indeterminate horizons, genitalia, anatomy, body hair, facial hair, breasts, and other secondary sex characteristics do not necessarily determine the site (or sight) of transgender, nonbinary, and gender-nonconforming subjects. In fact, there is resistance in indeterminate horizons, complicating the relation among body, world, medical rhetoric, and normative medical colloquialisms of making transgender bodies. Becoming flesh means to enter the world without being reduced to materiality and insisting on engaging in the world. Flesh becomes a relational byproduct of the relationship among self, the other, and the world, but not a simple resolution. Transgender, nonbinary, and gender-nonconforming subjects are often quickly reduced to the material, or how they "appear" to others in the world, and such visibility of the material can enact violence in the clinical encounter, on the street, in the bedroom, in the gay bar, and in other spaces in an always already entangled world. The material can be a locale of hypervisibility. That is, when we conceptualize the material and the ambiguity of being flesh, as Salamon shows us, being transgender, nonbinary, and gender nonconforming reveals the ways gendered and sexed truths do not have to adhere to a reduction of what is *seen* and produced as epistemological and ontological truth.

In *The Primacy of Perception*, Merleau-Ponty (1964) addresses the primary thesis of his *The Phenomenology of Perception* (2012). For Merleau-Ponty, the perceived world is paradoxical insofar as perception is paradoxical; it is in the atmosphere of paradox that we can better understand the perceived paradox that materiality represents perceptual truth in *site* and *sight*, unconcealing the implicit contradictions of being material. Briefly, I want to consider a conversation published between Merleau-Ponty and Émile Bréhier in *The Primacy of Perception*. Merleau-Ponty and Bréhier interrogate two things: (1) the other as an ethical subject in the world and (2) the problem of "seeing" and universal truths (1964, 30–31). In Bréhier's mind there is a serious danger in building premises that posit the Other in his relations, as well as in positing the Other in the world more generally. However, for Merleau-Ponty this becomes an ethical stake wherein he names the Other as an *ethical subject* in the world. And, he so eloquently asks, "How do we know someone is there before us unless we look? What do we see first of all, but corporeal experiences? How do these automata . . . become men for me? It is not the phenomenological method which creates this problem—though it does, in my view, allow us to better solve it" (1964, 30). Our phenomenologist is speaking on how the world is always already a positing of the Other because of the "I." When this "I" experiences a disagreement with the Other, there is no universality of the Other and the "I." When this "I" relationally experiences the Other, then, what "I" think "I" see, what "I" think to be true, what "I" claim to be universal for all beings, certainly, is complicated, troubled, and confounded by the relational Other. All of such takes place in an *atmosphere of ambiguity* in which gender (and sex) is neither real nor coherent, true nor false, here nor there, visible nor invisible. How are transgender, nonbinary, and gender-nonconforming individuals reduced to "corporeal experiences" in clinical encounters? What if what we see is not exactly who or what we think appears?

Materiality takes place in an atmosphere of visibility and invisibility incessantly filled with imagined possibilities. These imagined possibilities or indeterminate horizons enable us to think on the possibilities of gender and sex that inhabit time and space, seeking a livable way of being in the world and a more livable embodiment. To be clear, the intention here is not to ignore the *site* and *sight* of the body, but alternatively to ethically make sense of what precisely occurs when we are confronted with others and corporeal experiences amidst the everydayness of living a life. In a way, we can briefly recall Linda Alcoff's distinction between the public self and lived subjectivity (2006). The self we present to the world is seen, viewed, and judged by others, and oftentimes our lived subjectivity—how we experience ourselves—does not necessarily align with the image of this public self. In a similar vein, the site of the clinical encounter marks a place in time and space—a locale of ambiguity, visibility, invisibility, and rhetorical strategies that reconfigure gender's performativity. With phenomenology, we can come to think on the clinical encounter in which gender and sex are often conflated with flesh, and as we enter, entangle, and rub against this worldly flesh, the process of making gendered and sexed bodies unconceals the problematics of seeing the body as a medical site to be fixed and pathologized. In other words, phenomenology helps us chip away at the problem of reducing the *site* of materiality to *sight*, urging us to meet, in the relational atmosphere of (in)visiblity, embodiment in relation to the self, others, and objects. Reaching toward my self means to reach, bend, and move toward a "you." As I try to sketch in the following section, the biological and medical presumptions of testosterone administration suggest an expected appearance of masculinity and maleness.

TESTOSTERONE, MASCULINITY, MATTERING

The body as *site* and *sight* has provoked epic contributions from prominent philosophers and theorists of gender, sex, and sexuality, undoing gender and sex to reinscribe existing genders and identities. For instance, in writing using Merleau-Ponty, Salamon invites the reader to reconsider the possibilities of gender and sex, particularly for transgender subjectivity, beneath the material body and to consider instead how immaterial felt sense or psychic sense *and* bodily materiality are situated relationally in selves, others, and worlds. Important works on the rhetoric of medicine, science, gender, and sex, too, have engaged in like discussion because rhetorical practices in the clinical encounter are gendered; therein, the body becomes implicitly and explicitly sanctioned upon *site* and *sight* (Balsamo 1999; Cartwright 1995; Condit 2008; Derkatch and Segal 2005; Karkazis 2008; Waldby 1996, 2000). Such rhetorical strategies make bodies by which transgender, nonbinary, and gender-nonconforming bodies are both constructed and constrained by medical and healthcare discourses. To be clear, I am not contending that rhetoricians of health, medicine, and gender undertake projects *only* on gender and sex conflation in the clinical encounter, but rather I will not be commenting on those rhetoricians whose work focuses on health disparities and gender, the exclusion of women, queer, and transgender subjects from medical research or gendered patterns in health and disease. Instead, I extend my thinking toward how medical rhetoric of gendered and sexed materiality engenders epistemological and ontological truths of materiality.

The category gender became not only a diagnosis tool but also a clinical device when John Money developed it in 1955 with Anke Ehrhardt and Joan and John Hampson in order to modify or "fix" the visible body of intersex infants (Preciado 2013, 99). The categorical notion of gender unfolds comparative to a rhetorical device while the diagnosis process takes place in the clinical encounter, invariably an entangled world of subjects, Others, and somatechnologies. Indeed, surgical techniques along with hormone treatment quickly became a way to alter genitalia and materiality in the visual field wherein the body itself becomes a material discursive domain. Money deployed the category of gender to name a social role, moreover subjectivity. Thus, to be *male* and *female* coincides with being *masculine* and *feminine*—technological and medical functions whereby gender is sanctioned through sex and the converse. Preciado suggests that, with the category of gender, Money was able to deduce subjectivity through gender, conflating, as I contend, gender and sex onto the material matter of the body itself. That is, the body becomes the primary object in making visible both gender and sex through hormonal regulation and surgical techniques, fabricating subjectivity contingent upon coding and decoding technologies that make gender (and sex) visible to the medical eye. Medical rhetoric of gendered and sexed materiality continues to benefit from Money's deployment of gender, and such rhetorical strategies appear in contemporary transgender medical documents.

If one has been assigned female at birth and later seeks to alter the site and sight of the visible body through becoming-molecular, testosterone is one way to transmute the materiality of the body. In other words, altering one's gender through a biochemical process will change one's experience. For example, and respective to the limited space in this chapter, let us review one transgender medical digital document from the University of California, San Francisco's (UCSF) Center of Excellence for Transgender Health and UCSF Transgender Care program (note: this document meets WPATH standards of care). By analyzing this digital document, we can understand how medical rhetoric of gendered and sexed materiality comes to life. When perusing the guidelines (transcare.ucsf.edu/guidelines), one digitally stumbles upon a link that reads "Overview of masculinizing hormone therapy," specifically for female-to-male medical transition. Clicking on the link immediately initiates the perpetual conflation of gender and sex in the political materialization of the discursive body.[3] The introductory guidelines read as follows: "The goal of masculinizing hormone therapy is the development of male secondary sex characteristics, and suppression/minimization of female secondary sex characteristics. General effects include the development of facial hair, virilizing changes in voice, a redistribution of facial and body subcutaneous fat, increased muscle mass, increased body hair, change in sweat and odor patterns, frontal and temporal hairline recession, and possibly male pattern baldness. . . . Masculinizing hormone therapy may bring about changes in emotional and social functioning, though these can vary from person to person and stereotypes should be avoided" (Deutsch 2016). The subject-body undergoing masculinization is given a menu of testosterone self-administration methods to choose from: intramuscular testosterone injection, testosterone dermal patches, and testosterone creams. Pharmaceutical testosterone is a modern mimetic of testosterone that is secreted in the "human male" testicle. Reading the guidelines, the medical rhetoric of making a transgender body, then, mimics "male biological sex" insofar as the "female-to-male" patient undergoes masculinization to ensure the process of becoming "male" or "man." And as Preciado (2013) reminds us, with "the notion of gender, the medical discourse is unveiling its arbitrary foundations and its constructivist character, and at the same time opening the way for new forms of resistance and political action" (113). To make a transgender body means not to become a passive product in the clinical encounter but in fact a political materialization interface by which rhetorical strategies are deployed through guidelines and documentation marking what it means to *be* transgender.

We must take seriously the task of interrogating why it is precisely that female-to-male transgender patients are required to sign documentation that verifies their agreement to undergo masculinization. Do all transgender men want to be seen as masculine? Moreover, we must take seriously how this rhetorical strategy guised as a clinical device or diagnosis tool conceals gender and sex conflation and doubtlessly does not highlight the full potentiality of transgender, nonbinary, and gender-nonconforming embodiment. Consider the following example. Over a series of years, a subject-body marked female at birth reaches a particular phenomenological orientation toward medical transitioning; whether this includes both surgical and hormonal collaboration, only one of these somatechnologies, or moving among surgeries, hormone therapy, and other somatechnologies remains unknown. This subject-body has deliberated over medical transitioning and their perceived value of doing so. The subject-body, let's call them XY, enters the clinical site to seek options for top surgery and testosterone hormone therapy. XY makes it clear to the physician that they would like to take lower dosages of testosterone in order to get a sense of whether this is the direction they would like to take. XY cakes on pounds of foundation, glittery eyeshadow, the thickest mascara, lipstick, and luminous cheek highlighter. The physician gawks at XY in a curious way, wondering, "Does *she* really want to be a *man*?" Here we must pause and grapple with the perception of XY in the visual field. How is XY being seen and thus reduced to material norms? Prior to testosterone treatment and any surgical procedures, XY is deemed female until noted otherwise through a series of material, hormonal, and possibly surgical changes. Further, XY makes the claim to a male identity while refuting a masculinized gender. Is the patient deemed eligible for transgender health services and care? Are we moving beyond what is seen, affirming the complexity of being transgender, nonbinary, and gender nonconforming? More important, how is the patient treated in the clinical encounter?[4]

When transgender subject-bodies desire testosterone administration, the medical rhetoric of masculinization, testosterone, gender, and sex implodes in order to make a perceptible body that is socially valuable, politically normative, and understood as clearly legible for medical transitioning protocol—female-to-male. What would happen if we reimagined testosterone, considering why it matters for livable transgender, nonbinary, and gender-nonconforming embodiment? Do all subject-bodies undergoing testosterone hormone therapy self-conceptualize masculinity? Is a hormone known as *testosterone* interchangeable with a somafiction like masculinity? Preciado (2013) suggests that "masculinity is only one of the possible political (and nonbiological) by-products of the administration of testosterone. It is neither the only one nor, over the long term, the one that will dominate socially" (141). Preciado urges the reader, and I argue the subjects and others of the clinical encounter, to reimagine our conceptualizations of testosterone hormone adminis-tration. He goes on further to make the call that "testosterone isn't mas-culinity" (141). One cannot deny that bodily consumption of any phar-maceutically manufactured testosterone absolutely alters and generates perceptible changes to materiality. However, visible materiality does not expose consciousness nor self-conceptualization. Thus to make the call that masculinity is only *one* possibility of testosterone self-administration points to the myriad ways testosterone does not connote gender identity in a palpable nor visible way. Further, following the phenomenological tradition, testosterone can take on other meaningful understandings beyond a conventional masculinization of materiality, interrogating epistemological and ontological claims of the gendered and sexed body.

What is the point in this critique of testosterone as mattering to mas-culinity, especially in relation to the clinical encounter? In book 1 of *Rhetoric*, Aristotle describes the study of rhetoric as a study concerned with the myriad modalities of persuasion. He claims that "persuasion is a sort of demonstration" (Barnes 1984, 2153). Medical rhetoric demon-strates the most effective mode of becoming transgender, often exclud-ing nonbinary and gender-nonconforming subject-bodies through masculinization and feminization processes. One "acts" with speech and agreement to begin the process of masculinization, and in turn, the material body takes on the role of masculinity contingent upon a hor-mone, albeit a very powerful hormone. Judy Z. Segal (2008), building upon Aristotle's *Rhetoric*, imparts that "persuasion is a central element in many medical situations" (1). In this way, then, medical rhetoric of gen-der and sex perpetually conflates materiality as I have shown with one digital document for female-to-male transgender materiality. Specifically, medical rhetoric limits the possibilities of being transgender, underscor-ing gender's performativity. Further, Preciado (2013) interrogates the relation between masculinity and testosterone, arguing that "instantly, [the] testosterone turns me into something radically different from a cis-female. Even when the changes are socially *imperceptible*" (140; emphasis added). Those subject-bodies that refute medical rhetoric's strategizing to create a fictive perception of what is transgender reveal the medical conflation of gender and sex upon the body as *site* and *sight*.

What is *imperceptible* in the administration of hormones does not mean gender and sex must become perceptible/visible/palpable to constitute "real" gender and sex.

NARRATIVE MEDICINE RUMINATIONS

As Segal (2008) argues in *Health and the Rhetoric of Medicine*, rhetorical strategies in medicine and the power of persuasion persists. Rhetorical strategies and medical rhetoric do not occur as independent effects in the world, but rather medical rhetoric is a phenomenological encounter "in a world in which we act upon each other by influence" (2). Salamon's interpretation of Merleau-Ponty and flesh, in my view, speaks to the ways in which entering the clinical encounter means to enter a space wherein temporal and historical configurations of the body constitute contemporary medical treatment, medical history, patient charting, medical diagnoses, and overall health services and care. Medical rhetoric influences the felt sense of oneself, materiality, which treatments to agree to undergo, notions of health, notions of illness, and more. From a felt sense, then, ruminating on narrative medicine praxis imagines temporally and spatially phenomenological encounters in the clinical context and medicine's influence upon bodies and everyday human life. To end on ruminations of narrative medicine does not mean the purview of narrative medicine has failed in its mission of training physicians and other medical practitioners in "the narrative competence to recognize, absorb, interpret, and be moved by the stories of illness" (Charon 2006, vii). Instead of focusing on how "narrative vision is required in order to offer compassionate and effective care to the sick" (vii), I suggest making the imperative call to not only honor stories of illness but also to honor stories and narratives of becoming and being gendered and sexed. Surely individuals seek medical collaboration in times of sickness, and in other times neither in sickness nor with medical collaboration. In particular, illness has been a clinical device in historically sanctioning the making of gendered and sexed bodies. This chapter suggests that the goals of narrative medicine should honor stories of illness but also historical narratives that constrain the body in medical and illness experiences.

Transgender, nonbinary, and gender-nonconforming subject-bodies cannot be separated from Michel Foucault's (1994) archaeology of medical perception in *The Birth of the Clinic.* Foucault stresses how medical perception, medical rationality, and absolute scientific knowledge cognitively engender what is seen as epistemological truth, and in the case of gender and sex, ontological truth. He asserts, "The eye becomes the depository and source of clarity; it has the power to bring a truth to light that it receives only to the extent that is has brought it to light; as it opens, the eye first opens the truth: a flexion that marks the transition from the world of classical clarity" (xiii). Without a doubt, being able to look at a body and know how to take care of that body during illness, sickness, pain, and all forms of medical care is essential. However, various bodies have been pathologized, intended for correction, and subjected to the all-knowing medical eye and to normative modes of making subjectivity and bodies. Perhaps if narrative medicine's architecture intends to recognize, interpret, and absorb stories of illness, while also understanding stories of illness as cocreated in the clinical encounter, it is necessary for the purview of narrative medicine to not think only on stories of illness. Could we not argue that Foucault's *The Birth of the Clinic* traces master and cultural narratives of eighteenth- and nineteenth-century medical rhetoric, medical diagnoses, and the phenomena of medical epistemology?

Instead of primarily focusing on stories of illness, I suggest we collectively expand the purview of narrative medicine in order to ethically take seriously philosophies and critical theories of gender, sex, and sexuality, especially since bodily materiality and modes of nonnormative being are not distinct from medicine as such—a temporal and historical dissonance that has yet to fully be "past." Seeking medical collaboration as a queer/trans subject-body like illness "might trigger dissociation from life" (Charon 2006, 97). I do not mean to imply that queer and transgender subject-bodies are ill or that disorientation reveals a psychic disorder; rather, the clinical encounter can precipitate such dissociation when transgender, nonbinary, and gender-nonconforming subject-bodies seek transgender health care and services. In effect, this disorientation speaks to transgender livability, particularly the ways medical rhetoric and the clinical world can inhibit the making of a life for transgender beings. On the other hand, transgender, nonbinary, and gender-nonconforming subject-bodies will experience and encounter illness at some point in life, and therefore, competency and knowledge of gender and sex philosophy, theory, fiction, and nonfiction opens up the possibilities of narrative medicine—unforeseen and vulnerably open to the ethical subject, not merely a patient. Through narrative effort in gender and sex, we ought to take seriously an ethics of embodiment: *encounters with others and the impact this may have on recognizing transgender, nonbinary, and gender-nonconforming subjects.* The ethics of embodiment, then, understands that the reason for *seeing* the body is for *recognition*;

this does not mean to passively ignore what we see nor to wish away materiality in the visual field but for the body's *sight* to become a relational *site* of recognition and flesh. When we recognize our gendered and sexed lives are relational by-products of subjects, others, the world, medical rhetoric, and more, we are then better situated to realize an array of narrative medicine beyond the scope of illness. Ruminating on narrative medicine encourages us to ask What is health? insofar as transgender patients might enter the flesh of the clinical encounter without illness, and yet the potential to be perceived and stigmatized as "sick" or "ill" lingers.

What would narrative medicine of gender and sex look like? How can narratives of gender and sex expand the purview of narrative medicine? Can we consider reading philosophies and critical theories of gender and sex within the purview of narrative medicine? Doubtless, it reads as utopic to ruminate on narrative medicine in this way because to think on narrative medicine beyond stories of illness may read as a limit of its capital. However, to focus primarily on stories of illness presents the limitation of the possibilities of what narrative medicine can do for materiality, life, health, being, becoming, and death. In honor of queer theorist Jose Muñoz, this chapter, "Making Bodies," can be read as a performative critical analysis of gender's (and sex's) performativity and the relation to medical rhetoric that can often preclude other embodied forms of gender and sex. This short chapter "is meant to serve as something of a flight plan for a collective political becoming" (Muñoz 2009, 189). From shared interests in medical rhetoric, narrative medicine, embodiment, and gender and sex livability, we can arrive at the horizon of together becoming flesh and finally recognizing transgender, nonbinary, and gender-nonconforming individuals in all their multiplicity.

NOTES

1. The World Professional Association for Transgender Health (WPATH) is the primary professional association dedicated to treating and understanding dysphoria.
2. I thank a very special colleague from The Ohio State University, who will remain anonymous here for this formulation.
3. The University of California, San Francisco's Center of Excellence for Transgender Health follows WPATH's guidelines and standards of care. My questioning the role of masculinization through testosterone hormone therapy is not an attempt to undermine either organization. However, many transgender individuals take issue with the normalizing efforts and standards taken by WPATH. In 2017, transgender, nonbinary, and gender-nonconforming individuals protested the presence of the keynote speaker, Dr. Kenneth Zucker, at the annual conference due to his research on "gender confusion."

4.   This story, written by me from the many layers of my transgender experience in the exam room, concluded with the physician denying me, the transgender male patient, treatment because the doctor felt I did not meet all the masculinization standards. The doctor believed I was "more confused than the average gender dysphoric person." This kind of thinking, along with the normalization that stems from rhetorics that conflate masculinity with maleness, indeed can deny some transgender men and nonbinary and gender-nonconforming individuals access to testosterone hormone therapy. It was clear that a feminine-presenting person identifying as a transgender male did not seem possible in the eyes of this physician.

REFERENCES

Alcoff, Linda Martín. 2006. *Visible Identities: Race, Gender, and the Self*. New York: Oxford University Press.

Balsamo, Anne. 1999. *Technologies of the Gendered Body: Reading Cyborg Women*. Durham, NC: Duke University Press.

Barnes, Jonathan, ed. 1984. *The Complete Works of Aristotle: The Revised Oxford Translation*. Princeton, NJ: Princeton University Press.

Beauvoir, Simone de. 1953. *The Second Sex*. New York: Knopf.

Butler, Judith. 1990. *Gender Trouble: Feminism and the Subversion of Identity*. New York: Routledge.

Butler, Judith. 2011. *Bodies That Matter: On the Discursive Limits of Sex*. New York: Routledge.

Butler, Judith, and Liz Kotz. 1992. "The Body You Want: Liz Kotz Interviews Judith Butler." *Artforum* 31 (3): 82–89.

Cartwright, Lisa. 1995. *Screening the Body: Tracing Medicine's Visual Culture*. Minneapolis: University of Minnesota Press.

Charon, Rita. 2006. *Narrative Medicine: Honoring the Stories of Illness*. Oxford: Oxford University Press.

Condit, Celeste M. 2008. "Feminist Biologies: Revising Feminist Strategies and Biological Science." *Sex Roles* 59 (7–8): 492–503.

Derkatch, Colleen, and Judy Z. Segal. 2005. "Realms of Rhetoric in Health and Medicine." *University of Toronto Journal* 82 (2): 138–142.

Deutsch, Madeline B. 2016. "Overview of Masculizing Hormone Therapy." *Guidelines for the Primary Care of Transgender and Gender Nonbinary People*. USCF Transgender Care. https://transcare.ucsf.edu/guidelines.

Edelman, Lee. 2004. *No Future: Queer Theory and the Death Drive*. Durham, NC: Duke University Press.

Freeman, Elizabeth. 2010. *Time Binds: Queer temporalities, Queer Histories*. Durham, Duke University Press.

Foucault, Michel. 1994. *The Birth of the Clinic: An Archaeology of Medical Perception*. New York: Vintage Books.

Fausto-Sterling. 1997. How to Build a Man. In *The Gender/Sexuality Reader: Culture, History, Political Economy*, edited by Roger N. Lancaster, and Micaela D. Leonardo, 244–248. New York: Routledge.

Haraway, Donna J. 1991. "A Cyborg Manifesto: Science, Technology, and Socialist-Feminism in Late Twentieth Century." In *Simians, Cyborgs, and Women: The Reinvention of Nature*, by Donna Harraway, 149–181. New York: Routledge.

Karkazis, Katrina. 2008. *Fixing Sex: Intersex, Medical Authority, and Lived Experience*. Durham, NC: Duke University Press.

Lauretis, Teresa de. 1987. *Technologies of Gender: Essays on Theory, Film, and Fiction*. Bloomington: Indiana University Press.

Love, Heather. 2007. *Feeling Backward: Loss and the Politics of Queer History.* Cambridge, MA: Harvard University Press.

Merleau-Ponty, Maurice. 1964. *The Primacy of Perception: And Other Essays on Phenomenological Psychology, the Philosophy of Art, History and Politics.* Evanston, IL: Northwestern University Press.

Merleau-Ponty, Maurice. 2012. *Phenomenology of Perception.* Translated by Donald Landes. Hoboken, NJ: Taylor and Francis.

Muñoz, José Esteban. 2009. *Cruising Utopia: The Then and There of Queer Futurity.* New York: New York University Press.

Preciado, Paul B. 2013. *Testo Junkie: Sex, Drugs, and Biopolitics in the Pharmacopornographic Era.* New York: Feminist Press.

Salamon, Gayle. 2010. *Assuming a Body: Transgender and Rhetorics of Materiality.* New York: Columbia University Press.

Segal, Judy Z. 2005. *Health and the Rhetoric of Medicine.* Carbondale: Southern Illinois University Press.

Waldby, Catherine. 1996. *AIDS and the Body Politic: Biomedicine and Sexual Difference.* New York: Routledge.

Waldby, Catherine. 2000. *The Visible Human Project: Informatic Bodies and Posthuman Medicine.* New York: Routledge.

ABOUT THE AUTHORS

Mary K. Assad is a lecturer in the English department at Case Western Reserve University, where she teaches language courses for international students and serves as a first-year advisor. She is also an adjunct instructor at the Cleveland Institute of Art where she teaches a scientific writing course for biomedical art majors. Her research interests include rhetorics of health and medicine, rhetoric and composition, second language writing, and graphic novels and comics. She has presented her work at the Conference on College Composition and Communication, the College English Association Annual Conference, the Rhetoric Society of America Biennial Conference, and the National Communication Association Conference. She has published in the *CEA Forum* and the *Journal of Second Language Writing.*

Leslie R. Anglesey is an assistant professor in the Department of English at Sam Houston State University. Her research interests include rhetorical listening, feminist rhetorics, disability rhetorics, and composition theory and pedagogy. Leslie is a 2019 recipient of the CCCC Chairs' Memorial Scholarship. Her work has appeared in *The Peer Review* and *Works and Days.* She has presented her research at the Conference on College Composition and Communication, the Rhetoric Society of America Biennial Conference, and the International Writing Centers Association Annual Conference. Additional information about her research and teaching is available at www.leslieanglesey.com.

Beth L. Boser is an assistant professor in the Department of Communication Studies at the University of Wisconsin–La Crosse. Her current research centers on rhetorics of childbirth and motherhood and constructions of women's agency therein. One branch of this work investigates ways women are variously constrained and enabled by meanings created in and through motherhood discourses. Another explores childbirth advocacy, centering on home birth, midwife care, and other forms of resistance to medicalized birth. Her prior work appears in the edited volumes *Mediated Moms: Contemporary Challenges to the Motherhood Myth, Nasty Women and Bad Hombres: Gender and Race in the 2016 US Presidential Election, Recovering Argument,* and the journal *Rhetoric & Public Affairs.* She earned a PhD from the Annenberg School for Communication and Journalism at the University of Southern California.

Lillian Campbell is an assistant professor in the Department of English at Marquette University, where she teaches courses in academic and professional writing and rhetorical theory. Her research interests include rhetorics of health and medicine, feminist rhetorics, writing in the disciplines, and technical and professional communication. Drawing on a year of ethnographic fieldwork, her current research uses theories of embodiment, multimodal composing, and genre learning to explore how classroom clinical nursing simulations initiate students into the writing, talk, and action of the nursing field. This work is published or forthcoming in *Written Communication, Technical Communication Quarterly,* and the *Journal of Writing Research.*

Marleah Dean (PhD, Texas A&M University) is an associate professor at the University of South Florida and a collaborator-member of the Health Outcomes and Behavior Program at the Moffitt Cancer Center. Her research intersects health, interpersonal, and applied communication—emphasizing how communication can improve health outcomes among different healthcare stakeholders. Recently, her work investigates how patients, families, and healthcare providers exchange information, manage uncertainty, and make decisions regarding issues of hereditary cancer and genetic risk. Her publications can be found in outlets such as *Academic Medicine, Social Science & Medicine, Patient Education & Counseling, Qualitative Health Research, Health Communication,* the *Journal of Health Communication,* the *Journal of Applied Communication Research,* the *Journal of Genetic Counseling,* and *Supportive Care in Cancer.*

Lori Beth De Hertogh is an assistant professor in the School of Writing, Rhetoric and Technical Communication at James Madison University. Her work has appeared in the *Journal of Business and Technical Communication, Computers and Composition, Enculturation, Peitho, The Journal of Multimodal Rhetorics,* and *Composition Forum.* Additional information about her scholarship and teaching is available at www.loribethdehertogh.com.

Michelle F. Eble is an associate professor in the Department of English at East Carolina University, where she teaches technical and professional writing courses and research methods. Her research interests include technical writing theory and practice that incorporates social justice interventions as they relate to academic and scientific contexts. She is the coeditor of *Stories on Mentoring: Theory and Praxis* (Parlor Press, 2008), coauthor of *Primary Research and Writing: People, Places, Spaces* (Routledge, 2016), coeditor of *Reclaiming Accountability: Using the Work of Re/Accreditation and Large-Scale Assessment to Improve Writing Instruction and Writing Programs* (Utah State UP, 2016), and coeditor of *Key Theoretical Frameworks: Teaching Technical Communication in the 21st Century* (Utah State UP, 2018). She has also published in *Computers and Composition, Technical Communication, Technical Communication Quarterly, Present Tense,* and several edited collections. She serves as chair of ECU's Behavioral and Social Sciences Institutional Review Board and is past president of the Association of Teachers of Technical Writing (ATTW).

Erin A. Frost is an associate professor with the Department of English at East Carolina University. Her dissertation, *Theorizing an Apparent Feminism in Technical Communication,* won the 2015 Conference on College Composition and Communication's Outstanding Dissertation Award in Technical Communication. Her scholarly interests center on issues of gender and feminism in technical communication, most often as they manifest in health and environmental policy, risk communication, and teaching with technology. Her work has appeared in *Communication Design Quarterly, Computers and Composition,* the *Journal of Business and Technical Communication,* the *Journal of Technical Writing and Communication, Rhetoric Review, Technical Communication Quarterly, Programmatic Perspectives, Peitho,* and *Present Tense: A Journal of Rhetoric in Society.*

Dr. Leandra H. Hernández (PhD, Texas A&M University) is an assistant professor of communication studies at Utah Valley University. She utilizes Chicana feminist approaches to study Latina/o health, Latina/o journalism/media representations, and Latina/o cultural identities. She is the coauthor of *Challenging Reproductive Control and Gendered Violence in the Americas: Intersectionality, Power, and Struggles for Rights* with Dr. Sarah De Los Santos Upton, which was awarded the 2018 NCA Feminist & Women's Studies Division Bonnie Ritter Book Award. She is also the coeditor of *This Bridge We Call Communication: Anzaldúan Approaches to Theory, Method, and Praxis; Military Spouses with Graduate Degrees: Interdisciplinary Approaches to Thriving Amidst Uncertainty;* and the forthcoming volume *Latino/a Communication Studies: Theories, Methods, and Practice,* all with Lexington Books.

Her research on various health communication and media studies topics can be found in the journals *Communication Research, Women's Studies in Communication,* and *Women & Language.* As the coeditor of Lexington Books' series Lexington Studies in Health Communication, she enjoys collaborating with scholars on new and innovative health communication research projects. Furthermore, as the immediate past chair of the National Communication Association La Raza Caucus and Latina/o Communication Studies Division, she works to foster and support the study of Latina/o communication studies across the communication discipline.

Caitlin Leach is a clinical pharmacist and PhD student in women's studies at the University of Maryland, College Park. She completed her residency in community pharmacy at the University of Maryland School of Pharmacy and continues to teach Gender Affirming Therapeutics there as an invited content expert. Her work examines how clinical information, such as pharmaceutical data, can be redeployed from a critical, feminist perspective to challenge traditional biomedical conceptions of the normative body. Her broader research interests include feminist science and technology studies, critical medical studies, bioethics, and philosophy of the body.

Jordan Liz is an assistant professor of philosophy at San José State University. He specializes in philosophy of race, philosophy of medicine, and bioethics. More specifically, his work investigates the use of race within contemporary population genetics and biomedical science. It is concerned with the notion that racial groups—African, Caucasian, Asian, Native American, and Pacific Islander—correspond to discrete genetic clusters, and that these genetic differences may explain differences in disease prevalence by race. His work aims, first, to explicate the implicit presuppositions of this new genetic understanding of race, and second, to demonstrate how this contemporary medical discourse relates conceptually to similar discussion of race and disease throughout the nineteenth and twentieth centuries.

Cathryn Molloy is associate professor and director of undergraduate studies in James Madison University's School of Writing, Rhetoric and Technical Communication, where she teaches a variety of undergraduate and graduate courses. Her work has appeared in *Rhetoric Society Quarterly, Qualitative Inquiry, College English,* and *Rhetoric Review.* Cathryn serves as one of the assistant editors of the *Rhetoric of Health and Medicine* journal. She is the author of the book *Rhetorical Ethos in Health and Medicine: Patient Credibility, Stigma, and Misdiagnosis* and coeditor of the volume *Women's Health Advocacy: Rhetorical Ingenuity for the 21st Century.*

Miriam Mara is associate professor of English at Arizona State University. Her research interests include Irish literature and film, gender studies, and food studies, especially the fiction of Colum McCann, Nuala O'Faolain, Anne Enright, and Belinda McKeon. An additional research stream investigates medical discourse and cultural representations of health and illness, primarily in their treatment of gendered bodies. In all of these contexts, her work examines the intersections among landscapes, bodies, texts, and discourses. Her publications appear in *Technical Communication Quarterly, New Hibernia Review, Feminist Formations,* and *Nordic Irish Studies,* as well as in essay collections. Her book *Globalism and Gendering Cancer: Tracking the Trope of Oncogenic Women from the US to Kenya* (2020) investigates gendered understandings of cancer and their travel via the biomedical flows of globalism. The book partially developed out of research collected during a year as a Fulbright Scholar at Kenyatta University in Nairobi, Kenya.

Kerri K. Morris is an associate professor at Governors State University, where she directs writing across the curriculum and teaches writing and rhetoric courses. Her background is in historical rhetoric, with a special interest in the epideictic genre. She is currently focusing on rhetorics of health and the impacts of trauma on student writers and their teachers. She writes a blog for ChicagoNow, *Cancer Is Not a Gift* (http://www.chicagonow .com/cancer-is-not-a-gift/).

Maria Novotny is an assistant professor of English at the University of Wisconsin–Milwaukee. As a community-engaged scholar, she co-directs The ART of Infertility, which curates exhibits featuring patient perspectives of reproductive loss. Her research has been published in *Computers & Composition, Communication Design Quarterly, Harlot, Peitho, Reflections,* and *Technical Communication Quarterly.*

Sage B. Perdue is currently a graduate student in the Philosophy MA program at The George Washington University in Washington, DC. He/they also holds a master's degree in Interdisciplinary Humanities from the newest research university of the twenty-first century—the University of California Merced. Sage's philosophical areas of interest are in continental philosophy, feminist philosophy (especially feminist epistemology), philosophy of disability, and transgender studies.

Colleen A. Reilly is professor of English and faculty associate for the Centers for Teaching Excellence and Faculty Leadership at the University of North Carolina Wilmington. She teaches undergraduate courses in professional and technical writing, including Introduction to Professional Writing, Document Design, Writing about Science, Digital Composing, and Writing and Activism, and graduate courses in science writing; research methods; and genders, sexualities, and technologies. Reilly also served as the founding coordinator for an online postbaccalaureate certificate in science and medical writing designed to reach current UNCW students and working professionals. Recently, she has published articles and book chapters related to search engine optimization (SEO) and technical communication pedagogies, science communication pedagogies, gender and bioenhancement, privacy and surveillance in digital spaces, and entrepreneurship in technical communication programs.

Artist **Elizabeth Horn-Walker** is the cofounder and codirector of the international art, portraiture, and oral history project, The ART of infertility. With a degree in photography from the Art Institute of Pittsburgh, she works as a communications specialist for the University of Michigan Medical School's Department of Pathology, where she also manages the department's core imaging laboratory. Elizabeth serves on pathology's diversity, equity and inclusion committee as well as the Patients and Families Advisory Council. After her own infertility diagnosis, the focus of Elizabeth's artwork shifted from photography to using a variety of mediums to express her experiences with the disease. She also began documenting the lives of others with infertility through portraits and interviews in order to allow them healing through sharing their stories and to share those stories with medical practitioners and legislators, advocating for improvements to the care of those with the disease.

INDEX

activist/ism, 18, 188, 189, 192, 193, 196–200, 241, 244
advocacy, 18, 43, 55–58, 150, 192, 195, 201, 206–208, 215; patient advocacy, 30
American Heart Association (AHA), 18, 139, 171, 205, 207
androcentric, 4, 16, 121–123, 128, 134–135, 149
anorgasmia, 133–134
autonomy (bioethical tenets), 104, 110, 143, 171

Barad, Karen, 20n4, 84, 88–89, 98
beneficence, 172. *See also* bioethical tenets
bias, 7, 27, 28; cultural, 201; diagnostic, 9, 29, 33, 38; gender-based, 9, 17, 39, 171–173, 185–186, 200; racial, 189
bioethical tenets, 172. *See also* autonomy; justice
biomedicalization, 14, 16, 17
Black Women Do Breastfeed, 17–18, 188–204
bladder cancer, 17, 72, 157–168
breast cancer, 18, 159, 171–186; research on, 18, 172, 173, 223–236
breastfeeding, 13, 17–18, 188–201
Butler, Judith, 89, 257, 258

caregiving, 209–216
cancer, 10, 13, 28, 45, 56, 74, 89, 132, 134, 174–186, 214. *See also* bladder cancer; breast cancer
Charon, Rita, 71, 80, 267, 268
chronic pain, 68, 69, 72, 77
clitoris, 121, 122–124, 125–127, 130, 133
Comeau, Tammy Duerden, 171
counternarratives, 15, 46, 48, 197
critical imagination, 71

delayed diagnosis, 71–72, 79, 158, 160, 162
diffraction, 85, 88, 98
discursive practices, 68, 69, 191
disidentification, 158, 166
doctor-patient interaction. *See* patient-provider interaction

Diagnostic and Statistical Manual of Mental Disorders, The (DSM–5), 29, 31–32, 37, 40, 145
Dubriwny, Tasha, 10, 55, 171, 173, 193, 240, 242–244, 245, 248
dysmenorrhea, 67, 75

education, for health professionals, 9, 83, 105, 113, 128, 141, 167; for the public, 20n5, 58, 105, 152, 164, 167, 192, 215, 227–232
embodiment, 3, 6, 12, 17, 19, 92, 147, 151, 259, 262, 268, 269; gender and, 27, 141–142, 144, 256–258, 260, 265; race and, 148, 149
endometriosis, 16, 39, 44, 67–81
erectile dysfunction, 134
experiential data, 4, 12, 15
experiential knowledge, 14, 16, 28, 68, 79, 84, 101–102, 104–114, 240
evidence-based medicine, 12, 144

female genital cosmetic surgery (FGCS), 128, 130
female pelvic pain, 39, 68
female sexual dysfunction (FSD), 122, 127, 134, 144–148
Female Sexual Function Index (FSFI), 127

G-spot, 121, 122, 124–135
gender: gender binary, 141; genderqueer, 7, 139, 140, 141, 144, 257; gender roles, 7, 18, 86, 89–90, 94, 97–98, 103, 104, 111, 142, 151, 158, 216–218, 245
Groopman, James, 161, 165, 166–167
Go Red for Women (Go Red) campaign, 18, 139–140, 142, 143, 144, 164, 171, 205–218

health campaigns, 18, 173, 209, 215–217, 234
health disparity/ies, 3, 6, 10, 14, 18, 151, 157, 158, 188–193, 196, 197, 200, 201, 234, 263
heart attack, in women, 20n5, 32, 164, 211, 212, 214, 218n1, 218n4

heart disease, 9, 11, 18, 152–153, 171,
    205–206, 207, 208–210, 212–218
hematuria, 159, 161–162
Holloway, Karla, 171, 172
hysteria, 13, 16, 69, 121, 123, 134–135
hysterical woman, 39, 70

iatrogenic, 176, 181
identification, 12, 17, 38, 94, 95, 158,
    160–166
idioms of distress, 15, 29, 30, 33–35,
    36–40
individualization (of social/systemic prob-
    lems), 241, 244
inequality, 35, 152, 153
infertility: general, 13, 15–16, 43–62, 72,
    251; Art of Infertility, 44, 46, 48, 51–52,
    54, 59–60
intersectionality, 14, 16, 38, 39, 138–139,
    150–154, 172, 215
interventions (rhetorical), 19, 29, 62, 77,
    154
intra-action, 88–93, 96

Journal of the American Medical Association,
    141
justice, 12, 17, 154, 172; social justice, 149,
    152, 201. *See also* bioethical tenets

Kirsch, Gesa, 71
Komen, Susan, 171, 206

listening, 12, 17, 48, 67–81, 96, 98, 107,
    110; ethical, 29, 37–39; rhetorical, 15,
    37–38, 94–95, 158, 165–167

materiality, 19, 256–269
Mayo Clinic, 16, 17, 122, 130–135,
    172–186
menstruation, 17, 52, 72–76, 163, 167, 171
mental health, 19, 60, 191, 239
Merleau-Ponty, Maurice, 257–262, 267
metaphor, 4, 34, 101, 103, 108, 110, 138,
    157, 161–168, 171
metonymy, 165–166
motherhood, 45; ideals and expectations,
    45, 54, 164, 211, 239–253; feminism
    and, 56, 58; as metaphor, 163

narrative medicine, 16, 80–81, 257,
    267–270
nonbinary, xi, 7, 15, 19, 256–257, 259–270
nonmaleficence. *See* bioethical tenets
nonidentification, 17, 165, 167
nonnormative bodies, 57, 153, 256, 268
nursing (as occupation), 16, 83–99, 111

online communities, 189–201
orgasm, 16, 121–137, 176
overdiagnosis, 39, 176, 177

pain communication, 79; embodied expe-
    riences of, 8, 58; normalization of, 32,
    69, 71, 73, 127, 131; pain rating scale,
    74–77
pathogenesis, 68, 231
pathologizing/pathology: of experience,
    4, 8, 18, 32, 44, 46, 59, 62, 68–70, 190,
    197; of gender, 9, 45–46, 71, 122, 188;
    240–251
patient-centered, 61, 105, 110, 112, 113,
    141, 150
patient-physician interaction. *See* patient-
    provider interaction
patient-provider communication. *See*
    patient-provider interaction
patient-provider interaction, 16, 80, 101,
    103, 104, 110, 114, 158
patienthood, 14, 16, 17, 79, 139, 150, 154
performativity, 19, 89, 153, 257, 258, 262,
    266, 269
phenomenology, 257, 259–262
posthuman(ism), 89
postpartum, 19, 218, 240–253
pronatalism, 56–57
psychogenic symptoms, 15, 27–40
psychosomatic, 7, 27, 124

queer, 4, 7, 14, 15, 139–141, 144, 146, 147,
    148, 149, 257, 259, 260, 263, 268–269.
    See also gender: genderqueer

race and embodiment. *See* embodiment
Ratcliffe, Krista, 37, 94, 95, 98, 158, 161–
    166, 168
reproduction (human biological), 45–46,
    163
reproductive health, 20n6, 240
Royster, Jacqueline Jones, 71

screening, 172–178, 183–187
Segal, Judith, 12, 38, 145, 150, 159, 163,
    188, 191, 239, 263, 266, 267
self-help, 19, 218, 239–253
Selleck, Laurie G., 173
sexual dysfunction, 17, 122, 127, 131, 132,
    134, 138, 144–145, 148–150, 153
sexuality, 4, 84, 97, 121, 128, 134, 140,
    144–149
simulation, 16, 83–99
slavery, 151, 194–195
social media, 188–190, 192–203
social construction, 14, 16, 223, 250

somatic symptoms, 7, 27–28, 31, 35, 40
somatizations, 28–31, 33, 35, 36
stigma, 16, 40, 45–46, 58, 59, 134, 196,
    245, 252, 269
strategic contemplation, 71

technoscience, 4–6, 12, 15

transgender, 11, 19, 139, 138–154, 164,
    168, 256–270

urinary tract infection, 159, 160

vaginal orgasm, 16, 121, 124, 127
vaginally activated orgasm (VAO), 126